TRADITIONAL
JAPANESE
ACUPUNCTURE
FUNDAMENTALS OF
MERIDIAN THERAPY

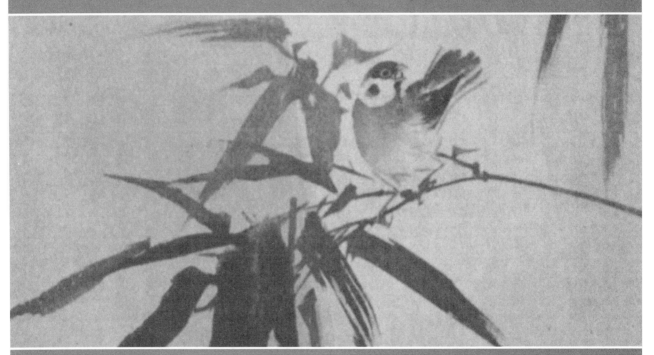

SOCIETY FOR TRADITIONAL
JAPANESE MEDICINE

T. KOEI KUWAHARA,
EDITORIAL SUPERVISOR
TRANSLATED BY JOSHUA MARGULIES

COMPLEMENTARY MEDICINE PRESS
Brookline Massachusetts and Taos New Mexico
2·0·0·3

Traditional Japanese Acupuncture
Fundamentals of Meridian Therapy

Nihon Shinkyu Igaku
Keiraku-chiryo Kisohen

The Society for Traditional Japanese Medicine

T. Koei Kuwahara, Editorial Supervisor
Translated by Joshua Margulies

©2003 T. Koei Kuwahara
ISBN 0-9673034-4-3

Library of Congress Cataloging-In-Publication Data

Traditional Japanese acupuncture : fundamentals of meridian therapy /
The Society of Traditional Japanese Medicine ; T. Koei Kuwahara,
editorial supervisor ; translated by Joshua Margulies.-- English ed.
        p. ; cm.
Includes index.
Translated from Japanese and/or Chinese, with some passages in Japanese and/or Chinese.
   ISBN 0-9673034-4-3 (pbk. : alk. paper)
   1. Acupuncture. 2. Medicine, Chinese--Japan.
   [DNLM: 1. Acupuncture Therapy. 2. Meridians. 3. Medicine, Chinese
Traditional--methods. WB 369 T763 2003a] I. Kuwahara, T. Koei (Taos
Koei) II. Society of Traditional Japanese Medicine. III. Title.
   RM184.T66 2003
   615.8'92'0952--dc22

                            2003017042

Cover design by Herb Rich III
Published by Complementary Medicine Press
Taos, New Mexico
Distributed by Redwing Book Company
www.redwingbooks.com

TABLE OF CONTENTS

TABLES AND ILLUSTRATIONS

Foreword to the Japanese Edition

This book is a text for learning the practice of traditional Japanese acupuncture.

Traditional Japanese acupuncture was developed over a long period of Japanese history into a unique medical system. Its foundation is the classical acupuncture texts that were gradually transmitted to Japan from China, where acupuncture was born more than two thousand years ago.

This medical system came into being in a time before reason, philosophy, and science were divided into specialized fields, and as such it holds a view entirely different from that of the scientific view of the Occident. It adopts the position of a diagnostic therapy system. In other words, it is a medical paradigm that considers a person's whole character and entire body, as well as their specific social context, in order to make a diagnosis and provide treatment. This stands in contrast to scientifically analyzing the human body. Thus, this form of medicine has a rich contemporary value as a kind of human science that looks closely at the overall human condition.

The acupuncture profession is one to be proud of, one to which practitioners devote their full strength. This work involves living and interacting in genuine human-to-human relationships with those who are suffering from disease.

Traditional Japanese medicine takes a humanistic approach to medicine and is more directly able to attain its goal by forming a treatment method through a unified consideration of an individual's mind, body, and lifestyle. The first step in learning this type of medicine begins with acquiring a deep understanding of yin and yang and of the five phases.

Without refining and improving our academic knowledge, our technical skills, and ourselves as human beings, as practitioners we will be of no use in the clinic. Therefore, although the Society of Traditional Japanese Medicine has previously focused on technical instruction such as pulse diagnosis and needling, with this new textbook we intend to teach and explain traditional Japanese medicine in a manner easily understood by all.

It is my anticipation that the members of the Society will closely read the text in conjunction with receiving practical training and that this will prove to be useful within their own practices.

Finally, I express my deep gratitude to the sages of old and to our more recent predecessors who strove with all their energy and spirit to revive, maintain, and develop traditional Japanese medicine. This book is dedicated to them.

March 1997

Okabe Somei, President

Society of Traditional Japanese Medicine

Introduction to the Japanese Edition

Komai Kazuo, MD, the editor-in-chief of the *Oriental Medical Journal*, encouraged acupuncturists across the country when he expressed his enthusiasm and hope for East Asian medicine in the January 1936 edition of the *Journal* as follows:

> The most important guide for the development of medicine, like a great beacon pointing the way into the future, lies in the study of the meridians. The foundation of this study is in the hands of acupuncturists, who can realize this ideal medicine through sincere service. Therefore, I earnestly hope that acupuncturists will recognize this truth and be inspired to strive towards the achievement of that goal.

Later, in the April 1938 monthly study meeting held at the Osaka Industrial Hall, attendees were greatly moved by the opening talk of the guest speaker, Yanagiya Sorei, in which he made his now-famous call: "Return to the classics!"

Yanagiya's plea was not simply a recitation of the idea that ancient equates with value and that therefore we should unconditionally accept the classics. Rather, his premise was that there is a need to reexamine the classics and to clinically test the knowledge gained therein in order to extract the truth. Accordingly, he emphasized that this work had to begin with a textual critique of the seminal texts.

Dr. Komai was deeply impressed by Yanagiya's point of view and by his great ambition for classical acupuncture. Therefore, in the same year, in the August edition of the Oriental Medical Journal, Dr. Komai announced, "Takeyama Shin'ichirō [a man in his company with whom he had built up a close friendship] has been made the director of the Tokyo Branch of the Oriental Medical Company and will oversee the development of programs for the retraining of acupuncturists." This course of action quickly gathered great momentum and lead to a progressive leap forward for classical acupuncture.

Since 1930, through the goodwill of Mr. Yamaguchi Enjiro, a merchant who sold medical supplies and acupuncture books in the town of Hongō-Haruki, Yanagiya had been allowed to use a separate building next to Mr. Yamaguchi's house as the meeting place for his own study group, the Society for the Study of Practical Acupuncture, where many people gathered to study under Yanagiya. Takeyama would often show up to gather information for articles. Before long he decided to make an organization that would work in close association with Yanagiya's group toward the same goal of furthering the study of classical acupuncture. To that end Takeyama employed Machida Masahiko (a relative of the herbalist Mr. Anzai Anshu) and gradually began working.

With the primary goal of promoting genuine study among acupuncturists, an informal gathering for young practitioners was held in 1939 at a restaurant called Hatsune in the Ōnegashi area of the Kyōbashi district in Tokyo. The day of the first meeting happened to be the day of the Doll's Festival on March 3 and so we called our group the Yayoi Freshmen Group, Yayoi being the old name for "March" in the lunar calendar.

The thirteen young practitioners who gathered were: Yanagiya Sorei, Okabe Sodō, Inoue Keiri, Konjiki Genmin, Aiba Jin, Ogura Shōdō, Matsuoka Takashi, Nakajima Muge, Yoshimori Mitsuki, Yatabe Yasuyuki, Tobe Sōhichiro, Nishizawa Seikei, and Okada Meiyu. The organizers were Takeyama Shin'ichirō, the director of the Oriental Medical Company's Tokyo Branch Office, and Machida Masahiko. Regular monthly study sessions were held. The youthful members of the Yayoi Group who drew together around Yanagiya were acupuncturists who shared the aim of advancement of learning. Later, the Yayoi Group became the body that gave birth to Meridian Therapy.

The Japanese word *shinjin* (新人), which literally means "new person" and which is translated as "freshmen" in the name "Yayoi Freshmen Group," connotes the meanings of reform and revolution.

The following summarizes the primary objective professed by the Yayoi Group for advancing the Meridian Therapy system:

To gain insight into deviations from the normal condition of the meridians, or more specifically, changes in the organs brought about by abnormalities in the meridians, which result from the combination of the effects of changes in the outside world (external pathogens) plus the accumulation of internal injuries due to the seven affects and which manifest in physical imbalance and cause changes in the meridian system that obstruct the circulation of ki, and are expressed as deficiency or excess.

That objective is met through the conduction of physical examinations to determine the pattern of imbalance by gathering information through the traditional four examinations of looking, listening, questioning, and palpation, with special emphasis placed on pulse diagnosis, and then further considering those findings in terms of the interconnections between the five phases.

Since the search for the pattern of imbalance transforms immediately into treatment, it is often said that the examination and the treatment are one and the same. Accordingly, the purpose of the examination is to ascertain any deficiency or excess in the meridians; it is not intended to diagnose disease in the terms of biomedicine. The system described in Chapter 69 of the *Nan Jing* (*Classic of Difficulties*) is such a treatment system. As a general rule in this system, points for what is considered the root treatment are chosen from among the distal five element points or command points. Furthermore, tonification and dispersion techniques are used together through the simultaneous application of what is considered the local treatment, which is conducted by locating treatment points by lightly palpating and gently pinching the skin at areas that reveal signs of the syndrome. These two aspects of the treatment go hand in hand. The special quality of Meridian Therapy is that it is a treatment system whereby one does not simply diagnose disease, but rather senses the flow within the meridians and the meridian's connection to the organs—in other words, takes into consideration the whole state of the patient and then uses acupuncture diagnostic and treatment methods to promote and restore health in suffering patients.

Once the objective of Meridian Therapy was solidified, the Yayoi Group held the Fourth Oriental Medical Company Conference in Kyoto and successfully presented its vision of the exceptional qualities in Meridian Therapy that made it the path of the future for acupuncture. The ideas were extremely well received, and the Group was greatly inspired to devotedly pursue further studies of the classics and advancements of the art.

Takeyama next had the Yayoi Group participate in the reorganization of the Oriental Medical Association in April of 1941. This was the objective they expressed:

We, the members, hereby reestablish the Oriental Medical Association and pledge to work in close cooperation with the Oriental Medical Company to establish reeducation programs for acupuncturists, to jointly engage in research and training, to revive the original spirit of the art of acupuncture, and to demonstrate its real potential as a treatment method.

Organization of the Oriental Medical Company

Headquarters: Oriental Medical Company, Tokiwa'ana-mura, Kurita-gun, Shiga-ken.

Chairman: Komai Kazuo, MD   Director: Ōhashi Isamu

Eastern Japan Chapter of the Oriental Medical Association

(Located at the Tokyo Branch Office of the Oriental Medical Company)
General Manager: Takeyama Shin'ichirō
Deputy Manager: Inoue Keiri
Education Department Director: Inoue Keiri
    Deputy Director: Nakamura Shinsaburō
Research Department Director: Okabe Sodō
    Deputy Director: Okada Meiyu
Organization Department Director:
    Nishizawa Seikei
    Deputy Director: Nakata Shūkō
General Affairs Department Director:
    Konjiki Genmin
    Deputy Director: Takeuchi Jōichirō
Planning Department Director: Aiba Jin
    Deputy Director: Gotō Shin'ichi
Accounting Department Director: Ogura
    Shōdō
    Deputy Director: Matsuoka Takashi
Records Department Director: Ono Bunkei
    Deputy Director: Takeda Isoji
Publication Department Director: Tobe
    Sōhichiro
    Deputy Director: Machida Masahiko
Administration Department Director:
    Nakamura Ryūhō
    Deputy Director: Shimizu Teiken
Advisors: Anzai Anshu, Yakazu Dōmei,
    Ōtsuka Keisetsu, Yanagiya Sorei, Jō
    Ikkaku, Shirota Bunshi

Western Japan Chapter of the Oriental Medical Association

(Located at the home of Higuchi
    Etsunosuke)
General Manager: Higuchi Etsunosuke
Deputy Manager: Hobo Yaichirō
Education Department Director: Hobo
    Yaichirō
    Deputy Director: Suehiro Takeru
Research Department Director: Kitamura
    Yukihiro
    Deputy Director: Ōshita Hiroshi
General Affairs Department Director:
    Higuchi Etsunosuke
    Deputy Director: Taniguchi Kiyosuke
Planning Department Director: Ohatsuse
    Norihisa
    Deputy Director: Kawasuki Katsukichi
Accounting Department Director: Sakamoto
    Shizuhiko
    Deputy Director: Kabayama Shigeyoshi
Records Department Director: Mizuno
    Shōsaku
    Deputy Director: Itasaka Ryōzō
Communication Department Director:
    Katayama Hideo
    Deputy Director: Toyama Tetsuaki
Advisors: Morita Kōmon, Matsumoto Gunji,
    Kooriyama Shichishi, Tatsui Fumitaka,
    Takino Kenshō, Yamamoto Shingo

① Establishment and Activities of the East-West Chapter

The East-West Chapter held a successful commemoration speech that was attended by many people and afforded a sharing of opinions.

Takeyama divided the Educational Department of the Eastern Japan Branch into four groups, headed by Okabe, Inoue, Nishizawa, and Ogura, respectively, and each group had a committee of five participants. Study meetings were held at appointed times every week at the homes of the leaders, and in this way the research work was split up. Later each group would make a presentation of its findings.

In order to further spread the popularity of Meridian Therapy, the Eastern Japan Chapter held two training sessions on Meridian Therapy.

Time:　　　　I.　　　Sunday nights, May to July 1942

　　　　　　　II.　　　Sunday nights, October to December 1942

Place:　Kinkei Hall (later Kudan Buddhist Hall), Hara-machi, Konishigawa, Tokyo

Lecture topics and presenters:

Principles of Meridian Therapy

　I. Okabe

　II. Inoue

Explanation of Proverbial Meanings from

the *Nan Jing*

　I. Inoue

　II. Okabe

A Compilation of Acupuncture Excerpts

　I. Ogura

　II. Nishizawa

Detailed Explanation of the Organs and

Meridians

　I. Nakamura

II. Okada

Precious Acupuncture Records

　I. Honma

　II. Ono

Nei Jing (*Su Wen*, *Ling Shu*)

　I and II. Yanagiya Sorei

Principles of Periods and Ki

　I. Takeyama Shin'ichirō

Five Phase Theory

I. Takeyama Shin'ichirō

Japanese Medical History

(Extra) Takeyama Shin'ichirō

② The Propagation of Meridian Therapy

With the establishment of Meridian Therapy, plans were then made to work toward propagating the system. The structure of Meridian Therapy had already been worked out, but it was at the following conference that the meat was really put on the bones, so to speak.

Presentations by Members of the Research Committee of Eastern Japan Chapter of the Oriental Medical Association, held at a lecture hall at Nihon University in Kanda, Tokyo:

The Issue of "Ki" in Meridian Therapy: Nakamura Shinsaburō, First Research Division

Areas of Pathogenic Ki Penetration into the Meridians and the Resultant Changes: Okada Meiyu, First Research Division

Factors that Influence the Pulse Quality: Honma Shōhaku, Second Research Division

Secrets of Acupuncture Abdominal Diagnosis: Ono Bunkei, Second Research Division

Principles of Tonification and Dispersion in Meridian Style Treatment: Yasuoka Nobuyasu, Third Research Division

Fourteen Needling Techniques from the *Nei Jing*: Suzuki Keimin, Third Research Division

Takeyama's comments on the day appeared in the Oriental Medical Journal: "We were very fortunate to have six research members from the Eastern Japan Chapter earnestly present the conclusions about Meridian Therapy that they reached by concentrating their full efforts."

To further the understanding of Meridian Therapy, the most urgent task was to devise a strategy for making pulse diagnosis easily comprehensible to all participants of the retraining programs. Takeyama called on Honma Shōhaku to find a way to address this task.

Honma developed a new approach. He chose three examples of Liver deficiency patterns from his files and denoted their transformations on staff notation paper. After conducting tests and revisions he then made a model diagram and reported confidently to Takeyama that he could clearly demonstrate floating or sinking, tight or soft, large or small pulses. Later, after Okabe, Inoue, Takeyama, and Honma had all extensively tested this startlingly clear Pulse Quality Diagram and were satisfied with the results, they decided to make it public.

The Pulse Quality Diagram, which collected all of the necessary conditions for comprehending how to take the pulse, brilliantly clarified the issue of making pulse taking understandable in studying, lectures, practical skills presentations, and journal reports of clinical trials.

(The above section contains quotes and paraphrases from *The Time of Showa Acupuncture* by Kamichi Sakae.)

③ **Appearance of the *Journal of Meridian Therapy***

The first issue of the *Journal of Meridian Therapy* appeared in April of 1965 and became established as one of the leading journals in the acupuncture world. It carries articles by distinguished teachers, reports of clinical trials by experts, and supports the literary activity of young practitioners and students.

In 1974, Okabe Sodō was installed as the first director of the Acupuncture Department. This was due to his instrumental role in establishing the East Asian Medicine Research Institute, which was located at the Kitazato Research Institute in Tokyo. Together with his son, Somei, Okabe worked hard on comprehensive studies of East Asian Medicine while also maintaining a treatment practice.

Moreover, the Meiji University of Oriental Medicine was opened in the Kansai region in 1983, thereby laying out a single systematic educational program for the study of East Asian medicine. With this, Japanese acupuncture came to hold a torch-bearing role in the world of acupuncture.

I do not feel it is an exaggeration to say that Traditional Japanese Acupuncture, a therapeutic system with a unified approach to diagnosis and treatment that has the outstanding features of a unique pulse diagnosis and strong tonification and dispersion techniques, has taken an historical step into the international arena in this century. Let us recognize Meridian Therapy as a guiding star, shining now and into the future.

March 1997

Okada Meiyu, Deputy Director, Society of Traditional Japanese Medicine

Preface to the English Edition

The printing of this book marks the English language edition of *Traditional Japanese Acupuncture: Fundamentals of Meridian Therapy* by the Society of Traditional Japanese Medicine. Years of effort went into constructing the theories that form the fundamental concepts of clinical acupuncture. Traditional Japanese acupuncture has largely been handed down through the generations by word of mouth. Not only acupuncture, but also all arts that involve technical skills have been passed down from hand to hand, from teacher to student. Even if we flatter ourselves that Japanese acupuncture is the best in the world in terms of technique, it cannot be widely transmitted to the world without a written record. It was with that understanding that we undertook the writing of *Traditional Japanese Acupuncture*.

In 1990, the 50th anniversary of the Society of Traditional Japanese Medicine, the Society began consolidating a wide range of opinions on the practice of traditional acupuncture in Japan. That was when the late Okabe Somei put forward the question: "Are we satisfied with Meridian Therapy [as it now is]?" An editorial committee was set up within the Society, and the book was completed over a ten-year period. The clinical skills of many clinical acupuncturists were formulated into theories and recorded in words. The process of working through problematic issues further systematized Meridian Therapy.

Twelve hundred years have passed since the propagation of Chinese acupuncture in Japan. The acupuncture that took root in Japan then underwent advancement and progression during the Edo Period. The technique of using an insertion tube was contrived, which allowed for acupuncture that matched the sensitive bodies of the Japanese people and also made possible treatment using shallow insertion. Practitioners became able to freely and painlessly tonify and disperse meridians and acupuncture points on the extremities. Meridian Therapy was developed from this tradition of Japanese acupuncture. Japanese acupuncture refers to the treatment style in which treatment that focuses on tonification and dispersion of essential points on the extremities is given by following the pattern of imbalance, which is determined through the Four Examinations (looking, listening (and smelling), questioning, and palpation). This English edition should become the most valuable book for anyone who wants to learn Japanese acupuncture.

Okada Akizō

President, Society of Traditional Japanese Medicine

November, 2002

Foreword to the English Edition

Traditional Chinese Medicine and Meridian Therapy

This book is titled *Traditional Japanese Acupuncture*, but its sources are the classical texts of Chinese traditional medicine, such as the *Su Wen* and *Ling Shu*. Nowadays many people think there is a fundamental difference between Traditional Chinese Medicine (TCM) and the Meridian Therapy of Japan. However, this is a misunderstanding. I would like to mention the basis for this misunderstanding as the foreword to this English edition of the present book.

For example, concerning the Liver, the *Su Wen* and *Ling Shu* say that the "Liver stores the blood," and that it works hard in the springtime. From this it is understood that the Liver, by the power of blood, functions in generation or creation during the springtime. However, it is also recorded that the Liver is tonified by sourness, and that sourness contains the functional property of gathering. These two points contradict each other, and many people continue to practice classical therapy while ignoring this contradiction.

For instance, the reason Meridian Therapists would focus on the pulse strength comparison diagnosis and think only about the meridians without saying anything about the physiology of the organs is because they could not resolve this contradiction. On the other hand, TCM acupuncturists make reference to the physiology of the organs, but when the time comes to give treatment, they do so while focusing on the acupuncture points. This as well is due to the inability to resolve the contradiction between the organs and the meridians.

To understand this without contradiction, you must think of it in the following way.

The Liver stores the blood. In the springtime it functions in generation or creation (in TCM this is called *shū xiè* or *free coursing*, although this term does not appear in the *Su Wen*) by the power of yang within the blood. However, generation cannot take place if there is an insufficiency of blood. That is why you encourage the gathering to the Liver of a lot of blood by tonifying the ki of gathering that is in the Liver channel (the ki that is tonified by sourness), which is in other words tonification of Liver deficiency.

The Lung can be used as another example. The Lung works hard in the autumn because there is a need to tighten or contract the skin in preparation for the upcoming cold. From this it can be understood that the Lung organ has the functional property of gathering. However, it is also said that spiciness tonifies the Lung, and that the Lung warms the body by circulating ki. Thus, it can be understood that the agency of warming by circulating ki and the functional property of releasing are in the Lung channel. That is why the Lung and Liver are in a controlling cycle relationship.

Moreover, the Heart works hard in the summer to release ki, but if it is too hot, the Heart suffers a burden. Therefore, to ensure that the Heart does not overwork, it is tightened or firmed by the lesser yin channel. The lesser yin Heart channel is connected to the lesser yin Kidney channel, and along with the fluids that are stored in the Kidney, holds the functions of reducing heat and tightening or firming. However, tightening and firming are yin functions. Because the property of yin is to be still and quiet, the body would not be able to function with only yin. It would also not be possible for the Kidney to perform its reproductive role. Therefore, just as there is yang within yin, there is yang ki within the Kidney. This is what the *Nan Jing* referred to as the *life gate*. The life gate acts as a counterpart to the yin function of the Kidney, and is the mainspring of all the body's activities.

It is because this kind of reciprocal functioning between the organs and the meridians was not understood that lopsided theories were framed by both TCM and Meridian Therapy. And, since both sides did not notice the contradiction, TCM and Meridian Therapy came to be considered as altogether different things. This is a quite lamentable fact. It is my hope that readers of this book will learn the correct traditional medical art. The door has been opened for you.

Ikeda Masakazu, Director of Education

Society of Traditional Japanese Medicine

Introduction to the English Edition

As the editorial supervisor of the English edition, I would like to express my gratitude at being able to publish *Traditional Japanese Acupuncture*.

First of all I would like to review the background of this text. Talk of publishing an English edition of the newly released textbook of the Society of Traditional Japanese Medicine began in 1999 at the Meridian Therapy Summer College. At that time Okabe Somei and I, along with Aizawa Ryō, were planning a lecture series for the year 2000 on the development and spread of traditional Japanese medicine through education; we referred to that program as the Boston Program.

Although I knew it was hardly possible that I myself could produce the English translation, I found myself answering yes that I would take on the task. Believing in President Okabe and his enthusiasm, I felt that perhaps it would be possible if I were to work together with friends who have strong English abilities.

Later, I started to solicit translation volunteers from among various friends in America, but there was a tendency for the work to fall into arrears and I was on the verge of being resigned to the fact that it could not be accomplished. I was worried that I was doing a grave disservice to the members of the Society by remaining in charge of this important project. Then, as I was considering sending my regrets that I could not continue with the translation, Okabe Somei, the president of the Society of Traditional Japanese Medicine, passed away on March 25, 2000. His passing was like a bolt out of the blue to Meridian Therapy and to all of us who knew him.

The Boston Program, which I mentioned above, was scheduled to start in March of the same year with Okada Akizō and to continue with Aizawa Ryō in April, Ikeda Masakazu in May, Shimada Ryūji in June, and Okabe Somei in July. I intended to have these five leading representatives of classical Japanese acupuncture give instruction here in Boston over a five-month period. However, it turned out that not only had Okabe Somei passed away, but Shimada Ryūji, the president of the Japan Traditional Acupuncture and Moxibustion Society, also had passed away. Thus, two of the central figures planned for the Program never made it to Boston.

Despite these interruptions in the schedule, the Boston Program finished with great success, thanks to the other instructors who showed great strength of heart and did not allow the light of their inheritance of Meridian Therapy to be dimmed.

However, I now had a problem. The person to whom I could give my resignation from the English translation project had passed away, and so to me it was as if I had been instructed in a will to see the project through to publication. At that time the translation had stopped after a rough draft had been made of only a few sections of the text. Just when I thought that it would be impossible to complete the translation, a strange thing happened. The person who would end up finishing the translation for me, Joshua Margulies, suddenly appeared, as if Okabe Sensei and Shimada Sensei had sent a savior from the other world to complete the translation. In complete contrast to the initial intention to have the translation done by volunteer friends, I thereafter made use of Joshua's skills, and that swiftly carried us to the stage of publication. Although the efforts of many were involved in the production of this text, I am ultimately and solely responsible for the translation and publication of this English edition.

Regarding the terminological choices, at first I thought that basic terminology and technical jargon that is difficult to translate into English should be written in Japanese transliteration, since this is a book intended for the learning of Japanese acupuncture. However, as we went through the text we made efforts to translate nearly all the basic vocabulary into English. My reasoning was that to learn Japanese acupuncture, which is so deeply entwined with the traditional East Asian point of view and way of thinking, native English speakers should not be impeded by foreign jargon while using this text, since the language that has roots running deep into someone's being provides the easiest path to understanding.

Nevertheless, there are rewards to be gained through the study of language, and thus we have introduced a fair amount of Japanese terminology and provided appendices that cover specialized vocabulary for those who are interested in pursuing such study. In some cases where common English translations for specialized terms already existed, we continued the use of those terms. In other cases when there was no comparable concept in the English language, we attempted to add explanations of the new terms as they were introduced in the text. We also appended a glossary to the text for readers curious about terminology.

Shimada Sensei had an influence on my thoughts concerning these matters when we were talking about the contents of his proposed lectures to be given during the Boston Program. As is well known, Shimada Sensei was a leading figure in opening the path of research into East Asian classical medicine in Japan after World War II, and was also known for his brilliant mind and his 35 years of clinical experience born of research into classical acupuncture. The topic of his lecture for the Boston Program was to be the interpretation of the classics, and we planned for him to speak about the significance of traditional medicine and ways to pass it on to later generations. The original motive of such thinking can, I believe, be partially attributed to the query answered by Takeyama Shin'ichirō, in his quote on the opening page of Chapter 1 of the present text.

As our predecessors have said, it is my sincere hope that everyone, including myself, will realize the essence of humankind, will learn and make use of the fundamental nature of traditional medicine, which is based upon that essence, and will thereby gain happiness.

Finally, I would like to express my appreciation to everyone who was indispensable to the production of this book. Thank you all very much. Acknowledgments must be given to Professor Takeshi Kokubo who gave kind assistance with working out some of the more obscure passages in the Japanese. Zhenzhen Zhang kindly assisted with the Chinese pronunciation of the technical terms that are included in the appendices. John Mince-Ennis, Trish Sommeling, Charles Homonnay-Preyer, and Michael Helme all proofread the text. Rough drafts of sections from chapters 4, 7, and 8, made by Ichiro Shoji, Sayuri Miura, and Seiko Maki, were all appreciated for speeding the completion of this work. Particular notice must be given to Esther Rockett, whose published translation of sections from this work concerning abdominal diagnosis, pulse diagnosis, and treatment methods, arranged according to patterns of imbalance, was used as a welcome reference. Of course, appreciation must also be given to the many instructors of the Society of Traditional Japanese Medicine for kindly clarifying our numerous questions that arose in the course of editing the text. Sincere thanks also go to Robert Felt, our publisher, and Martha Fielding, our layout editor, without whose continuing support this book would not have come to fruition. Again, my deepest thanks to all those who were involved, including of course all those whose names are not mentioned here.

T. Koei Kuwahara

January 2003

Translator's Preface

The deepest roots of traditional Japanese acupuncture are firmly imbedded in the ancient Chinese medical texts. This explains the considerable overlap in the technical vocabulary in use in Japan and China, as well as Korea, in what is more broadly referred to as traditional East Asian medicine. Nonetheless, because this text is an introduction to Japanese-style acupuncture, we have favored translating technical terminology into English over using transliterations of the Chinese pronunciations, even when such transliterations are in common use. In a very few cases the transliteration of the Japanese pronunciation has been used throughout the text, such as the prime example of using *ki* instead of the Chinese pronunciation, *qi*.

Although Japanese is not used as the working vocabulary in the body of the text, we have introduced the Japanese for a large number of technical terms, in which cases both the characters and transliterations are provided.

To accommodate students who are more familiar with Chinese, as well as to facilitate cross referencing to Chinese medical dictionaries, the list of traditional East Asian medical terms given in Appendix 1 includes the Chinese pinyin in addition to characters, Japanese transliteration, the English translations used in this book, and also alternative English translations in use by other translators. This list is neither exhaustive in number of terms included, nor in providing all alternative English translations, but I hope it will be of use to those who are interested in broadening their studies by acquiring, or at least becoming familiar with, the source language vocabulary for traditional Japanese acupuncture. For those inspired students who also wish to study modern medical terms in Japanese, Appendix 2 offers a selection of such terminology that is gathered from the main text.

All Japanese personal names have been given in Japanese order—that is, surname followed by given name. The exceptions to this rule are the names of T. Koei Kuwahara, the Editorial Supervisor of the English edition, and of Ichiro Shoji, Sayuri Miura, and Seiko Maki, who were mentioned in the acknowledgments by T. Koei Kuwahara. Concerning orthography, the Hepburn system has been used for the transliteration of Japanese with the exception that diacriticals have been left off of commonly known place names, such as Tokyo.

Joshua Margulies

Boston, Massachusetts, 2003

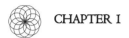 CHAPTER I

Principles of Meridian Therapy

経 絡 治 療 総 論

Nowadays there are various schools of thought that govern the practice of acupuncture. Some treatments are based on modern (i.e., Western) medical concepts, some on traditional Chinese medical (i.e., TCM) ideas, and some on the classical theories. Meridian Therapy, or *Keiraku Chiryō* (経絡治療), as explained in this book, is an acupuncture method based on the classical theories.

Acupuncture was developed in an era before the introduction of modern medicine. Therefore, it is only natural for it to take shape based on the classical theories and in this form demonstrate its true power.

Until the Meiji Restoration, which marked the ushering in of the modern era to Japan in 1868, all medical treatment followed the classical paradigm. Meridian Therapy, being based on the classics, was therefore initially called classical therapy or classical acupuncture. So, why did it end up being called Meridian Therapy? Takeyama Shin'ichirō explained it thus:

> Bearing the torch and carrying on traditions that have been handed down from a people means to comprehend the essence of those traditions, to make use of them in the present, and to then pass them on to the next generation. ... It was our intention to understand the essence of the acupuncture classics, with emphasis paid to the *Su Wen (Basic Questions), Ling Shu (Vital Axis),* and *Nan Jing (Classic of Difficulties),* and

to revive [these medical traditions] in contemporary Japan by grasping the East Asian way of thinking and points of view that serve as the supporting pillar of the clinical system. Thus, [having done so], in lieu of calling it classical acupuncture, we gave this traditional acupuncture system the new name Meridian Therapy. *(Takeyama, 1971.)*

Our predecessors understood the essence of these traditions, and in order to make the most of them in this age and to pass them on to the next generation, they advocated a revival of this classical medical art, which they called by the new name Meridian Therapy. There is another reason for choosing the name Meridian Therapy, and to understand this we must turn our gaze back to the eve of its birth.

1.1   The Development of Meridian Therapy 経絡治療の成り立ち

1.1.1   On the Eve of the Birth of Meridian Therapy

① The Campaign Against Kampo and Acupuncture

The new Meiji government (est. 1868) resolved to thoroughly modernize Japan by westernizing the whole country. Herbal medicine and acupuncture were put on the list of the old fashioned and outdated. Based partly on the perspective that they neither qualified as preventive medicine nor were useful on the battlefield, the old traditions were abandoned and there was a rush to introduce Western medicine. As early as 1875 a law was enacted that set down the rules of medical examinations, and in 1876 exams were administered throughout the country to all physicians who wished to practice.

Then, although there were many twists and turns along the way, with the proclamation of the Physicians Licensure Law in 1883 it became mandatory for all prospective physicians to learn Western medicine. It was announced in 1874 that "those who take acupuncture or moxibustion as their trade, having not received instruction in internal medicine and surgery, may not practice." This represented for all practical purposes a ban against acupuncture.

Movements for the survival of traditional medicine began to pop up all across the country in opposition to the government's campaign against kampo and acupuncture. These movements developed into a major campaign when the Onchi Association of Tokyo, the Hakuai Association of Aichi, the San'iku Association of Kyoto, and the Harusame

Association of Kumamoto organized conjointly. The majority of the protesters were herbalists, but they were joined by a number of acupuncturists as well. "Within the Onchi Association alone there were over 100 acupuncturists." *(Kamichi, 1985)*

However, after the Sino-Japanese War (1894–1895) there was a rapid decline in the movement for the survival of traditional medicine. The reason for this is not clear, but it was probably due in part to the widespread tendency to support westernization after winning the war. It was thought that kampo and acupuncture were powerless to help those who were wounded in battle.

The last president of the Onchi Association, Asai Kokkan, sobbed bitter tears in front of his ancestors' graves as he informed them of his helplessness as he witnessed the loss of the traditional art. He passed away in 1902.

② Acupoint Therapy

Acupuncture survived despite all the pressures against it. Kamichi commented:

> The government was in such a rush to introduce Western medicine that it tried to do away with kampo, acupuncture, and anma massage all at a single blow. However, acupuncture and anma massage survived for no other reason than that they were the conventional occupations of the blind.

> Then, in August of 1911, more than ten years after all the excitement caused by the movements for the survival of traditional medicine had subsided, the government, in apparent recognition of the demands made by acupuncturists from across the country, issued the Regulatory Rules for Acupuncture and Moxibustion Businesses (Ministry of Home Affairs Order XI). These rules, which took effect in January of 1912, promoted the systematization of acupuncture.

> Acupuncture treatment is effective when applied, as it should be, on the basis of its original theories. But the government attempted to alter this foundation by dressing up traditional medicine for battle in the Western medical arena, much like doing sumo wrestling on a baseball field—a rather strange sight! In other words, it tried to interpret acupuncture through the theories of cellular pathology, and the first thing it took hold of was the arrangement of acupuncture points. *(Kamichi, 1985)*

Keiketsu (経穴), the standard name in Japanese for acupuncture points, was changed to *koketsu* (孔穴), and these "revised acupuncture points" were placed in a new arrangement of

221 points spread across the body. This was an attempt, as Kamichi pointed out, to explain acupuncture from the perspective of cellular pathology. As a result of these developments the concepts of the meridian (classical therapy) approach fell into disuse, and acupoint therapy became the mainstream system. This was also the genesis of the acupuncture style that is practiced by the so-called "science faction."

③ The Beginnings of Meridian Therapy

At this time there were practitioners who, in fact, purported to practice secret methods or methods passed down solely within their family. But most of these people were practicing acupoint therapy. The reality of the matter was that they were simply "inserting needles where the patient indicated" he or she was experiencing pain, as pointed out by Ono Bunkei in his talk given at the Fiftieth Anniversary Lecture of The Society of Traditional Japanese Medicine on January 13, 1990. However, that is not to say that treatment based on the meridian system had completely disappeared. The famous Yagishita Katsunosuke was practicing a therapy that adjusted the flow of the meridians, and Wagi Tessai also used a system based on the meridians; he treated the meridian therapy advocator Inoue Keiri for swollen cervical lymph glands and caries of the ribs.

While the acupuncture points are indeed given their due importance within the classical acupuncture systems, it is not reliable to give treatment based on a system whereby each individual acupuncture point has been designated the main point of treatment for a specific symptom (often a symptom or disease as seen from the modern medical perspective). Without accumulating considerable experience or relying on old family traditions or secrets, talk of a systematic treatment method is only a fanciful tale. Those novices who could not genuinely fall back on family or secret teachings must not have had the remotest idea what to do when they came face to face with real patients. In such a time it is no wonder there were people who began to question the trend of discarding the classical systems with their rich tradition, all the more so considering that there were still leaders who were practicing the traditional systems. Having decided to spread these old traditions and pass them on to the next generation, Takeyama started using the name Meridian Therapy with the implied meaning that it was *not* acupoint therapy.

1.1.2　The Birth of Meridian Therapy and Its Fifty-Year Journey Hence

①　The Birth of Meridian Therapy

In 1927 Yanagiya Sorei opened the Sorei School with his famous plea, "Return to the classics!" Later, around 1933–1934, Okabe Sodō and Inoue Keiri, along with others who would later become the leading players in the Meridian Therapy group, gathered around Yanagiya. With the help of Takeyama Shin'ichirō they launched the Yayoi Freshmen Group (新人弥生会 *Shinjin Yayoi Kai*), which later became the parent organization of the Society of Traditional Japanese Medicine (経絡治療学会　*Keiraku Chiryō Gakkai*). The Yayoi Group was founded in 1939, and as early as 1940, the Summer Conference on Acupuncture and Herbal Medicine was held at the Kyoto Municipal Medical College. Yet, "at that time we were still exploring meridian therapy-type treatments, and did not yet have a unified treatment system." *(Kamichi, 1985)* However, by the time of the conference the following year, Meridian Therapy had developed into such a modality.

②　Meridian Therapy Fifty Years Later

Half a century has passed since those early days, and in tracing the changes Meridian Therapy went through, there emerges a history of simplification. The study of the classics that started at the Sorei School was of a considerably high level. It is obvious from looking at the Oriental Medical Journal that the members used to stay up all night discussing, sorting out, and systematizing Meridian Therapy. Then, with the accumulation of clinical experience and other contributing factors, they gradually refined the system, simplifying it in such a way that diagnoses could be made without asking too many questions and treatments could be given in stylized patterns. The following points can be considered as contributing factors to the simplification of Meridian Therapy.

First, concerns that it was too advanced and difficult to understand because of complicated content had to be addressed in order to demystify and establish Meridian Therapy as a new academic system. It is likely there were worries that even if one understood the classical principles, suddenly having to deal with pulse position/pulse quality diagnosis or obscure and difficult concepts would be too much to handle for both those who were learning it and those who were teaching it. It would be easier to demystify and establish Meridian Therapy if both the theories and techniques were simple and easy to understand.

The second factor was the diversity within Meridian Therapy. Each meridian therapist brings his or her own individuality to the system. For example, even just within pulse diagnosis there is a subtle difference between practitioners in the way they position their fingers on the pulse and their understandings of the depths for the superficial and deep levels.

The third factor is related to the second. In fact it is easier for each practitioner to develop his or her own unique clinical system when the foundational theories and techniques are simple.

The fourth factor concerns changes in the environment that surrounds acupuncture. Due to advancements in contemporary medicine and improvements in health standards, acupuncture is no longer used as much as it once was to treat acute illnesses. In actuality, contemporary medicine and traditional East Asian medicine have come to hold claim over separate turfs. Moreover, with the growth of industry and the increasing complexity of society, the structure of illness in the present age has changed such that most patients present with deficient-type patterns of imbalance, as explained in the East Asian medical system. Clinical acupuncture has had no other choice but to respond and adapt to these changes in the environment.

The culmination of these past fifty years can be summed up in the development of the following principles:

- The affirmation of the existence of the meridians.
- The view that all diseases will manifest as a change in the meridians.
- Changes in the meridians, whether deficient or excess, are grasped by focusing on the pulse strength comparison diagnosis.
- Focusing on the patterns of imbalance (証 *shō*) that are of the yin deficiency type. These are deficiency of the Liver, Spleen, Lung, and Kidney.
- The splitting of treatment into root treatment and local treatment, although these are performed simultaneously and have equal value.
- Basing the treatment theory on the rule that says to tonify deficiency and disperse excess.
- Focusing on tonification, using extremely shallow insertion and retained needles, or no insertion at all.
- Standardization of the root treatment methods.

1.1.3   The Future of Meridian Therapy

As previously noted, Meridian Therapy was simplified over the past half century. That simplification was important, but it brought with it two problems. One is an increase in the number of voices, particularly among young people, calling for an explanation of the fundamental theories of Meridian Therapy.

The other is that, since Meridian Therapy now has a greater than fifty-year history after initially being brought forward, it must be further improved and developed, and not simply maintained as an unchanging therapeutic system. Moreover, there are those who wonder if perhaps Meridian Therapy had too hasty a start, having been put into practice without being fully worked out. That has given rise to people from within the Meridian Therapy community itself calling for the improvement and development of the Meridian Therapy treatment system. However, there are reservations as to whether there is really any validity to the claim that Meridian Therapy has some defective points today or that it had too hasty a start.

① Problems in Meridian Therapy

Kamichi Sakae pointed out various problems when he said:

> Before the birth of Meridian Therapy, acupuncture was mainly used as pain therapy that was simply the insertion of needles at places of discomfort. Of course, the needling of distal points did occur, but it is safe to say that there was no utilization of the five phase points nor needling that made use of the meridians. With that in mind, the establishment of a treatment system that was consistent from diagnosis through to treatment was of great significance from the standpoint of clinical practice. That is not to say that [Meridian Therapy] no longer needs to be enhanced or investigated. *(Kamichi, 1985)*

Other people have pointed out the following problems, which are only briefly mentioned here for lack of space.

- Meridian Therapy should more fully adopt pulse quality diagnosis.
- Instead of mechanically choosing KI-10 and LR-8 as points for Liver deficiency, more thought should be given to wider point selection methods.
- There is a need to make etiologies and pathologies clear.

- There is talk of root treatment and local treatment, but if local treatment is not actually effecting the healing, is root treatment obsolete?
- When taking the pulse, is one examining the meridians or the organs? Are they not separate?

② Solutions to the Problems and a New Beginning

All these concerns are satisfactorily answered in this book. Moreover, as to the question of whether the founders of Meridian Therapy made too hasty a start, leaving these problems unresolved, we do not believe they did so.

For example, Inoue Keiri made clear the relationship between root treatment and local treatment on the tape of his lecture about the *Nan Jing (Classic of Difficulties)*.

At the Fifth Oriental Medicine Conference (1941), Takeyama Shin'ichirō said:

> Meridian Therapy corrects imbalances in the body by feeling for changes in the meridians through diagnostic techniques peculiar to acupuncture and by adjusting those changes. This is possible because changes within the five zang organs and six fu organs manifest as [perceptible] phenomena in the meridians. In other words, one can approach the essence by grasping the manifestation.

In 1940, at a time when people were saying that Meridian Therapy was not yet clearly formed, Okabe Sodō made the following comments in his speech "Concerning the relationship between pulse diagnosis and the meridians in the clinical setting" at the summer conference held at the Kyoto Municipal Medical College.

> The meridians and acupuncture points are the root of acupuncture; they are the basis. Acupuncture was established on the foundation of the meridians and acupuncture points. Therefore, it is only after one has thoroughly studied the meridians and acupuncture points that one is able to give accurate treatment. The aspects in which acupuncture is superior to other treatment systems lies within the meridians and acupuncture points and the related [understanding of] pathology and diagnostic techniques, as well as the needling and moxibustion [that is given] based on these.

Okabe further described 24 pulse qualities and the methods of tonification and dispersion used to treat them. At the same time, he explained what kinds of symptom patterns correspond to the various combinations of pulse qualities that can be found in the six pulse positions.

Based on the above facts, we believe that the founders of Meridian Therapy commanded a full understanding of their field. Claims and allegations that Meridian Therapy had too hasty a start and that it still harbored problems spring from previously mentioned factors which led to the simplification of Meridian Therapy. This is different from saying that there is a defect within Meridian Therapy itself.

Nonetheless, the circumstances today are different from what they used to be. There is an abundance of information about acupuncture, especially books on Traditional Chinese Medicine (TCM). It is easy to get hold of seminal works, and has become simple to understand them with the help of explanatory guidebooks. Therefore, along with providing answers to the problems mentioned above, we must conform to the times by giving explanations and theoretical concepts in as thorough a manner as possible so that even beginners will be able to satisfactorily understand the material.

Finally, as concerns the future of Meridian Therapy, it is important that we all give more attention to the areas that are criticized. Also, since there is a valid concern that recently Meridian Therapy has become just a name and that people are rampantly practicing so-called acupoint therapy, one should understand even those things that were not taught by our predecessors, and then pass down that information to the next generation. Efforts should be made to read the classical texts such as the *Su Wen*, *Ling Shu*, and *Nan Jing*, as well as those books listed in the bibliography that have been translated into English.

1.2 What is Meridian Therapy? 経絡治療とは

1.2.1 Kinds of Tools and Their Usage

① Needle Materials

In ancient China needles were mainly made of animal bones, bamboo, copper, and iron. Gold and silver needles appeared from the time of the Early Han dynasty (206 B.C.E.–8 C.E.).

Contemporary needles are mainly made of gold, silver, and stainless steel.

② Kinds of Needles

In the *Ling Shu (Vital Axis)*, nine different needles are categorized and explained according to their different uses.

Today the most commonly used needle is the *gōshin* needle (毫鍼 filiform needle). It comes in various lengths such as 40mm and 30mm, and practitioners should use the length of needle that has the best feel. In addition there are other needles used such as the *taishin* (大鍼 big needle), *chōshin* (長鍼 long needle), *teishin* (鍉鍼 blunt needle), *enrishin* (員利鍼 round-sharp needle), *sanryōshin* (三稜鍼 three-edged needle), *kyūtōshin* (灸頭鍼 moxa-on-the-handle needle), *chōheishin* (長柄鍼 long-handled needle), and *hifushin* (皮膚鍼 touching needle).

The Nine Needles of the *Ling Shu*

Zanshin (鑱鍼 chisel needle). Length: 1.6 *cùn*. A sharp-pointed needle with a big head. It is used to disperse yang ki.

Enshin (員鍼 round needle). Length: 1.6 *cùn*. The tip has an egg shape. It is used to massage between the channels and to disperse ki without cutting the flesh.

Teishin (鍉鍼 blunt needle). Length: 3.5 *cùn*. The tip resembles the sharpness of millet. It is used mainly to press the meridians and thereby send ki [to the needed areas].

Hōshin (鋒鍼 lance needle). Length: 1.6 *cùn*. It has a three-edged blade and is used to dispel chronic diseases.

Hishin (鈹鍼 sword needle). Length: 4 *cùn*. Width: 0.25 *cùn*. It resembles a double-edged sword and is used to drain pus.

Enrishin (員利鍼 round-sharp needle). Length: 1.6 *cùn*. As thin as the hair of a yak, and round and sharp, its body is a little big. It is used to disperse fulminant ki.

Gōshin (毫鍼 filiform needle). Length: 3.6 *cùn*. It is sharp and resembles the proboscis of a mosquito or horsefly. It is used to treat painful numbness (*bi* syndrome) by giving a nourishing stimulation through very softly and gently inserting the needle and then retaining it for a long time.

Chōshin (長鍼 long needle). Length: 7 *cùn*. The tip is sharp and the body is thin. It can be used to treat deep numbness (*bi* syndrome).

Taishin (大鍼 big needle). Length: 4 *cùn*. It is tipped like a stick and the point is slightly round. It is used to drain water from the joints.

---

③ Needle Usage

When using the filiform needle, it is common to use an insertion tube when needling. However, no insertion tube is used with the long-handled needle. Since an insertion tube cannot be used with the *taishin* or *chōshin* needles, they have their own needling methods. Needling is not difficult for beginners when using an insertion tube. However, it is painful and easy for ki to leak when needling is done poorly or without a tube, and it is possible for accidents to happen when inexperienced people use the *taishin* or *chōshin* needles.

④ Moxa-on-the-Handle Needle *Kyūtōshin* 灸頭鍼

The *kyūtōshin*, or a needle on which moxa is burned on the handle, is effective for treating chronic chills or pain since it has the ability to warm deep areas, but it must be used with caution so as not to cause burns. However, if you simply warm the surface of the skin because you are worried about burns, it is likely that you will not achieve the expected results.

⑤ Warming Moxibustion *Onkyū* 温灸

Moxibustion includes methods whereby the moxa is burned directly on the skin and methods that are used to warm just an area. There are various methods of performing warming moxibustion, such as removing the moxa once it gets hot or burning the moxa on top of garlic, salt, or ginger. Of course, the method to be used is determined by the symptom pattern.

It is good to use coarse moxa for warming moxibustion and moxa-on-the-handle needle. If you use high quality moxa that is very dry, the burning time is too quick and often the desired result is not attained. Care should be taken with warming moxibustion as well, so as not to burn the patient.

⑥ Direct Moxibustion *Tōnetsukyū* 透熱灸

Some people have reservations about applying direct moxibustion since it is burned directly on the skin and thus leaves a scar, but it is very effective depending on the condition. However, it is important that the size and hardness of the moxa be uniform. High-quality bleached moxa that is very dry should be used.

1.2.2 Training for Examination and Treatment

① Warm, Soft Hands

Acupuncturists should have warm and soft hands and fingers. It is said that Okabe Sodō's hands and fingers were as soft as an infant's skin. It is easier to feel ki and project ki when one has warm, soft hands. Also, with such hands you will naturally be able to correctly locate acupuncture points and will be able to painlessly needle the points.

Cold and wet hands are the worst hands for an acupuncturist to have. People with such hands can make them warmer and softer by practicing anma massage. Touching skin as much as possible is the best practice for making good acupuncture hands.

② Needling Practice

Even for those with soft hands it is important to practice needling. First, you should practice needling a soft wooden board without using an insertion tube. This will help in making a sturdy supporting hand (*oshide* 押手), which is important because the supporting hand of many beginners is too loose, making their needling technique painful and allowing ki to leak out.

Next you should practice needling fruit that is floating in water. This will ensure that your supporting hand does not become too strong or heavy, which is important since it is not effective to have excessive strength in the supporting hand when doing tonification.

③ Practice Pulse Diagnosis and Abdominal Diagnosis

Of course, developing warm, soft hands is the first step, but it is also very important to acquire a lot of experience with pulse diagnosis and abdominal diagnosis. At the same time it is good to build a habit of always making a mental note of the relation between what you observe in the pulse or the abdomen and the symptom pattern and pathology. For example, remember which pulses occur when someone is constipated or having diarrhea. It takes more than just an idle examination of the pulse in order to improve as a practitioner.

④ Study Under a Good Teacher *Shishō* 師匠

Traditionally, when people wished to learn a skill or acquire a profession the best method was to apprentice to a good teacher and learn through observation. It is the same even with games such as golf, *go* (a Japanese board game of strategy), and *shōgi* (Japanese chess).

Hence there is no reason that acupuncturists alone can become professionals as soon as they graduate from school.

The section that introduced problems facing Meridian Therapy mentioned that there are people who say that learning pulse diagnosis is too difficult. But this is a big misunderstanding. Persons of this type have given up becoming professionals.

Certainly it is not easy to learn pulse diagnosis and the other skills of an acupuncturist. That is precisely why it is important to become an apprentice, to study everything that your teacher says, to observe treatments, and to follow your teacher's example. However, who will make a good teacher for someone depends on the student. Finding a good teacher involves a bit of luck and whether or not the teacher and student hit it off with each other. Therefore, it is good to trust your intuition and go with the teacher that makes you feel comfortable. If you do that your path should naturally open up before you.

> Those who are slow and soft in speech, have good dexterity, and are clear-headed should be made to practice acupuncture. ... Those who have hard fingernails and poison in their hands (i.e., who are ruthless in nature), and who are apt to hurt others should be made to massage accumulations (積 Jpn: *shaku*, Chn: *jī*) and control [i.e., treat] bi-syndromes (痺) ... [In order to discover] who has poison in their hands, as a test have [the person] handle a turtle. Put the turtle under a dish, and have [the person] press the top [of the dish]. The turtle will die in fifty days [if the person has poison in their hands], and will still be alive in fifty days if the person has sweet hands [i.e., is merciful in nature]. (*Ling Shu*, Chapter 73)

1.2.3 Definition of Meridian Therapy

Meridian Therapy is a traditional medical system that grasps all diseases as a condition of deficiency or excess of ki or blood in the meridians, and then uses the techniques of acupuncture to tonify or disperse that deficiency or excess in order to bring about healing. It is also known as the *zuishō* (随証) treatment method, which means treatment is given by following the pattern of imbalance.

In order to put the above definition into practice in the clinic, you must understand and master the following points.

① The flow of the meridians and the location of the acupuncture points, as well as the methods for locating the points and point selection theory.

② Foundational concepts, yin/yang and five phases theory, deficiency and excess theory.

③ Physiology (i.e., visceral manifestation 蔵象 *zōshō*) as described in Meridian Therapy, in other words the functioning of the organs, ki, blood, and fluids.

④ The etiological factors that generate deficiency and excess, and the resultant symptom pattern and pathologies.

⑤ Diagnostic techniques, such as pulse diagnosis and abdominal diagnosis.

⑥ Tonification and dispersion techniques, such as needling and moxibustion.

Understanding these points means that you are able to determine the pattern of imbalance and carry out treatments.

As an example, suppose you are examining a patient with low back pain. Upon asking the reason for the pain, the patient tells you that it came on after carrying some heavy bags. From this you know that the etiological factor is fatigue, a non-endogenous/non-exogenous factor (see Chapter 5). You then consider the possibility of Liver deficiency because the Liver controls the sinews (muscles) and the muscles in the lower back are experiencing pain. (The organs and the pathologies are related.)

Next, when you take the pulse you find that there is deficiency at the deep level in the middle and proximal positions on the left wrist, and that the pulse is clearly felt when the artery is only lightly touched. This means that there is deficiency in the Liver and Kidney, and that ki has collected in the yang meridians. (Yin and yang and the five phases are related.) This calls for tonification of KI-10 and LR-8, and for additional local tonification or dispersion if there is a condition of deficiency or excess in the lumbar muscles. (Tonification and dispersion, point location, and point selection theory are related.)

The points outlined above may appear to be simple, but in actual practice it is often difficult to judge the number of needles and the depth of insertion needed for individual patients. Therefore, you must consider the prognosis and how much needling to give by taking into account the person's build, sex, and physical constitution (these are related to observational diagnosis), as well as the presenting symptom pattern and its relation to the pulse.

For example, it is difficult for a solidly built person who has a weak pulse to get well. You cannot use deep needling on such a person, and it is also important to use only a few needles. When you can clearly make these distinctions, your patients will no longer become exhausted from overstimulation during treatment. If you can correctly grasp the pattern of imbalance there is no problem, but this is an area where beginners often become confused and make mistakes. The vital importance of grasping the pattern of imbalance cannot be overemphasized. You should keep this in mind as you read this text.

Finally, the table below gives a list of the main patterns of imbalance that are seen in the practice of Meridian Therapy.

Table 1–1: Patterns of Imbalance
Liver deficiency heat pattern (肝虚熱証 *Kan-Kyo Nesshō*)
Liver deficiency cold pattern (肝虚寒証 *Kan-Kyo Kanshō*)
Spleen deficiency heat pattern (脾虚熱証 *Hi-Kyo Nesshō*)
Spleen deficiency yang ming channel excess heat pattern (脾虚陽明経実熱証 *Hi-Kyo Yōmeikei-Jitsu Nesshō*)
Spleen deficiency Stomach excess heat pattern (脾虚胃実熱証 *Hi-Kyo I-Jitsu Nesshō*)
Spleen deficiency Stomach deficiency heat pattern (脾虚胃虚熱証 *Hi-Kyo I-Kyo Nesshō*)
Spleen deficiency cold pattern (脾虚寒証 *Hi-Kyo Kanshō*)
Spleen deficiency Liver excess heat pattern (脾虚肝実熱証 *Hi-Kyo Kan-Jitsu Neshhō*)
Spleen deficiency Liver excess pattern (脾虚肝実証 *Hi-Kyo Kan-Jitsu Shō*)
Lung deficiency yang channel excess heat pattern (肺虚陽経実熱証 *Hai-Kyo Yōkei-Jitsu Nesshō*)
Lung deficiency cold pattern (肺虚寒証 *Hai-Kyo Kanshō*)
Lung deficiency Liver excess pattern (肺虚肝実証 *Hai-Kyo Kan-Jitsu Shō*)
Kidney deficiency heat pattern (腎虚熱証 *Jin-Kyo Nesshō*)
Kidney deficiency cold pattern (腎虚寒証 *Jin-Kyo Kanshō*)

1.3   The Philosophical Background of Meridian Therapy

経絡治療の哲学的背景

Many sections of the *Su Wen (Elementary Questions), Ling Shu (Vital Axis),* and *Nan Jing (Classic of Difficulties)* are explained in terms of yin and yang, the five phases, Daoist thought, mountain sage thought, and the concept of the correlation of heaven (i.e., the universe) and humans. These concepts among others are briefly explained below, as they are useful for understanding Meridian Therapy.

1.3.1   Yin and Yang

In Japanese, we often speak of yin and yang and the five phases together as one phrase, but the concept of yin and yang and that of the five phases theory developed separately. In particular, the concept of yin and yang is exceptionally old. The concept is commonly thought to have derived from divination practices such as those related to the *Yi Jing (Classic of Changes)*. Certainly the best way to gain an understanding of yin and yang is to study the changes described in the *Yi Jing*, but here we will give a brief introduction.

The concept of yin and yang is an attempt to comprehend all phenomena and worldly material and as being composed of two polar states: yin, which has qualities such as feminine, negative, hidden, dark, and soft, and yang, which has qualities such as masculine, positive, obvious, light, and hard.

①   Classifications of Yin and Yang

All material and phenomena can be divided into either yin or yang. However, there is nothing that is purely the one or the other. In other words, there is always some yang within yin and some yin within yang. This is a fundamental concept of yin and yang theory.

Table 1–2: Classifications of Yin and Yang						
Yang	Heaven	Sun	Fire	Sunny weather	Man	Spring & Summer	Day
Yin	Earth	Moon	Water	Rainy weather	Woman	Fall & Winter	Night

Yin exists within yin, and yang exists within yang. From dawn until midday is [the time of] the yang of heaven, and is yang within yang. From midday until sunset is [the time of] the yang of heaven, and is yin within yang. From dusk until the cock's crow is [the time of] the yin of heaven, and is yin within yin. From the cock's crow until dawn is [the time of] the yin of heaven, and is yang within yin. *[Su Wen, Chapter 4]*

② **Functions and Characteristics of Yin and Yang**

Table 1–3: Functions and Characteristics of Yin and Yang								
Yang	Warming	Movement	Softening	Drying	Opening	Diffusing	Emerging	Ascending
Yin	Cooling	Stillness	Firming	Moistening	Closing	Gathering	Entering	Descending

These characteristics and functions of yin and yang do not work independently, but rather are relative to each other. Here are some principal concepts of yin and yang.

- Yin and yang continuously maintain balance by alternating and circulating.
- If one becomes strong, the other becomes weak.
- If yin increases to the extreme it will transform into yang; if yang increases to the extreme it will transform into yin.

This is easy to understand if you think about the seasons. After the extreme yin of winter, or what is called yin within yin, the seasons gradually change into spring and then into summer. After the extreme yang of summer, or yang within yang, the seasons start to change towards autumn and then back to winter. When winter goes to the extreme, spring will follow again, and the cycle continues.

While all living things, all of nature, and all phenomena can be classified into yin or yang aspects, at the same time everything follows the laws of nature mentioned above, continually transforming, endlessly rising and falling with the flow of yin and yang. The disruption of this harmonious condition causes natural disasters and is the root of sickness. In Japanese, the phrase *ten no kyoja* (天の虚邪), which means that heaven is deficient and that there is an outbreak of pathogenic or evil ki, is used to describe this situation. In other words, the ki of the heavens becomes weak, causing a disturbance in the homeostasis between the solar system and the Earth, which in turn can lead to illness in people.

Diagram 1–1: The Waxing and Waning and Circulation of Yin and Yang

Season	Vernal Equinox	Summer Solstice	Autumnal Equinox	Winter Solstice
Time of Day	Sunrise	Midday	Sunset	Nighttime
Amount of Yang Ki		Yang Ki		
Amount of Yin Ki			Yin Ki	

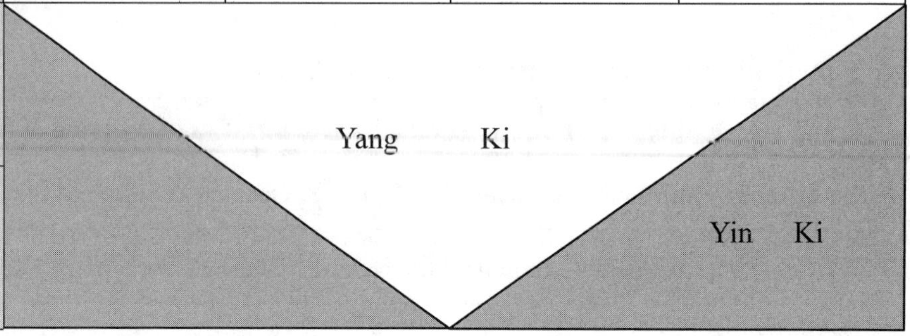

1.3.2 Five Phases Theory *Gogyō* 五行説

The five phases theory is a concept that divides everything into five categories of elements: wood, fire, earth, metal, and water. It is said that all phenomena can be explained in terms of two relationships among these five phases: the generative cycle and the controlling cycle.

Wood (木 Moku). This refers to wood in the sense of a living tree. It corresponds to the direction of east and the season of spring. Spring is the time when things are generated or created, and generation/creation is a quality of the wood phase. It is associated with the color green, a rancid smell, and a sour taste. The associated grain, fruit, and domestic animal are wheat, plum, and dog.

Fire (火 Ka). This refers to a flaming fire. It corresponds to the direction of south and the season of summer. Summer is the time when things flourish, and growth is a quality of the fire phase. It is associated with the color red, a burnt smell, and a bitter taste. The corresponding grain, fruit, and domestic animal are millet, apricot, and sheep.

Earth (土 Do). This refers to earth and sand and clay. It corresponds to the central position and the season of midsummer between summer and autumn. Midsummer is a time when things change, and change is a quality of the earth phase. It is associated with the color yellow, a fragrant smell, and a sweet taste. The corresponding grain, fruit, and domestic animal are barnyard grass, jujube, and cow.

Metal (金 Kin). This refers to metallic objects. It corresponds to the direction of west and the season of autumn. Autumn is the time when things gather, pulling their energy in and concentrating it, and coming to fruition is a quality of the metal phase. It is associated with the color white, a fleshy smell, and a pungent taste. The corresponding grain, fruit, and domestic animal are rice, peach, and horse.

Water (水 Sui). This refers to all things in liquid form. It corresponds to the direction of north and the season of winter. Winter is a time when things hide, and the condition of being hidden is a quality of the water phase. It is associated with the color black, a rotten smell, and a salty taste. The corresponding grain, fruit, and domestic animal are beans, chestnut, and pig.

Spring, summer, autumn, and winter are the only seasons, which means only four seasonal phases. However, the addition of midsummer is what gives five seasonal phases. Actually, the Japanese word *doyō* (土用), which is used to refer to midsummer, means the transitional periods between all the seasons. The 18 days before the beginning of summer is the spring *doyō*, the 18 days before the beginning of autumn is the summer *doyō* or midsummer, the 18 days before the beginning of winter is the autumn *doyō*, and the 18 days before the beginning of spring is the winter *doyō*. These transitional *doyō* periods are controlled by the ki of the earth phase. The summer *doyō* period is the time when the functional properties of the earth phase are most in need, and that is why it was added as one of the seasons of the five phases.

① **The Generative Cycle of the Five Phases** *Gogyō no Sōsei Kankei* 五行の相生関係

One of the relationships between the five phases is the generative cycle, which is also known as the engendering cycle, or the parent-child cycle. This relationship states that wood generates fire, fire generates earth, earth generates metal, metal generates water, and water generates wood. This is usually explained as: burning wood makes fire; burning a fire out completely leaves behind ash (i.e., earth); metal ore is found in earth; adding heat to metal makes liquid (i.e., water); and giving water to a tree generates the growth of wood.

② **The Controlling Cycle of the Five Phases** *Gogyō no Sōkoku Kankei* 五行の相剋関係

The five phases are also in a controlling cycle with each other. Controlling implies holding sway over, causing trouble for, or taking something away from the relational phase.

Wood controls earth, earth controls water, water controls fire, fire controls metal, and metal controls wood. This is usually explained as: wood sucks up the nutrients from the earth; earth dams up water; water extinguishes fire; fire melts metal; and metal cuts wood.

Diagram 1–2: Generative and Controlling Cycles

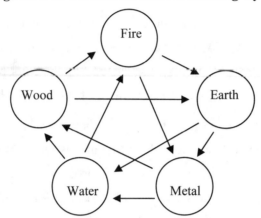

1.3.3 Ki and the Meridians *Ki to Keiraku* 気と経絡

The meridians (経絡 *keiraku*) are the most critical concept in forming the basis of Meridian Therapy. Ki and blood circulate through the meridians. Ki and blood are divided by functional properties and expressed as defensive ki, nutritive ki, blood, fluids, essence, and spirit. Lumped together they can be explained as the workings (*hataraki*) of ki.

Ki and the meridians cannot be seen with the eyes. There are some people who deny their existence because they cannot see them. However, from the clinical point of view one can adequately sense the existence of the meridians. Because it is the same with ki, in the clinic the practitioner gives treatments while maintaining an awareness of ki. As such, ki and the meridians are neither philosophical concepts nor constructs of the mind. They are facts that can be recognized within the clinic. If you are going to try to understand ki and the meridians, the only way to do so is to practice therapy that is thoroughly traditional. That is the quickest way. Comparing meridian therapy to Western medicine or looking at it from the Western medical perspective is like watching sumo wrestling while thinking about the rules of Olympic-style wrestling. That is not to say that one is superior to the other, but that they are completely different systems.

1.3.4 Other Concepts

① Daoist Thought

Daoist thought is one of the ancient Chinese systems of thought. It came about during the later half of the Zhōu Dynasty, in a time known as the Spring and Autumn period (770–402 B.C.E.). Daoism is the school of thought founded on the concept of *Dao* or the *Way*, as given by Laozi in the seminal work attributed to him, the *Dàodéjīng*. Daoist thought is also highly influenced by Zhuangzi, and is also known as Lao-Zhuang Thought, giving credit to both authors. Many phrases seen in the *Su Wen (Elementary Questions)* are very similar to passages in the *Dàodéjīng*.

> In ancient times the sages taught [the following] to the people below them:
>
> There are times [and methods] for warding off those pathogenic influences that weaken and harm [the body]. True ki will follow [the person who is in] a condition of serenity and satisfaction and a state of emptiness. If one preserves one's essence and spirit internally, how can illness occur?
>
> Therefore, ki will flow smoothly through those who temper their ambition [i.e., give up ambitions that are beyond their reach], have few desires, have contented hearts and fear nothing, and do not work so hard as to become fatigued. [Such people] can have all their wants satisfied. In other words, the people will be simple like an uncarved block of wood because they will enjoy [whatever] food [they have], will be content with [whatever] position [they hold], will be happy with their lots [in life], and will not be concerned about social status. In such a state, no temptation will divert their eyes, and no carnal desire will mislead their hearts. They will have nothing to worry about even though they may have differences in intelligence, knowledge, or character. Thus, they will be in tune with the Dao.
>
> It is because people used to cultivate virtue and did not diverge from such a life that they were able to live past 100 years of age without becoming decrepit. (*Su Wen*, Chapter 1)

② Mountain Sage Thought

The mountain sages referred to here are people in ancient China who aimed at attaining immortality. They reasoned that good health was required in order to attain immortality. If sickness arose, treatment was necessary. One of the treatment methods they used was acupuncture. The *Su Wen* also contains passages that are concerned with mountain sage thought.

> In ancient times the Yellow Emperor was born a child prodigy. From infancy he had a command of language, and he was wise and upright from the time he was very young. As he grew he showed himself to be honest, sincere, and comprehending. When he grew up he became emperor and [eventually] rose to heaven [as an immortal]. [*Su Wen*, Chapter 1]

③ Concept of the Correlation of Heaven and Humankind

This concept says that there is an intricate correlation between the natural world and universe and the human body. The reason for the rise in this kind of thought is related to the Daoist thought and mountain sage thought just mentioned.

This concept holds that if one lives in harmony with the rhythm of the natural world then he will be healthy, but if one goes against this natural rhythm then he will become ill. So, the question is, just what is this natural rhythm? Naturally, as the air becomes drier, the human body will also dry out, or as the humidity rises, the level of water in the body will also rise. If you understand the natural rhythm, you will also understand the close relationship between the natural world and the human body. There are many passages in the classics concerning this relationship.

> The Yellow Emperor stated, "Among the myriad things covered by Heaven and supported by Earth, nothing is more precious than humans. Humans are made to live by the qi of Heaven and Earth, and to grow in accord with the laws of the four seasons." … Qibo said, "Humans are born of the Earth and connected to Heaven. [In other words,] humans are made by the intercourse of the qi of Heaven and Earth. If humans adapt to and follow the laws of the four seasons, then Heaven and Earth will be like a mother and father, [caring for them affectionately.]" … *(Su Wen*, Chapter 25)

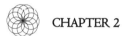

CHAPTER 2

Introduction to the Basics

基 礎 概 論

In this introduction to the basics we will take a look at yin and yang, the five phases, ki, blood, fluids, and deficiency and excess. You should make yourself familiar with these concepts before reading the rest of this textbook as they are related to the organs, etiology, pathology, patterns of imbalance, diagnosis, and treatment. However, they can be somewhat difficult to understand in the beginning. Sometimes it is easier to understand one concept once you have grasped a different one, so you should study further even if there are points that do not make sense at first.

2.1　Yin and Yang in Treatment　　治療における陰陽

2.1.1　Yin and Yang Divisions of the Body (Yin and Yang of the Diseased Area)

Just as we divided nature up into yin and yang aspects, so too can the human body be divided. These divisions can be organized as shown in Table 2–1 (page 24).

Yin and yang are relative characteristics; the designation depends on what is being compared. Thus, something that is designated as yin in one case can change to yang when the thing it is being compared to changes and vice versa. In Meridian Therapy, all illnesses are treated based on an understanding of the transformations in yin and yang ki (deficiency or excess, heat or cold) occurring within the yin and yang areas of the body (meridians). It follows that all areas and points of the body, as well as ki, blood, and fluids, have either yin or yang aspects. Where there is a yin aspect, there is a corresponding yang aspect. Where there is a yang aspect, there is a corresponding yin aspect. Assigning a position as belonging to either a yin or a yang aspect in this way is based on the fact that a particular area has more or less yin ki or yang ki *relative* to other areas.

Table 2 –1 Yin and Yang Divisions of the Body (Yin and Yang of the Diseased Area)	
Yin	**Yang**
Lower Body	Upper Body
Trunk	Extremities
Three Yin Channels	Three Yang Channels
Flesh, Sinews, and Bone	Skin, Hair, and Blood Vessels
Abdomen	Back
Zang Organs	Fu Organs
Kidney	Heart
Liver	Lung
Spleen	Stomach
Blood	Ki
Fluids	Blood

2.1.2 Functions of Yin and Yang (Physiology of Yin and Yang)

Each part of the body is designated as having either a yin or a yang characteristic, yet each of those areas has both yin ki and yang ki. At the same time, they also have the yin ki and yang ki that is circulated through the meridians. Yin ki and yang ki have the following properties and functions.

① The Functions and Properties of Yin Ki

Yin ki has, among others, the following functions: to firm; to shorten; to pull down; to gather; to store; to bear (as in childbearing); to cool (something that has heat); to tranquilize.

Things in liquid form belong to the yin aspect. Therefore, materials such as bodily fluids and blood have yin functions and properties.

② The Functions and Properties of Yang Ki

Some functions of yang ki are: to spread out; to extend; to rise; to diffuse; to dry; to heat; to remove cold, to activate something that has become stagnant. However, sometimes when yang ki becomes hyperactive it diffuses so much that it actually acts to cool things down. Chapter 5 of the *Su Wen* expresses this concept as "yang kills" or "weakening the ki of a vigorous fire (壮火 Jpn: *sōka*, Chn: *zhuàng huǒ*)."

Moreover, while blood has a liquid form that gives it a yin quality such as cooling, it also has yang ki and works to warm the body. This difference in function depends on the location. Blood that is in a yang part of the body works as yang while blood that is in a yin part of the body works as yin.

③ Yin Leads, Yang Follows

The founders of Meridian Therapy used the phrase, "yin leads, yang follows." This expresses the fact that sickness results from yin deficiency, and hence that should be the practitioner's first concern when determining the pattern of imbalance.

Again, Chapter 5 of the *Su Wen* says, "Yin is internal and is the guardian of yang; yang is superficial and is the regulator of yin." Chapter 3 says, "Yin stores the essence and prepares it for use; yang sets up a strong guard from the outside."

"Yin is internal and is the guardian of yang," means that if yin securely stores ki, blood, and fluids and makes proper use of them, then the yang areas (the superficial level) of the body will not be influenced by external pathogens. In other words, the functioning of yang ki will be activated when there is sufficient ki, blood, and fluids. As moderate amounts of yang ki are released from the surface, it triggers the opening and closing of the pores of the skin, which when open allow for the release of heat as the body becomes active and when closed allow for defense from external pathogens. Therefore, yang is said to be at the superficial level, to protect the outside, and to be the regulator of yin. These are important qualities of yin and yang.

④ **The Waxing and Waning, Alternation, and Circulation of Yin and Yang**

Yin and yang wax and wane, alternating between each other just as the four seasons transform one into the other in a continuous circulatory pattern. This rule can also be seen within the example of a single day. Yang ki gradually waxes as the sun rises in the morning. It reaches a peak during the midday, and then as the sun leans into the west, yang ki wanes and yin ki emerges. During the night yin ki becomes the most active, but then gives way to yang ki again the next morning.

This kind of interchange or alternation between yin and yang also takes place within the human body and logically follows the natural flow of yin and yang. Thus, in the morning we open our eyes and become active as yang ki emerges. Our pores are triggered to open as yang ki is released through the skin. Yang ki is then pulled in at night, and yin ki takes over, closing the pores and protecting the body from the influence of external pathogens.

Yin and yang ki and blood are generated in the Spleen and Stomach and then circulate in the meridians by first rising up to the chest and then going via the yin channels of the hands to the tips of the fingers. From there they travel in the yang channels of the hands, rising up to the head and releasing moderate amounts of ki. Next, while still releasing ki, the path descends to the feet via the yang channels and then enters the inside of the body by way of the yin channels of the feet. Throughout this circulatory pattern, yang ki is plentiful at the superficial levels and limited at the deep levels during the daytime, and yin ki is plentiful at the superficial levels while during the nighttime yang ki is plentiful at the deep levels.

2.2　The Five Phases in Treatment　　治療における五行

Just as the natural world was divided into the five phases, the parts and functions of the human body, etiology, pathology, and patterns of imbalance, are also classified into five phases, centering on the five zang organs (五臓 *gozō*). This is more easily understood in conjunction with explanations of visceral manifestations and symptom patterns, and thus details will be introduced here and given more attention in later Chapters. Table 2–2 lists some of the attributes and relations of the five phases (五行 *gogyō*), and Table 2–3 on page 30 lists acupuncture points classified by five-phases groupings.

The five zang organs as well as the five phases are in generative and controlling cycles with each other. That point has already been briefly touched upon, but with not enough detail to make it useful in the clinic. Your understanding concerning these matters will deepen later when we cover visceral manifestations.

Table 2–2: Attributes of the Five Phases					
Five Phases	**Wood**	**Fire**	**Earth**	**Metal**	**Water**
Five Zang Organs	Liver	Heart	Spleen	Lung	Kidney
Five Fu Organs	Gallbladder	Small Intestine	Stomach	Large Intestine	Bladder
Five Essences	Ethereal Soul	Spirit	Intention and Wisdom	Corporeal Soul	Will
Five Principal Parts	Sinews and Fascia	Blood Vessels	Flesh	Skin and (Body) Hair	Bone Marrow
Five Orifices	Eyes	Tongue	Mouth	Nose	Ears
Five Minds	Anger	Joy	Pensiveness/ Thought	Sorrow/ Anxiety	Fear
Five Accessory Parts	Nails	Facial Color	Lips	Body Hair	Head Hair
Five Flavors	Sour	Bitter	Sweet	Pungent/ Spicy	Salty
Five Odors	Rancid	Burnt	Fragrant	Fleshy	Rotten
Five Voices	Shouting	Laughing	Singing	Wailing	Groaning

2.2.1 Generative Cycle Relationships *Sōsei Kankei* 相生関係

Note that the names of the organs do not designate those specific anatomical organs but rather an overall function associated with these organs as understood in acupuncture theory.

① The Liver Generates the Heart

The blood that is produced by the Spleen and Stomach is stored in the Liver. It is sent from there to the Heart through the channels, and it functions in combination with ancestral ki (宗気 Jpn: *sōki*, Chn: *zōng qì*) and nutritive ki (栄気 Jpn: *eiki*, Chn: *róng qì*) (see below) to make the Heart active. This relationship is expressed by saying that the Liver generates the Heart.

② The Heart Generates the Spleen

The Heart is rich in ceaselessly active yang ki. The Spleen function is activated when it receives this yang ki from the Heart, and thus it is said that the Heart generates the Spleen.

③ The Spleen Generates the Lung

The Spleen commands the Stomach and Intestines to produce ki, blood, and fluids. The ki and blood are then sent throughout the body by the circulation of Lung ki. Of course, the ki that is needed by the Lung is also produced by the Spleen and Stomach. Thus, it is said that the Spleen generates the Lung.

④ The Lung Generates the Kidney

The Kidney is an organ rich in fluids. But, fluids cannot move by themselves. They are circulated throughout the body by ki that is sent from the Lung. This means that the Lung generates the Kidney.

⑤ The Kidney Generates the Liver

The Kidney is rich in fluids. These fluids moisten the blood that is stored in the Liver. Without the fluid component, blood cannot circulate throughout the body. Therefore it is said that the Kidney generates the Liver.

2.2.2 Controlling Cycle Relationships *Sōkoku Kankei* 相剋関係

Recall that "controlling" implies holding sway over, causing trouble for, or taking away from the relational phase.

① The Liver Controls the Spleen

The Liver stores the blood, which is produced by the Spleen. The blood is, to be precise, moved by Lung ki and Liver ki. But, it is generally thought of as the Liver *taking blood away from* the Spleen in order to store it. This relationship is explained as the Liver controlling the Spleen.

② The Spleen Controls the Kidney

The Kidney is an organ rich in fluids. The Spleen causes the production of ki, blood, and fluids by using the yang ki that it receives from the Heart and the fluids that it *takes away from* the Kidney to activate the Stomach and Intestines. Thus, it is said that the Spleen controls the Kidney.

③ The Kidney Controls the Heart

The Kidney is rich in yin ki. It is strong when yin ki hardens together with fluids, but that is not enough to make it function. It is only with the addition of yang ki from the Heart that comes via the Pericardium that the Kidney begins to function. In other words, the Kidney is always reliant on yang ki from the Heart. So, it is said that the Kidney controls the Heart.

④ The Heart Controls the Lung

The Heart governs the channels and is responsible for circulating the blood. It is also rich in the ceaselessly active yang ki. However, because blood cannot circulate by itself, there is a need for ki. That ki comes from Lung ki. Also, without the yang ki of the Heart being circulated away by Lung ki, too much heat would accumulate in the chest. Thus, it is said that the Heart controls the Lung.

⑤ The Lung Controls the Liver

The Liver stores the blood, and the Lung circulates ki. Blood moves, nourishing the organs and meridians, because of the circulation of Lung ki. The more the Lung ki circulates, the more the blood of the Liver is consumed. Thus it is said that the Lung controls the Liver.

Table 2–3a: Yin Channel Five Phase Points						
Meridian	**Well Wood Point**	**Spring Fire Point**	**Stream Earth Point**	**River Metal Point**	**Uniting Water Point**	**Source Point**
Liver/Wood	LR-1	LR-2	LR-3	LR-4	LR-8	LR-3
Heart/Fire	HT-9	HT-8	HT-7	HT-4	HT-3	HT-7
Spleen/Earth	SP-1	SP-2	SP-3	SP-5	SP-9	SP-3
Lung/Metal	LU-11	LU-10	LU-9	LU-8	LU-5	LU-9
Kidney/Water	KI-1	KI-2	KI-3	KI-7	KI-10	KI-3
Pericardium/Fire	PC-9	PC-8	PC-7	PC-5	PC-3	PC-7
Table 2–3b: Yang Channel Five Phase Points						
Meridian	**Well Metal Point**	**Spring Water Point**	**Stream Wood Point**	**River Fire Point**	**Uniting Earth Point**	**Source Point**
Gallbladder/ Wood	GB-44	GB-43	GB-41	GB-38	GB-34	GB-40
Small Intestine/ Fire	SI-1	SI-2	SI-3	SI-5	SI-8	SI-4
Stomach/ Earth	ST-45	ST-44	ST-43	ST-41	ST-36	ST-42
Large Intestine/ Metal	LI-1	LI-2	LI-3	LI-5	LI-11	LI-4
Bladder/ Water	BL-67	BL-66	BL-65	BL-60	BL-40	BL-64
Triple Warmer/ Fire	TW-1	TW-2	TW-3	TW-6	TW-10	TW-4

2.3   Ki, Blood, and Fluids   気・血・津液

Meridian Therapy could be called "ki medicine." The body maintains health by the appropriate circulation and diffusion of ki. All of its parts are moistened and nourished by the blood and fluids that are moved throughout the body by ki. Sickness occurs when there is an excess (実 *jitsu*) or deficiency (虚 *kyo*) of ki.

All bodily functions can be explained as the workings of ki. However, this concept is usually further refined and explained with the more specific terms: ki, blood, fluids, defensive ki, nutritive ki, spirit ki, source ki, ancestral ki, and essential ki. Bcause these concepts can be difficult for beginners to understand, a technical explanation of these terms will be given in the following section.

2.3.1 Prenatal Ki *Senten no Ki* 先天の気

People are born with essence (精 Jpn: *sei*, Chn: *jīng*) that they received from their parents. That essence is called prenatal or constitutional essence, and it is stored in the Kidney. This essence of the Kidney generates spirit (神 Jpn: *shin*, Chn: *shén*), otherwise known as yang ki of the Heart. The yang ki of the Heart goes to the Lower Warmer and merges with Kidney essence. The result is called prenatal ki or yang ki of the life gate (命門 Jpn: *meimon*, Chn: *mìng mén*).

Prenatal ki is the driving force for the production of postnatal ki (i.e., the ki, blood, and fluids obtained through the digestion and absorption of food and drink). The ki, blood, and fluids produced in this way become the fluids of the Kidney and the yang ki of the Heart, thereby supplementing the prenatal ki. Therefore the yang ki of the life gate is the product of the combination of prenatal and postnatal ki.

Hence, prenatal ki generates postnatal ki, and postnatal ki supplements prenatal ki. However, there is another explanation of their relationship.

Chapter 8 of the *Nan Jing* (*Classic of Difficulties*) says that even if the postnatal ki is abundant and the pulse is normal, if the prenatal ki is exhausted, death will follow. According to this explanation it is not possible to supplement prenatal ki with postnatal ki. And certainly there are individuals who are born with a strong physical constitution and individuals who are weak or sickly from birth.

When a person is weak or sickly from birth, it means that the prenatal ki of this individual was weak from the time of birth. If the prenatal ki is weak, then the production of postnatal ki will also be weak. It follows then that there will only be a little ki, blood, and fluids produced that can supplement the prenatal ki. That is why these individuals are weak and sickly.

The origin of life is called essence. (*Ling Shu*, Chapter 8)

When people are born [they] first produce essence. (*Ling Shu*, Chapter 10)

The body is completed by the blending of the true ki of heaven [i.e., prenatal ki] with the ki of grains [i.e., postnatal ki]. (*Ling Shu,* Chapter 75)

2.3.2 Postnatal Ki *Kōten no Ki* 後天の気

Food and drink are digested, absorbed, and processed through the functions of the Spleen and Stomach that produce postnatal essence.

Ki, blood, and fluids are formed by the combination of postnatal essence and the heavenly ki brought in by the Lung. This is called postnatal ki. Postnatal ki includes ancestral ki, defensive ki, nutritive ki, blood, and fluids.

① Ancestral Ki *Sōki* 宗気

Chapter 71 of the *Ling Shu* says, "When the five grains enter the Stomach they split into three paths, becoming dregs (i.e., a chymous substance), fluids, and ancestral ki. Thereupon, the ancestral ki accumulates in the chest, emerges into the throat, and drives respiration by passing through the Heart channel."

Thus, ancestral ki is the driving force behind breathing. It is also the foundational ki used by the Lung to circulate blood and ki. When the Lung circulates ki there are no urination problems. Therefore, it is said that ancestral ki also has the function of controlling urination by descending to the Bladder and combining with the source ki (原気 Jpn: *genki*, Chn: *yuán qì*) of the Triple Warmer.

② Defensive Ki (Guarding the Exterior) *Eki* 衛気

Defensive ki (Chn: *wèi qì*) is the ki that is extracted by the yang ki of the life gate from the dregs (chyme) of food and drink as they pass from the Small Intestine to the Large Intestine. Defensive ki is one type of postnatal ki, and is continuously active, which means it is yang ki. The name used for defensive ki changes depending on where it goes. In the Stomach it becomes Stomach yang ki. In the Lung it becomes Lung ki. In the Kidney it is called the yang ki of the life gate. In other words, it circulates throughout the whole body.

During the daytime, defensive ki patrols the skin and between the muscles, controls the opening and closing of the pores, regulates the proper release of yang ki from the body, and thereby protects the body from temperature changes in the external world. In the event that the body receives some stimulation from the outside world, defensive ki gathers at the affected site and closes and opens the pores accordingly. In these cases, if the defensive ki is deficient, the pores will be left open, which makes it easy for sweat to leave the body, or the pores will remain closed, which makes it difficult for sweat to leave the body. If sweat cannot escape, the defensive ki that collects in the area will stagnate and cause an outbreak of heat.

During the nighttime defensive ki enters the interior via the Kidney channel and circulates around the organs. Defensive ki that goes to the Heart mixes with yang ki of the blood and becomes the sovereign fire (君火 Jpn: *kunka*; Chn: *jūn huǒ*) which is spirit. The sovereign fire turns into the ministerial fire (相火 Jpn: *sōka*; Chn: *xiāng huǒ*) and descends to the Lower Warmer where it mixes with Kidney essence and becomes yang ki of the life gate. This is also called true ki (真気 Jpn: *shinki*; Chn: *zhēn qì*). When the function of the yang ki of the life gate is emphasized, it is also called source ki of the Triple Warmer. (See page 122, diagram 4–3)

> [The character of] defensive ki is swift and valiant; it unceasingly patrols the four limbs, between the muscles, and through the skin. In the daytime it travels through the yang aspect [of the body], and in the nighttime it travels through the yin aspect [of the body]. It usually goes to the five zang and six fu organs from the spaces between the muscles along the foot lesser yin channel. (*Ling Shu*, Chapter 71)

③ Nutritive Ki and Blood (Guarding the Interior) *Eiki to Ketsu* 栄気と血

Nutritive ki comes from digested and absorbed food and drink.

> The dregs [chyme] of food is digested, the water vaporized, and the essence removed. The [essence] then ascends and pours into the Lung channel. There it is transformed into blood and spontaneously travels to all the channels and vessels, and with this the physical body is made [as a gift from Heaven]. There is nothing more valuable than this. It is called nutritive ki. (*Ling Shu*, Chapter 18)

According to this passage, nutritive ki and blood are the same thing. That is why the *Nan Jing* uses the phrase "nutritive blood." Therefore the idea was developed that since nutritive blood circulates in the channels, if you can adjust the deficiency and excess in the channels, then you would also be able to adjust the blood.

However, because symptom patterns that are associated with blood can appear as either heat-type or cold-type conditions, from the clinical point of view it is useful to think of the ki that drives the circulation of blood as nutritive ki, and to specify blood as yin and nutritive ki as yang.

The above quotation from the *Ling Shu* says further:

> The Yellow Emperor said, "How is it that blood and ki have different names, yet are of the same category?" Qibo answered, "Nutritive and defensive ki are essential ki, and blood is spirit ki, so blood and ki have different names but belong to the same category."

Belonging to the same category yet having different names means that there is a difference in their functions.

Nutritive ki is also known as constructive ki (営気 Jpn: *eiki*, Chn: *yíng qì*), but this book will use the name "nutritive ki" throughout the text.

④ Fluids *Shineki* 津液

The *Nan Jing* does not mention fluids because it considers fluids to be included in blood. However, actual examination of the symptom pattern reveals many illnesses with water (i.e., fluid) stagnation. Abnormal liquid (or pathological liquid) results from the stagnation of fluids. Therefore, it is also useful to acquire an understanding of the fluids.

Ki and blood are made from fluids, but fluids themselves have unique functions. In the *Ling Shu* it is pointed out that the first character that composes the Chinese word for fluids (津液 Jpn: *shineki*; Chn: *jīn yè*) denotes yang fluids and the second character denotes more yin fluids. It also said that fluids have a yang-type function.

Moreover, since fluids are included in the blood, their function cannot be separated from that of the blood, and thus they also have a yin-type function. Both blood and fluids have the yin-type function of moistening each part of the body.

> Food and drink enter [the body through] the mouth. They have five tastes that pour into the [four] seas, respectively. Fluids [produced from food and drink] are distributed through each of the paths [in the body]. Thus, when ki is emitted from the Triple Warmer it warms the flesh and enriches the skin. The fluid [that is released from the skin in this way] is called the lighter/thin/yang fluid, and the fluid that is not released but stays [in the body] is called the heavier/thick/yin fluid. (*Ling Shu*, Chapter 36)

2.3.3 Essential Ki *Seiki* 精気

The term essence, or essential ki, has an especially broad definition. In the narrow sense, essence is the substance that is stored in the Kidney, and essential ki is the ki that is stored in each of the five zang organs. In the broad sense, essence is called the original substance from which prenatal ki develops. Here we will stick with the explanation that essential ki is ki of the five zang organs.

① Ethereal Soul *Kon* 魂

The ethereal soul is essential ki that is stored in the Liver. It has positive/active and intentional/deliberate functional properties since it is mixed together with the blood that is stored in the Liver.

② Spirit *Shin* 神

Spirit has two meanings. In the narrow sense it refers to essential ki that is stored in the Heart. If there is a deficiency of this kind of spirit the person will die. But, before that happens they will experience an unstable psyche, or will suffer from dementia, derangement, or unconsciousness.

In the broad sense, spirit is explained in this quote from Chapter 32 of the *Ling Shu*. "If the five zang organs are balanced and the blood vessels are harmonized and effective, then the essence-spirit will reside [within the body]. Thus, spirit is essential ki of water and grains." In terms of the pulse this corresponds to Stomach ki, and indicates luster in terms of the skin. (See Chapter 8, section 2.1 for an explanation on Stomach ki, and Chapter 7, section 1.1 for the importance of luster.)

However, spirit does not exist independently. If the form is sound, then the spirit will flourish, and if the spirit flourishes, then the form will be enhanced. Form belongs to yin, and spirit belongs to yang.

③ Intention and Wisdom *I to Chi* 意と智

Intention and wisdom are essential ki that is stored in the Spleen. They are ki that are related to memory and cognition.

④ Corporeal Soul *Haku* 魄

The corporeal soul is essential ki that is stored in the Lung. In terms of the activities of the psyche, it is related to vigor or vitality.

The corporeal soul can be said to be the same as ancestral ki. It is the ki that collects in the chest and is the driving power for respiration and the circulation of blood. This is also called yang ki of the chest or ki of the chest center (CV-17).

⑤ Essence and Will *Sei to Shi* 精と志

Essence is the ki that is stored in the Kidney and, as noted above, is also called prenatal ki in the sense that it is the source of the life force. Since essential ki has a yin ki function, when the essence is sturdy, the fluids in the Kidney will be abundant. Will is included in essence and is the ki that causes things to be executed in a continuous manner.

2.4   Deficiency and Excess   虚 実

In Meridian Therapy the techniques of tonification and dispersion are used to treat deficiency and excess. Thus, treatment cannot be given unless one is able to distinguish between deficiency and excess in terms of symptom patterns, and of course in terms of pathology. This section will present the definitions of deficiency and excess and arrange them into classifications. In the wide sense, deficiency refers to a deficiency of correct (also known as right) ki (正気 Jpn: *seiki*; Chn: *zhèng qì*), and excess refers to an excess of pathogenic (also known as evil) ki (邪気 *jaki, xié qì*). However, there is a lot of depth behind these meanings.

2.4.1 Essential Ki Deficiency *Seiki no Kyo* 精気の虚

> The five zang organs are in charge of storing the essence, which should not be injured. If the essence is injured, the [body's] defenses will be lost, resulting in yin deficiency. (*Ling Shu*, Chapter 8)

> The Yellow Emperor said, "All illnesses are caused by deficiency and excess. You [Qibo] just said there are five surpluses and five insufficiencies. How do they come about?" Qibo answered, "They all arise from [disharmonies in] the five zang organs." (*Su Wen*, Chapter 62)

> Being deprived of essential ki results in deficiency. (*Su Wen*, Chapter 28)

As is understood from the above quotations, disease stems from deficiency of essential ki of the five zang organs. That is why the pattern of imbalance in Meridian Therapy is expressed as deficiency of the organs and meridians.

However, in actuality deficiency of essential ki alone cannot be called illness. Deficiency of essential ki simply manifests as a degree of weariness. If some kind of etiological factor comes into play at this junction, then this situation is compounded by the addition of a deficiency of ki, blood, or fluids of the organs to the already present essential ki deficiency. When the condition develops to this stage, a clear symptom pattern will appear. This is called pathological deficiency. When there is an outbreak of pathological deficiency, in many cases cold or heat symptom patterns will also manifest.

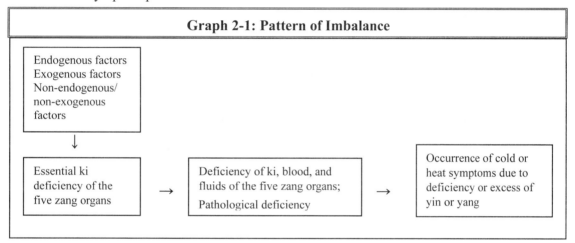

Graph 2-1: Pattern of Imbalance

Endogenous factors
Exogenous factors
Non-endogenous/
non-exogenous
factors
↓
Essential ki deficiency of the five zang organs → Deficiency of ki, blood, and fluids of the five zang organs; Pathological deficiency → Occurrence of cold or heat symptoms due to deficiency or excess of yin or yang

Looking at the above graph, the first point to note is that although there is a box that says "essential ki deficiency of the five zang organs," there are *no* illnesses caused by an occurrence of essential ki deficiency of the Heart. Or, in other words, there is no Heart deficiency pattern. This will be explained later.

The etiological factors were separated into endogenous, exogenous, or miscellaneous (neither endogenous nor exogenous) factors, and depending on which factor contributes to the development of the illness, there will be evident differences in the pathology and symptom patterns.

First, when there is only essential ki deficiency, disease will occur upon the addition of pathogenic ki and may cause changes in ki, blood, and fluids.

Second, when endogenous factors or non-endogenous/non-exogenous factors are introduced to a condition of essential ki deficiency, the deficiency can spread to the ki, blood, and fluids of the five zang organs and thereby cause illness. Also, the addition of exogenous factors to such a condition can also cause disease.

However, in all cases there is no doubt that because the disease starts with essential ki deficiency, the practitioner's first attention should be given to finding and tonifying the deficient yin channel, which will allow for the simultaneous tonification of insufficient ki, blood, and fluids. Beyond that, one only needs to determine whether or not any dispersion is necessary.

Another way of expressing pathological deficiency is by saying deficiency of ki, blood, or fluids. The Liver stores blood. The Kidney stores fluids. The Lung stores ki. And it is the Spleen that produces all of them. Therefore, ki, blood, or fluid deficiency is related to organ deficiency of the organ to which it is most intimately related, as explained below.

Finally, when there is an outbreak of heat or cold due to pathological deficiency, that heat or cold can spread out and affect other organs and meridians, causing the manifestation of specific symptoms. All these areas must be treated in addition to the primary yin deficiency. The problem the practitioner faces at that time is deciding the number of needles to use and the depth of needle insertion. In order to make this determination, you have to be able to distinguish deficiency and excess in cold and heat symptom patterns. More will be explained about this later.

2.4.2 Pathological Deficiency *Byōri no Kyo* 病理の虚

This section will present an organ-focused explanation of deficiency, since illness is caused by essential ki deficiency of yin and deficiency of the other essences stored by the organs.

① Liver Deficiency *Kan Kyo* 肝虚

The essential ki of the Liver is called the ethereal soul. The Liver stores the blood, and the blood stores the ethereal soul. Thus, essential ki deficiency of the Liver means the same thing as deficiency of Liver blood. Therefore, Liver deficiency should be thought of as blood deficiency. It is not possible to have just ki deficiency of the Liver.

When the blood that is stored in the Liver becomes deficient, either cold or heat symptom patterns will manifest depending on the pathology. These two possibilities are called Liver deficiency cold patterns and Liver deficiency heat patterns.

② Heart Deficiency *Shin Kyo* 心虚

There is <u>no</u> Heart deficiency. The Heart stores the essential ki known as spirit. It is also continuously active and is an organ with a rich abundance of yang ki. If either of these were to become deficient, death would follow. Thus, there is no pattern of Heart deficiency.

However, it is possible for the Heart to be affected by cold or heat and to display symptom patterns accordingly. In these cases the Heart receives heat or cold that is generated by the deficiency of other organs.

③ Spleen Deficiency *Hi Kyo* 脾虚

The Spleen holds the essential ki known as intention and wisdom. At the same time it also maintains the ki, blood, and fluids. Therefore, it follows that in Spleen deficiency there can be ki deficiency of the Spleen, blood deficiency of the Spleen, or fluid deficiency of the Spleen. However, in making general distinctions based on pathology, there can be either a Spleen deficiency cold pattern or a Spleen deficiency heat pattern.

④ Lung Deficiency *Hai Kyo* 肺虚

The Lung stores the corporeal soul. At the same time, it controls ki. Thus essential ki of the Lung should be thought of as equal to Lung ki, and Lung deficiency should be thought of as meaning the same thing as ki deficiency.

When the Lung becomes deficient there will be an outbreak of heat or cold. However, since the Lung controls the external surface of the body (the *hyō* 表 external/yang-type areas), the cold or heat symptom patterns that manifests with the deficiency of Lung ki will develop in the yang channels.

⑤ Kidney Deficiency *Jin Kyo* 腎虚

The Kidney stores both the essential ki known as will and the fluids. Essential ki and fluids are mixed together. Therefore, in a number of cases, essential ki deficiency of the Kidney will be accompanied by deficiency of fluids. However, in some cases, deficiency of essential ki produces the primary symptom pattern, and in other cases deficiency of fluids produces the primary symptom pattern. Moreover, there are also cases when deficiency of yang ki of the life gate produces the primary symptom pattern. These conditions are arranged under the designations of Kidney deficiency cold patterns, and Kidney deficiency heat patterns.

⑥ **Fu Organ Deficiency** *Fu Kyo* 腑虚

Since the zang organs control the fu organs, if a zang organ becomes deficient, the corresponding or paired fu organ can also become deficient. This happens because the fu organs receive cold that was generated by the pathological deficiency. The pulse will be either sinking and weak or floating with decreased power.

2.4.3 The Definition and Categories of Excess

In one sense, if deficiency occurs, then excess will also occur. Chapter 29 of the *Su Wen* says, "The way of yang is [to become] excess, and the way of yin is [to become] deficient." This is one principle of excess, which is a condition of full and stagnated blood or heat.

As noted above, cold and heat are generated when pathological deficiency is caused by the addition of blood deficiency or fluid deficiency to a condition of essential ki deficiency. Cold and heat naturally spread to other organs and meridians. Organs and meridians that receive cold at this time will not develop excesses. However, areas that receive heat can develop excesses. When observing this condition using the pulse position/pulse quality diagnosis, excess can be determined because the position that receives the heat will be stronger. Heat will also be revealed in the symptom pattern. The different possible conditions can be categorized by organ correspondence as follows.

① **Fu Organ Excess** *Fu Jitsu* 腑実

Fu organs correspond to individual zang organs and can receive heat and become excess when the associated zang organ becomes deficient and generates heat. For example, if the Spleen is deficient, then the Stomach will develop a condition of excess heat. This condition can develop so far as to become heat in the meridian. Or, heat from the deficiency of other zang organs can send off "sparks" of heat. For example, heat caused by a deficiency of fluids in the Spleen can spread to the Gallbladder channel or to the Gallbladder itself. There are also cases where the heat tries to enter a zang organ. Or, there are even times when a fu organ receives heat at the same time that a zang organ receives it. For example, the Gallbladder often receives excess-type heat when there is a condition of Liver excess heat.

② Liver Excess *Kan Jitsu* 肝実

There are three types of Liver excess. The first is a condition of heat invading and stagnating in the Liver at the same time that the Spleen has a deficiency of fluids. This condition is called Spleen deficiency Liver excess heat.

The second condition arises when the Liver becomes excess due to a stagnation of blood that was caused by heat, even though the Liver heat itself has dissipated. This is called Spleen deficiency Liver excess. People who constitutionally tend to have considerable blood stasis are prone to getting Spleen deficiency Liver excess.

The third condition is one in which blood stagnates in the Liver due to a lack of moisture caused by a deficiency of fluids in the Kidney that occurs simultaneously with poor circulation of Lung ki. This is called Lung deficiency Liver excess.

③ Heart Excess *Shin Jitsu* 心実

There is *no* Heart excess. However, it is possible for heat to increase in the Heart. Therefore, it would not be impossible to refer to such a condition as excess, but it is called Heart heat. This heat spreads to the Heart from heat generated by a deficiency in the Kidney, Liver, or Spleen.

④ Spleen Excess *Hi Jitsu* 脾実

The Spleen does not become excess since it does not retain heat. However, it does receive heat that is generated in other areas. But, were the Spleen to fully take on this heat, death would ensue. Therefore, the Spleen normally diverts the heat back to the fu organs (usually the Stomach). (Refer to Chapter 4 of the *Ling Shu.*) Nonetheless, there are cases when heat in the greater yin channel attempts to penetrate to the Spleen.

⑤ Lung Excess *Hai Jitsu* 肺実

The Lung, like the fu organs, comes into contact with external ki (i.e., air), and has pores that are used by defensive ki. Therefore, the Lung can also become stagnant and full. This condition occurs when heat generated in the yang channels by external pathogens strikes inward or when heat generated by the deficiency of a zang organ strikes inward.

⑥ Kidney Excess *Jin Jitsu* 腎実

The Kidney does not become excess due to stagnant heat since it is rich in fluids. If heat increases in the Kidney the fluids will simply absorb the heat by evaporating. However, if there is a further increase in heat, the fluids will dry up and the Kidney position in the pulse (left proximal) will become hard. Because this condition can sometimes be seen in an excess pulse, there are people who use the expression "Kidney excess." But the pathology is utimately an insufficiency of fluids, so this condition is really one of Kidney deficiency.

2.4.4 Deficiency and Excess in Symptom Patterns

Imagine a case where there is blood deficiency of the Liver (Liver deficiency pattern) and an outbreak of heat. The heat will spread to other organs or meridians. If it goes to meridians in the head, back, or abdomen and obstructs the circulation of ki or blood in those areas, pain will appear there. At the same time it can cause the formation of pain on pressure (i.e., points at which pain is elicited by palpation), indurations, and depressions. These formations are the manifestations of deficiency and excess in the symptom patterns, and must be treated as well. Naturally, pain on pressure, indurations, and depressions must be identified as either deficient or excess and treated accordingly with tonification or dispersion.

The symptom patterns, pulse quality, and palpation are used as the basis for differentiating deficiency and excess. Watery bowel movements, frequent urination, and excessive sweating are usually signs of deficiency, and a lack of these unbalanced fluid signs usually indicates excess. If the pulse quality shows excess, then there should be many other signs of excess. If the pulse quality shows deficiency, then there should be many other signs of deficiency. An increase in pain when pressing on the body is a sign of excess. Deficiency is indicated if pressing on the body feels good.

In cases of acute febrile diseases, the symptom pattern and pulse quality are the main concern when determining the appropriate tonification and/or dispersion. But in cases of chronic disorders, the results of the palpation examination take precedence.

There is a difference in meaning between the tonification and dispersion used to treat the deficiency and excess of cold and heat symptom patterns and that used to treat the deficiency and excess related to pathology. Tonification and dispersion methods used for pathological deficiency and excess are part of the *root treatment*. Those used for deficiency and excess in the local symptom pattern are part of the *local treatment*.

A person can have three [kinds of] deficiency and three [kinds of] excess. What does that mean?

It is thus: Deficiency and excess [can be found] in the pulse, in the [course and condition of] illness, and in the examination [of the patient]. As for deficiency and excess in the pulses, a soggy pulse indicates deficiency and a firm pulse indicates excess. As for deficiency and excess in the [course and condition of] an illness: an illness that [arises inside and] moves toward the outside indicates deficiency and an illness that moves from the outside [invading into the body] indicates excess; deficiency is indicated if [the patient] speaks [a lot], and excess is indicated if [the patient] does not speak [much]; a chronic [slowly progressing] [illness] indicates deficiency, and an acute [quickly progressing] [illness] indicates excess.

As for the examination [of the patient]: [when touching the patient,] softness indicates deficiency and hardness indicates excess; itchiness indicates deficiency and pain indicates excess; [a condition of] external pain and internal comfort indicates external excess and internal deficiency and [a condition of] internal pain and external comfort indicates internal excess and external deficiency. (*Nan Jing*, Chapter 48)

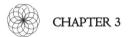 CHAPTER 3

The Flow of the Meridians
経 絡 の 流 注

As was mentioned in Chapter 2, defensive ki and nutritive ki (blood) circulate through the meridians. If deficiency or excess occurs in the circulation of ki, blood, or fluids, it will cause the appearance of definite pathological conditions and symptom patterns. In Meridian Therapy, these disharmonies are adjusted by the use of techniques called tonification and dispersion. To that end, you must master diagnosis and become skillful in tonification and dispersion techniques. Since acupuncture techniques are used on the meridians and acupuncture points, you cannot give treatments unless you become thoroughly familiar with their functions and flow.

In the classics, the meridians were expressed with various names including conduit, channel, network vessel, and grandchild vessel. Meridian is the general term. These more precise words also indicated the depth of the meridian. Starting from the surface of the skin, the order of depth is grandchild vessel, network vessel, and channel. The channels are connected to the organs. Actually the skin and body hair hold the first position in the order because they contain the pores and are thus continuously protecting the body from external pathogens by circulating defensive ki. Thus, skin and body hair can also be used as treatment locations. (Refer to Chapter 56 of the *Su Wen.*)

3.1.1 Meridian Classifications

① Twelve Channels *Jūni Keimyaku* 十二経脈

The twelve channels are divided into six yin channels and six yang channels. The yin channels connect to the Liver, Heart, Spleen, Lung, Kidney, and Pericardium. The yang channels connect to the Gallbladder, Small Intestine, Stomach, Large Intestine, Bladder, and Triple Warmer. The yin and yang channels are in paired relationships with each other like the two faces of a coin, one being external (*hyō* 表), which refers to the yang areas or surface of the body), and the other being internal (*ri* 裏), which refers to the yin areas or deep parts of the body). In the internal areas are the yin channels that connect to the zang organs and run close to the fu organs. The yang channels run close to the surface of the body in the external areas and connect to the fu organs.

Table 3–1: Classification of the Twelve Channels			
Internal	**External**	**Internal**	**External**
Channels of the Hand		**Channels of the Foot**	
Hand Greater Yin Lung Channel	Hand Yang Brightness Large Intestine Channel	Foot Greater Yin Spleen Channel	Foot Yang Brightness Stomach Channel
Hand Lesser Yin Heart Channel	Hand Greater Yang Small Intestine Channel	Foot Lesser Yin Kidney Channel	Foot Greater Yang Bladder Channel
Hand Reverting Yin Pericardium Channel	Hand Lesser Yang Triple Warmer Channel	Foot Reverting Yin Liver Channel	Foot Lesser Yang Gallbladder Channel

There are two of each channel—one on each side of the body. For example, there is a left Lung channel and a right Lung channel. For the purpose of introducing the different channels, the text in the following sections will mostly present them as if talking about only one side of the body.

The six yin and six yang channels are divided between the designations of hand and foot. The three hand yin channels go from the chest to the hand, and then connect with the hand yang channels, which go to the head. The channels that receive the flow from the hand yang channels become the foot yang channels and go to the feet. The yang channels that went to the feet connect to the foot yin channels. The foot yin channels rise up while wrapping around the organs. This is the circulation of ki and blood throughout the body.

② Eight Extraordinary Vessels *Kikei Hachimyaku* 奇経八脈

There are eight extraordinary vessels. Unlike the twelve channels, the eight extraordinary vessels do not have rules of circulation; rather, they have a completely different system of movement. This will be further explained later.

③ Fifteen Network Vessels *Jūgo Rakumyaku* 十五絡脈

When the conception vessel and the governing vessel are added to the twelve channels, the group is called the fourteen channels. From each of the fourteen channels extend the network vessels. When the great network vessel of the Spleen is counted, the group is called the fifteen network vessels.

The network vessels of the twelve channels diverge from the primary channel distal to the elbows and knees, and form paths of interconnection along the surface of the body between the yin and yang channels.

The network vessels of the conception vessel are distributed in the abdomen. The network vessels of the governing vessel are distributed in the back. The great network vessel of the Spleen is distributed near the free ribs. Through these network vessels, the unification and connections of the body are strengthened.

④ Twelve Divergent Channels *Jūni Keibetsu* 十二経別

The twelve divergent channels are branches of the twelve channels. Their circulation goes from the four extremities and enters the internal organs, and then reemerges at the nape of the neck. Compared to the network vessels, the divergent channels go deeper and are longer. They are in paired relationships with each other and are pathways that strengthen the interrelationship between the yin and yang channels by making connections between them in both directions.

The yang divergent channels rejoin their primary channel, but the yin divergent channels do not. Instead, they join the yang channel that is their paired channel.

⑤ Twelve Channel Sinews *Jūni Keikin* 十二経筋

Channel sinews should be thought of as sinews that follow the flow of the channels. Thus, they arise from the ends of the four extremities and travel through the joints and muscles, but they do not enter the internal organs.

Low back pain or muscular pain (including the condition that is known in Japan as "fifty-year-old's shoulder") are said to be disorders of the channel sinews. There is no need to give them special consideration because if you improve the flow of the meridians, channel sinew disorders will also heal. Still, the places where the channel sinews become knotted and hard are naturally areas to be treated. Moreover, being familiar with the symptom patterns of the channel sinews is often quite useful.

⑥ Twelve Water Channels *Jūni Keisui* 十二経水

The term "water channels" emphasizes the management and functions of water. Naturally, if the circulation of ki and blood deteriorates, movement in the water channels will likewise deteriorate. Therefore, conditions arising mainly from the occurrence of water stasis are referred to in the classics by such names as "damp syndrome," "blood syndrome," "water ki syndrome," and "phlegm retention" If you tonify and disperse the deficiency and excess of the meridians in accordance with the Meridian Therapy method, conditions such as "water ki syndrome" and "blood syndrome" should also heal. Nonetheless, from the perspective of understanding pathological conditions, it is a good idea be able to diagnosis these conditions.

> The twelve water channels receive water and distribute it. The five zang organs combine and store the spirit, ki, and the corporeal and ethereal souls. The six fu organs receive food [and they] process and distribute [the essence]. … The channels receive blood [produced from the essence of the food] and distribute it to nourish [the body].   (*Ling Shu*, Chapter 12)

> The twelve channels [allow for the maintenance of] human life, are [the places where] disease [can arise], are the [places where] treatment [can be given], and are

the origin of disease. They are the places [where beginners] start their studies and the place where proficient practitioners continue to focus their attention. (*Ling Shu*, Chapter 11)

⑦ Vessel Length

Chapter 17 of the *Ling Shu* and Chapter 23 of the *Nan Jing* describe the length of the vessels. Selected passages are gives here as a reference.

The three hand yang channels reach from the hands to the head and are 5 *chǐ*[1] long, totaling 3 *zhàng* for both the left and right sides.

The three hand yin channels reach from the hands to the chest and are *3 chǐ 5 cùn* long, totaling 2 *zhàng* 1 *chǐ* for both the left and right sides.

The three foot yang channels reach from the feet to the head and are 8 *chǐ* long, totaling 4 *zhàng* 8 *chǐ* for both the left and right sides.

The three foot yin channels reach from the feet to the thorax and are 6 *chǐ* 5 *cùn* long, totaling 3 *zhàng* 9 *chǐ* for both the left and right sides.

The heel vessel reaches from the feet to the eyes and is 7 *chǐ* 5 *cùn* long, totaling 1 *zhàng* 5 *chǐ* for both the left and right sides.

The governing vessel and conception vessel are each 4 *chǐ* 5 *cùn* long, totaling 9 *chǐ*.

3.1.2 The Functions of the Meridians

① The Meridians are Circulation Paths for Ki, Blood, Nutritive Ki, and Defensive Ki

Chapter 47 of the *Ling Shu says*, "The vessels circulate blood and ki, and [thereby] nourish yin and yang." They do this without missing a nook or cranny throughout the whole body. Therefore, the meridians function as paths for bringing nutrients to the yin and yang areas and to the organs.

---

[1] Note: One *chǐ* is approximately one foot

② The Relationship Between the Meridians and the Organs

Ki, blood, and fluids are made by the Spleen and Stomach and are sent to each zang organ by Lung ki and the channels. Thus, this leads to blood being stored in the Liver, fluids being stored in the Kidney, and ki being stored in the Lung. Of course, the Spleen also receives benefit from this.

The ki, blood, and fluids that go to each organ become the driving force behind their functioning. However, their functional properties cannot be put into effect without the channels, since it is the channels that transport the ki, blood, and fluids to each area controlled by a zang organ, such as the fu organs, muscles, or bone. The malfunctioning of the organs will therefore show up as a change in the channels, and deterioration in the flow of the channels will have an effect on the organs. Thus, the channels and organs are very closely related. A deeper understanding of this fact can be gained by studying physiology and pathology.

> The yin channels nourish the zang organs and the yang channels nourish the fu organs, [circulating ceaselessly] like a circle, which has no beginning and no end. The ki that flows [through these channels] fills [the body], pouring into the internal organs and moistening the skin. (*Ling Shu*, Chapter 17)

③ The Different Amounts of Ki and Blood in Each Channel

The classics say there are different amounts of ki and blood flowing in each of the channels. This is noted here since it is useful to know this when performing tonification or dispersion. There is a slight difference in the descriptions given in the *Su Wen* and *Ling Shu*, and in the table below we have chosen the explanation found in Chapter 24 of the *Su Wen*.

The proper needling depth for each channel is given in Chapter 12 of the *Ling Shu*. There are theories that compare the needling depth to the depth and size of the channel, but since we feel that it is related more to the amounts of ki and blood in the channels, we will give these two facts together in the table below. Note that the depths given are for the foot channels. Depths for the hand channels are all 2 *fēn*.

Table 3–2: Needling Depth for the Channels from *Su Wen* Chapter 24		
Channel	**Amount of Blood and Ki**	**Needling Depth**
Greater Yang Channel	Much blood and little ki	5 *fēn*
Yang Brightness Channel	Much blood and much ki	6 *fēn*
Lesser Yang Channel	Little blood and much ki	4 *fēn*
Lesser Yin Channel	Little blood and much ki	2 *fēn*
Greater Yin Channel	Little blood and much ki	3 *fēn*
Reverting Yin Channel	Much blood and little ki	1 *fēn*

Note: 1 *fēn* is 1/10 of a *cùn*.

3.1.3 Concerning Acupuncture Points

Acupuncture treatment consists of adjusting deficiency and excess in the meridians, and this is done at the acupuncture points. Acupuncture points are also called ki gates and ki points, and in the classics these are recorded as being the places that diverge from the network vessels. More accurately, acupuncture points can be thought of as the network vessels themselves because the network vessels are close to the skin.

According to one classical text it says that the grandchild network vessels, which are considerably shallower and smaller than the network vessels, can also be used as treatment locations. Further, many points along the line marking the thin gap between muscles can also be used as acupuncture points. Even the skin and body hair, which are even shallower than the grandchild vessels, can be used as treatment locations. This is reasonable considering that the skin and body hair are always conducting defensive ki. In any case, all parts of the body have the potential to respond as an acupuncture point. Therefore, after learning the information presented in the textbooks, it is critical that you learn to adapt to the clinical circumstances in determining the treatment locations; and there is no other way to do this than to make the tips of your fingers sensitive.

3.1.4 Categories and Functions of Acupuncture Points

Among the acupuncture points there are some that are particularly important, such as the five phases points, which overlap with the five transport points. These particularly important points are introduced below.

① **The Five Transport Points of the Yin Channels** *Goyuketsu* 陰経の五兪穴

The five transport points overlap with the five phase points—that is, they are divided among the five phases of wood, fire, earth, metal, and water. (See Table 2–3, page 30)

According to the first Chapter of the *Ling Shu*, each of the acupuncture points has its own function. Here we will append a few thoughts to the descriptions from the *Ling Shu*.

Well-wood point(s) *Sei-moku-ketsu* 井木穴

"The place that puts forth [ki] is the well [point]."

These points tend to make good dispersion points since they are points from which ki easily comes forth. Moreover, the flavor of the wood phase is sour, which has the functional property of gathering. Thus, the well-wood points also have the functional property of gathering. Therefore, they are effective in treating swelling and tenderness in the hypochondriac region by gathering together the congested material and pulling it down to the Lower Warmer.

Spring-fire point(s) *Ei-ka-ketsu* 榮火穴

"The place that trickles is the spring [point]."

"Trickle" most likely means that ki easily flows out, so naturally these points make good dispersion points. The flavor of the fire phase is bitter, which has the functional properties of firming in the sense of formation and cooling in the sense of controlling the expulsion of heat. Because the spring-fire-points have the same functional properties, they are effective in treating body heat.

Stream-earth point(s) *Yu-do-ketsu* 兪土穴

"The place that pours is the stream [point]."

This should be thought of as the spot where ki is poured or sent inside the body. In other words the stream-earth points possess the characteristic of the Spleen—that is, of sending nourishment into the body. On yin meridians they are the same as the source points. Naturally, they make good tonification points. The flavor of the earth phase is sweet. Sweetness works on the Spleen and Stomach to increase blood and fluids. The stream-earth-points have the same functional property. Therefore, they are effective in treating illnesses related to food and fatigue. Moreover, the stream-earth points should be used when the joints hurt and the body becomes heavy and languid due to Spleen or Stomach deficiency.

River-metal point(s) *Kei-kin-ketsu* 経金穴

"The place that sets [ki] in motion [activates ki] is the river [point]."

These points are thought to be more active than the stream-earth points in encouraging the circulation of ki. Naturally they are used for tonification. The flavor of the metal phase is pungent/spicy, which has the functional properties of tonifying and releasing yang ki. The river-metal points have the same functional properties. Therefore, they are effective in treating wheezing and coughing as well as chills and fever.

Uniting-water point(s) *Gō-sui-ketsu* 合水穴

"The place that enters is the uniting [point]."

The word "enter" gives the sense of the place where ki goes into the organs, or of the place where ki that is floating on the surface goes inside the body. These entry places are the uniting points. Moreover, the water-points have the same functional property as the Kidney—that of firming and forming. Therefore, they are effective in treating the leaking of fluids and counterflowing ki.

② Source Points *Genketsu* 原穴

Source points are places "to be treated when the patient has an illness of the five zang organs or six fu organs." (*Ling Shu*, Chapter 1) The term "source" is also "an honorific name for the Triple Warmer." (*Nan Jing*, Chapter 66) Therefore, it is a rule that the corresponding source point should be selected for treatment for each channel when there is are symptom patterns related to that organ.

Source points are the same as stream-earth points in yin meridians. This is due to the relation between the Triple Warmer source ki and the Spleen and Stomach. When cold patterns are seen in the clinic, the Triple Warmer source ki must be tonified while also increasing the postnatal ki, and thus the source points should be used for this.

For example, rather than using the point selection descriptions from *Nan Jing* Chapter 69 (as is usual in Meridian Therapy) when there is a case of a Liver deficiency cold pattern, it is usually effective to concentrate on tonifying the stream-earth points such as KI-3 and LR-3. For the source points refer to Table 2–3 on page 30.

③ Cleft (Accumulation) Points *Geki* 郄穴

Each channel has a cleft point. Cleft points are effective for use when there is a sudden presentation of a symptom pattern. Note, however, that they are often used as dispersion points in the yang channels and as tonification points in the yin channels.

④ Network Points *Rakuketsu* 絡穴

Network points are located at the connection sites between the yin channels and the yang channels. Thus they are used as tonification points when both yin and yang are deficient. For example, LR-5 is used in conjunction with KI-3 and LR-3 for a Liver deficiency cold pattern.

⑤ Back Transport Points *Haibu Yuketsu* 背部兪穴

Back transport points reflect deficiency or excess according to the cold and heat symptom patterns of each pattern of imbalance. For example, BL-18 (the Liver back transport point) will show deficiency or excess in cases of a Liver deficiency heat pattern. Therefore, whereas back points are normally used for local treatment, since the pulse can be adjusted by tonifying or dispersing only the back transport points of the related organs, and the flow of channel ki can be improved by such, in this text the back transport points are given the name *root treatment supplementary points* and are distinguished from local treatment points.

⑥ Alarm Points *Boketsu* 募穴

Widespread–type needling (*sanshin* technique) and retention of the needle are techniques often used on alarm points. There are two purposes for such needling. First, the pulse will become clearer when widespread–type needling is used, to focus on the alarm points of the chest and abdomen, as this causes improvement of the circulation of stomach ki. Second, similar to the back transport points, alarm points can be used in local treatment. However, since these points have different qualities from most other points located on the chest and abdomen, they are separately classified as root treatment supplementary points.

⑦ Eight Meeting Points *Hassōketsu* 八会穴

The eight meeting points are recorded in Chapter 45 of the *Nan Jing*.

Fu organ meeting point	CV-12	Zang organ meeting point	LR-13
Sinews meeting point	GB-34	Marrow meeting point	GB-38
Blood meeting point	BL-17	Bone meeting point	BL-11
Vessels meeting point	LU-9	Ki meeting point	CV-17

These points are used when there is an abundance of heat. For instance, if heat caused by the pattern of imbalance spreads to the fu organs, then the fu organ meeting point (CV-12) should be used. Or, the sinew meeting point (GB-34) should be used in the case of muscle aches, and the bone meeting point (BL-11) used in the case of bone diseases. Additionally, the vessels meeting point (LU-9) can be tonified to clarify a pulse that is difficult to read, or the blood meeting point (BL-17) can be used when there is a symptom pattern related to the blood.

⑧ Four Command Points *Shisōketsu* 四総穴

Like other points, the four command points are effective when their use is differentiated according to the patterns of imbalance.

- Conditions of the head and nape: LU-7
- Conditions of the face and mouth: LI-4
- Conditions of the abdomen: ST-36
- Conditions of the back: BL-40

Pain on pressure is often found at LU-7 when the patient is experiencing a headache. Pain on pressure tends to appear at LI-4 or along the Large Intestine channel when the patient has a toothache or other condition of the face. ST-36 should be used in conjunction with other points for any condition of the abdomen, and BL-40 should always be used for low back pain. These are the ways to differentiate points depending on the patterns of imbalance.

	Meridian/Organ	Cleft Point	Network Point	Alarm Point	Back Transport Point
	Table 3–3: Meridian Cleft, Network, Alarm, and Back Transport Points				
Yin	Liver	LR-6	LR-5	LR-14	BL-18
	Pericardium	PC-4	PC-6	CV-17	BL-14
	Heart	HT-6	HT-5	CV-14	BL-15
	Spleen	SP-8	SP-4	LR-13	BL-20
	Lung	LU-6	LU-7	LU-1	BL-13
	Kidney	KI-5	KI-4	GB-25	BL-23
Yang	Gallbladder	GB-36	GB-37	GB-24	BL-19
	Triple Warmer	TW-7	TW-5	CV-5	BL-22
	Small Intestine	SI-6	SI-7	CV-4	BL-27
	Stomach	ST-34	ST-40	CV-12	BL-21
	Large Intestine	LI-7	LI-6	ST-25	BL-25
	Bladder	BL-63	BL-58	CV-3	BL-28

3.2 Hand Greater Yin Lung Channel 手の太陰肺経

The following descriptions of the flow of the meridians are based on the classical texts.

3.2.1 Flow of the Greater Yin Lung Channel *Tai'in Haikei no Ruchū* 太陰肺経の流注

The Lung or hand greater yin channel starts at the Middle Warmer (CV-12). It descends and loops around the Large Intestine (CV-9), then ascends upward and crosses the cardia (upper orifice of the stomach) (CV-13). It passes through the diaphragm and joins with the Lung. Then it emerges laterally to the brachial tubes (LU-1, LU-2) and skirts the axilla. It descends the anterior aspect of the upper arm through LU-3 and LU-4. It runs laterally to the lesser yin (Heart) channel and the Heart governing (Pericardium) channel. It crosses the transverse cubital crease through LU-5, descends the forearm through LU-6, passes over the medial corner of the styloid process of the radius at LU-7, enters the area of the radial pulse at LU-8 and LU-9, moves inferiorly down the thenar eminence of the palm passing through LU-10, and emerges at LU-11 at the tip of the thumb.

The branch diverges slightly proximal to the wrist at LU-7, immediately emerges along the lateral side of the index finger (near the Large Intestine channel), and ends at the tip of the finger.

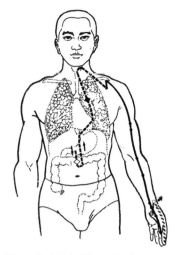

Figure 3–1: Main Channel and Connecting Vessel of the Lung

3.2.2 Connecting Vessel of the Lung *Haikei no Betsuraku* 肺経の別絡

The connecting vessel of the hand greater yin Lung channel is called "Broken Sequence" (LU-7). It starts between the muscles slightly proximal to the wrist. It runs parallel to the greater yin channel and then immediately diverges to enter the palm where it spreads and enters LU-10. From there it connects to the Large Intestine channel.

3.2.3 Divergent Channel of the Lung *Haikei no Keibetsu* 肺経の経別

The hand greater yin Lung channel sends off a divergent channel (from LU-1) that passes medial to the lesser yin channel (Heart channel) and GB-22. It then goes deep and runs through the Lung. It spreads and goes to the Large Intestine. From the Lung it again ascends to emerge at ST-12, and then crosses the throat to converge with the yang brightness (Large Intestine) channel.

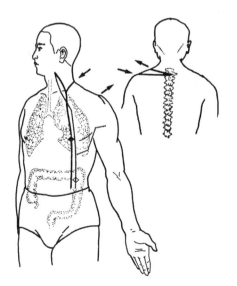

Figure 3–2: Divergent Channel of the Lung

3.2.4 Channel Sinews of the Lung *Haikei no Keikin* 肺経の経筋

The channel sinews of the hand greater yin Lung channel start at the tip of the thumb. They ascend the thumb and gather proximal to the thenar eminence of the palm. They then pass laterally to the area of the radial pulse, ascend through the forearm, and gather at the transverse cubital crease. They ascend through the medial aspect of the upper arm, through the axilla, emerge at the supraclavicular fossa (ST-12) and gather at the anterior prominence of the shoulder. They return and gather at ST-12. They then descend to gather internally at the chest where they spread and pass through the cardiac orifice area, from which they descend again to the area of the free ribs.

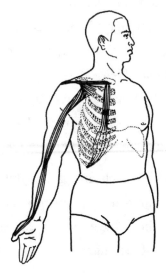

Figure 3–3: Channel Sinews of the Lung

3.2.5 Explanation

① According to the explanation given in the classic Chinese text *Elaborations of the Fourteen Meridians* (*Shísì-jīng Fāhuī* 十四経発揮), the section of the Lung channel that rises from CV-9 to the cardia flows on the posterior side of the Kidney channel. However, another explanation gives it as flowing on the medial side of the Kidney channel. If it flows on the medial side of the Kidney channel, then it is between the Kidney channel and the Conception Vessel.

② It is clear that the Lung channel is related to the Conception Vessel and that it mixes with the Liver channel at CV-12. Moreover, it has connections with the Spleen, Stomach, Large Intestine, and Kidney channels.

③ Naturally the Lung channel is used to treat respiratory diseases, but it can also be used to treat Large Intestine disorders and Kidney deficiency. It can even be used for emotional depression, since it circulates ki.

④ The areas of the Lung channel that most easily become excess are LU-1, LU-3, LU-4, and LU-6. LU-1 tends to reflect the accumulation of heat in the chest. LU-1, LU-3, and LU-4 often develop stiff lumps when the patient is experiencing fifty-year-old's shoulder. Pain on pressure is often elicited at LU-6 when the patient has hemorrhoids or pneumonia.

⑤ LU-5, LU-7, LU-8, and LU-9 tend to reflect deficiency in the Lung channel. Among this group, LU-5 and LU-7 tend to reveal pain on pressure, and LU-7 even more so if it shifts

---

slightly proximal. LU-9 and LU-8 do not generally reveal pain on pressure, but rather they often leak their ki.

⑥ Because the divergent channel extends all the way to the throat, treating the Lung channel can heal sore throat.

⑦ The flow of the channel sinews passes through ST-12 and the area of the free ribs, but the Lung channel itself does not. The areas where the channel sinews gather tend to exhibit pain on pressure and develop indurations.

3.3　Hand Yang Brightness Large Intestine Channel　手の陽明大腸経

3.3.1　Flow of the Yang Brightness Large Intestine Channel
Yōmei Daichōkei no Ruchū (陽明大腸経の流注)

The Large Intestine or hand yang brightness channel starts at the distal end of the index finger at LI-1. It ascends along the posterior lateral edge of the finger, passes through LI-2 and LI-3, and then continues up through LI-4 between the first and second metacarpal bones. It then goes through the carpal joint at LI-5 and continues along the posterior margin of the forearm, passing through LI-6, LI-7, LI-8, LI-9, LI-10, and reaching LI-11 at the lateral edge of the transverse cubital crease. It then ascends along the lateral margin of the upper arm passing through LI-12, LI-13, and LI-14 up to LI-15 at the acromioclavicular joint. Passing through LI-16, it then crosses over the shoulder to GV-14 on the spine and returns over the shoulder to ST-12 at the supraclavicular fossa. From there it wraps around the Lung and descends to join with the Large Intestine.

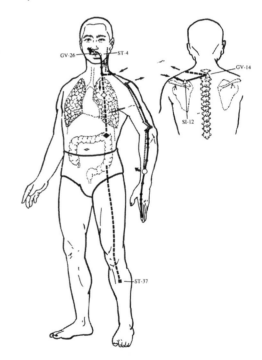

Figure 3–4: Main Channel and Connecting Vessel of the Large Intestine

A branch ascends from ST-12 along the neck, passing through LI-17 and LI-18. It then traverses the cheek and enters the lower teeth and gums. It curves back around the mouth, going through ST-4, and crosses the midline of the body (the conception vessel), the channel from the right side of the body going left and the channel from the left side of the body going right. It then ascends to the nostril at LI-20, where it connects with the yang brightness Stomach channel.

3.3.2 Connecting Vessel of the Large Intestine *Daichōkei no Betsuraku* (大腸経の別絡)

The connecting vessel of the hand yang brightness Large Intestine channel is called "Veering Passageway" (LI-6). It diverges from the primary channel at LI-6, three cùn proximal to the wrist, and enters the greater yin (Lung) channel. A branch ascends the arm, passes through LI-15, and connects to the cheek and teeth. Another branch enters the ear and joins the ancestral vessel.

3.3.3 Divergent Channel of the Large Intestine *Daichōkei no Keibetsu* (大腸経の経別)

The divergent channel of the hand yang brightness Large Intestine channel runs from the hand to the shoulder at LI-15. From there a branch crosses over to GV-14 and then runs through the Lung and joins with the Large Intestine. Another branch ascends from LI-15 through ST-12 to the throat, where it rejoins the yang brightness (Large Intestine) channel.

3.3.4 Channel Sinews of the Large Intestine *Daichōkei no Keikin* (大腸経の経筋)

The channel sinews of the hand yang brightness Large Intestine channel start at the tip of the index finger and gather at the wrist. They then ascend along the posterior lateral aspect of the forearm and gather at the lateral aspect of the elbow. They continue ascending and gather on the shoulder at LI-15.

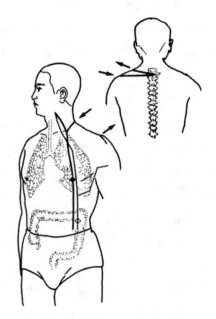

Figure 3–5: Divergent Channel of the Large Intestine

From there a branch passes over the scapula and attaches to the spine (i.e., to both sides of the Governing Vessel). The primary path continues ascending to the neck from LI-15. From there, a branch ascends the cheek at the mandible and gathers inferior to the eyes. Again, the primary path ascends, emerging in front of the greater yang (Small Intestine) channel, and for the pathway coming from the left it ascends the left side of the face, circles over the head, and descends to the right mandible.

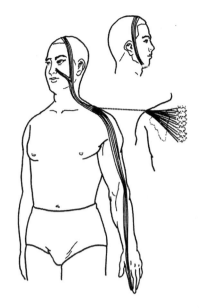

Figure 3–6: Channel Sinews of the Large Intestine

3.3.5 Explanation

① The whole of the Large Intestine channel tends to display heat and often develops indurations, especially at LI-4, LI-5, LI-7, LI-10, LI-14, and LI-15. LI-14 is connected to TW-13, so understandably the whole area around the deltoid muscle tends to become stiff. Attention should be paid here especially in cases of fifty-year-old's shoulder.

② LI-6 and LI-11 are the two points that tend to become deficient on the Large Intestine channel.

③ The Large Intestine channel and other yang channels flow into GV-14 and ST-12. Because they tend to reveal illnesses of the yang meridians they make good treatment points.

④ Because the Large Intestine channel flows along the sternocleidomastoid muscle, there are patients in whom this area becomes stiff.

⑤ The right path of the Large Intestine channel ascends the left side of the body, and the left path ascends the right side of the body. It is a good idea to make practical use of this flow when treating toothaches or Bell's palsy. Moreover, you should also treat the Large Intestine channel for cases such as eczema around the mouth. The Large Intestine channel is also often used for skin diseases and for illnesses of the eyes and nose.

⑥ The Large Intestine channel is connected with the Stomach channel, which is also part of the yang brightness channel. Therefore, there are times when it is useful to think about the whole yang brightness channel when you are trying to understand the symptom pattern.

⑦ The yang brightness channel is rich in both ki and blood, and thus it tends to accumulate heat. It also takes the brunt of the burden when using the arms and leg. Therefore, the Large Intestine channel should be treated when a person has a stiff shoulder from overuse of the arms, and the Stomach channel should be treated when a person has overused the legs.

⑧ Although the primary channel does not flow to the throat or ears, the connecting vessel and divergent channel are connected to these areas. Therefore, there are patients whose tympanitis or sore throat has gotten better through treatment of the yang brightness channel.

⑨ The channel sinews run along the area where the cord of a helmet would be when the helmet is tied onto the head. Parts of the Large Intestine channel and Stomach channel run though this area, but it can be valuable to explain certain conditions of this area in terms of the channel sinews. For example, when the arms are used too much, this area becomes painful.

The channel sinews also run from the scapula to the spine. However, it is not known exactly how far they go. Our experience has shown that they go at least to BL-13 or possibly medial to BL-13. This is because when the shoulders become stiff with overuse of the arms or when patients complain of toothaches or headaches, these areas tend to exhibit pain on pressure.

3.4   Foot Yang Brightness Stomach Channel   足の陽明胃経

3.4.1 Flow of the Yang Brightness Stomach Channel *Yōmei Ikei no Ruchū* 陽明胃経の流注

The Stomach or foot yang brightness channel starts at the nose and ascends to the root of the nose. It then enters the nearby greater yang channel at BL-1, and descends lateral to the nose through ST-1, ST-2, and ST-3. It enters the upper gums and then turns to curve around to the corner of the mouth, passing through ST-4. It continues to circle around the lips and descends to CV-24, where the left and right channels meet. Drawing back, it follows the angle of the mandible, passing through ST-5 and ST-6, and then ascends anterior to the ear through ST-7. It crosses the Gallbladder channel at GB-3, passes through GB-6, GB-5, GB-4, and ST-8 along the hairline, and ends at GV-24 on the forehead.

From anterior to ST-5 a branch descends to ST-9, passes through ST-10 and ST-11 on the throat, and enters ST-12. It descends through the diaphragm, joins with the Stomach at CV-13 and CV-12, and then connects to the Spleen.

The primary channel descends from ST-12 medial to the mammillary line, passing through ST-13, ST-14, ST-15, ST-16, ST-17, and ST-18. It continues to descend while passing through ST-19, ST-20, ST-21, ST-22, ST-23, and ST-24, goes by the navel, then descends through ST-25, ST-26, ST-27, ST-28, and ST-29, and enters ST-30.

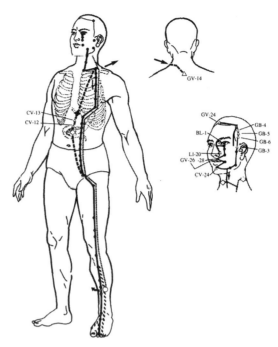

Figure 3–7: Main Channel and Connecting Vessel of the Stomach

A branch starts at the pylorus [the lower orifice of the stomach] near CV-10 and descends internally through the abdomen to rejoin the main channel at ST-30. From there it descends through ST-31 and on to ST-32. Then it descends to the patella, passing through ST-33, ST-34, and ST-35. It continues to descend along the shin, passing through ST-36, ST-37, ST-38, and ST-39. Then it descends through ST-41 and ST-42 on the dorsum of the foot, passes through ST-43 and ST-44 intermediate to the second and third toes, and ends at ST-45 at the lateral tip of the second toe.

A branch diverges from ST-36, descends through ST-40, and enters the lateral side of the third toe.

Another branch diverges from ST-42 on the dorsum of the foot, enters the big toe, and exits at the tip, where it meets the Spleen channel.

3.4.2 Connecting Vessel of the Stomach *Ikei no Betsuraku* 胃経の別絡

The connecting vessel of the foot yang brightness Stomach channel is called "Bountiful Bulge" (ST-40). It starts at ST-40, 8 *cùn* superior to the lateral malleolus, and connects to the foot greater yin Spleen channel.

A branch ascends along the lateral edge of the tibia, going all the way up to encircle the nape of the neck, where it meets the ki of other meridians, and then descends to wrap around the throat.

3.4.3 Divergent Channel of the Stomach *Ikei no Keibetsu* 胃経の経別

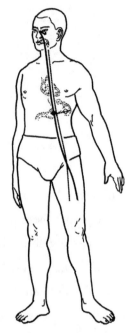

Figure 3–8: Divergent Channel of the Stomach

The divergent channel of the foot yang brightness Stomach channel ascends from the thigh, enters deep into the abdomen, and joins with the Stomach. It spreads and goes to the Spleen, and then ascends through the Heart. It continues to ascend through the throat, exits through the mouth, and ascends to the brow. It then returns down to connect with the eyes and join the primary channel of the foot yang brightness Stomach channel.

3.4.4 Channel Sinews of the Stomach *Ikei no Keikin* 胃経の経筋

The channel sinews of the foot yang brightness Stomach channel start at the second, third, and fourth toes and gather at the proximal end of the dorsum of the foot. They ascend laterally at an angle, increase over the fibula, and gather lateral to the knee at GB-34. They then ascend vertically and gather lateral to the hip joint. Then they ascend around the lateral side of the chest and connect to the spine.

The main path ascends from the dorsum of the foot over the tibia and gathers at the knee.

A branch diverges from the knee and gathers at GB-34 on the lateral side of the fibula, where it joins the lesser yang pathway.

The main path continues to ascend from the knee up through ST-32 on the thigh and gathers at the groin. It gathers in the genital area at CV-2, ascends through the abdomen, and continues to ascend and gather at ST-12. It ascends the neck, passes by the mouth, goes up to the zygomatic area, and descends to gather at the nose. Then it ascends again to meet the greater yang channel. The greater yang channel is superior to the eyes, and the yang brightness channel is inferior to the eyes.

A branch diverges from the cheek and gathers anterior to the ears.

3.4.5 Explanation

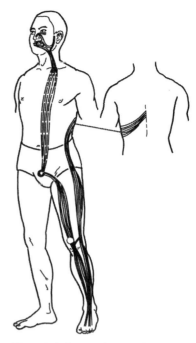

Figure 3–9: Channel Sinews of the Stomach

① One section of the Stomach channel on the face flows in the same path as that of the Large Intestine channel. Moreover, it is also connected to the Bladder channel, Gallbladder channel, and Governing Vessel, as well as to the eyes, nose, ears, teeth, mouth, and throat. Acupuncture points on the Stomach channel are often used when there is a heat pattern in these areas or when there is Bell's Palsy. Use of the Stomach channel is also effective in treating headache due to surplus heat in the yang brightness channel.

② The acupuncture points in the thoracic and abdominal areas are also important points. In particular, notice that there are connections to CV-13, CV-12, and CV-10.

When there is a problem in the Spleen or Stomach, the points from ST-19 to ST-25 tend to show pain on pressure, resistance, or depressions. Particularly, ST-21 will always show deficiency when there is a gastric ulcer. Moreover, when there is a duodenal ulcer or pancreatitis, ST-24 and ST-25 will reveal pain on pressure and there will be spontaneous pain [i.e., pain felt without elicitation by palpation or movement] in those areas. When there is blood stasis, the area between ST-25 and ST-27 or ST-28 (see Figure 7–8, page 229) will always show resistance and pain on pressure.

③ Since the Stomach channel tends to show heat patterns, the acupuncture points going down the lower limb tend to reveal pain on pressure, especially ST-36, ST-37, ST-39, and ST-44.

④ Chapter 2 of the *Ling Shu* says, "… ST-37 is three *cùn* inferior to ST-36, and ST-39 is three *cùn* inferior to ST-37. The Large Intestine belongs to the former [ST-37] and the Small Intestine belongs to the latter [ST-39]." Therefore, ST-37 should be used for treatment when there is heat in the Large Intestine, and ST-39 should be used when there is heat in the Small Intestine. For example, ST-37 should be used when there is appendicitis.

⑤ Generally, signs appear on the yang brightness channel when there is an abundance of heat. They also tend to appear in healthy people who are able to bear heat in the Stomach. Although all the reference books say that the yang brightness Stomach channel is effective for treatment of diarrhea and stomachaches, no signs will be apparent in cases of Spleen deficiency unless there is heat in the Stomach or yang brightness channel.

⑥ The connecting vessels of the Stomach channel run all the way to the nape of the neck. Thus, there will be sharp pain at the nape of the neck along with pain in the greater yang channel when there is febrile disease.

⑦ Note that the channel sinews of the Stomach channel go from the dorsum of the foot to GB-34 and to the knee. When there is sciatica, pain on pressure along the Gallbladder channel below GB-34 will naturally reverberate in the Stomach channel and at times go as far as SP-2 and SP-3. Moreover, it can be effective to treat GB-30 when there is pain in the knee joint. The channel sinews of the Stomach channel go from GB-34 to the lateral side of the chest, but probably only as far as LR-13. It is thought that from there they go around to the back and connect to the medial side of BL-20 and BL-21. The channel sinews connect to the external reproductive organs at about the area of CV-2, and the connections are to what are termed ancestral sinews/sexual organs. If one engages in excessive sexual intercourse the ancestral sinews will become weak and the essence power will diminish.

3.5.1 Flow of the Greater Yin Spleen Channel *Tai'in Hikei no Ruchū* 太陰脾経の流注

The Spleen or foot greater yin channel starts at SP-1 on the tip of the big toe. It follows the medial aspect of the foot, passing through SP-2 along the border between the red and white skin, and then through SP-3 and SP-4, slightly inferior to the first metacarpal bone. It ascends passing through SP-5 anterior to the medial malleolus, then ascends the medial aspect of the lower leg posterior to the tibia, passing through SP-6, SP-7, SP-8, and SP-9. At eight *cùn* superior to the medial malleolus, it crosses to run anterior to the reverting yin Liver channel. It then ascends the anteriomedial aspect of the knee and thigh, passing through SP-10 and SP-11, and then ascends to enter the abdomen. After passing through SP-12 and SP-13 it meets CV-3 and CV-4 and then meets CV-10 after first passing through SP-14 and SP-15. A branch runs deep to the primary channel, and after passing through CV-12 and CV-10, it joins with the Spleen and then connects to the Stomach. The primary

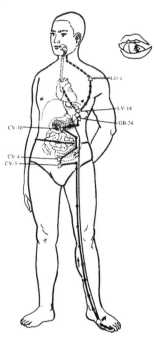

Figure 3–10: Main Channel and Connecting Vessel of the Spleen

channel ascends from SP-16 and passes through GB-24, LR-14, and the diaphragm. After touching SP-17, SP-18, SP-19, SP-20, and SP-21, it goes to the Lung channel at LU-1. It then travels up past the throat to connect with and spread around the lower surface of the root of the tongue.

A branch diverts from the Stomach (between SP-16 and CV-10), ascends through the diaphragm, and pours into the center of the Heart (CV-17). From there it continues in the Heart channel.

3.5.2 Connecting Vessel of the Spleen *Hikei no Betsuraku* 脾経の別絡

The connecting vessel of the foot greater yin Spleen channel is called "Yellow Emperor" (SP-3). It diverges one *cùn* proximal to the head of the

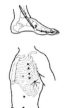

Figure 3–11: Great Connecting Vessel of the Spleen

first metatarsal bone and runs with the yang brightness channel. A branch enters internally to connect to the intestines and Stomach.

3.5.3 Divergent Channel of the Spleen *Hikei no Keibetsu* 脾経の経別

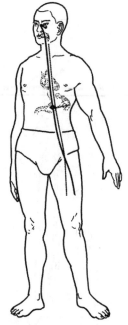

Figure 3–12: Divergent Channel of the Spleen

The divergent channel of the foot greater yin Spleen channel diverges from the primary channel on the thigh and runs together with a branch of the yang brightness Stomach channel. It ascends to the throat then passes into the tongue.

3.5.4 Channel Sinews of the Spleen *Hikei no Keikin* 脾経の経筋

The channel sinews of the foot greater yin Spleen channel start at the medial tip of the big toe and ascend to gather at the medial malleolus. The primary path ascends to connect to the medial side of the knee and then ascends the inner thigh to gather in the genital area. It then ascends the abdomen to gather at the navel, passes through the internal abdomen, gathers at the ribs, and spreads throughout the chest. Branches go deep to connect to the spine.

3.5.5 Explanation

① The Spleen channel has many connections with other channels simply because it is the controller of ki and blood production.

② The abdominal portions of the Spleen channel, the Conception Vessel, and the Stomach channel comprise an important diagnostic area for abdominal diagnosis.

③ SP-6 and SP-10 are both diagnostic points and treatment points for gynecological problems. Because these points will reveal signs of both blood deficiency and blood stasis, it is important to be able to distinguish between blood stasis (Liver excess) and blood deficiency (Liver deficiency) (see Figures 7–8

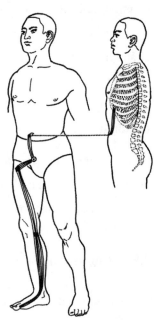

Figure 3–13: Channel Sinews of the Spleen

and 7–9, page 229). CV-4 and CV-3 are also related to such conditions because they are meeting points between the Spleen channel and the Conception Vessel.

④ SP-4, SP-5, and SP-6 are often used for digestive tract problems. If these points show signs of imbalance, then the points BL-20, BL-21, and BL-22 will always be deficient concurrently.

If moxibustion is to be applied to SP-6 during pregnancy it should be done after the fifth month. SP-6 is used to ensure an easy delivery, and BL-67 is used in cases of breech birth or difficult deliveries.

⑤ The Spleen channel on the lower limbs tends to exhibit pain on pressure. Healing will be slow if there are depressions along the Spleen channel here.

⑥ The channel sinews of the Spleen channel go to the genital areas the same as the Stomach channel. They also connect to the spine—most likely medial to BL-20.

⑦ The channel sinews run along the medial side of the knee. But, they are closer to the patella than to the Liver channel.

⑧ When there is abdominal pain due to Spleen deficiency, the patient will feel better if moxa is burned on top of salt poured into the navel since the channel sinews gather at the navel.

3.6   Hand Lesser Yin Heart Channel   手の少陰心経

3.6.1 Flow of the Lesser Yin Heart Channel *Shōin Shinkei no Ruchū* 少陰心経の流注

The Heart or lesser yin channel starts in the Heart. It emerges with the network vessel of the Heart and descends through the diaphragm to connect with the Small Intestine two *cùn* above the navel at CV-10.

A branch leaves the Heart and ascends lateral to the Conception Vessel line, passing along the throat and connecting to the eyes at the inner canthus.

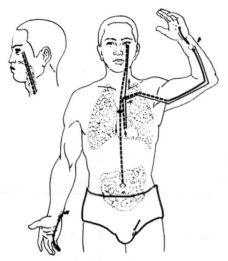

Figure 3–14: Main Channel and Connecting Vessel of the Heart

The primary channel leaves the Heart and ascends through the Lung. It then descends to emerge in the axilla at HT-1. It continues to descend along the medial aspect of the upper arm (the posteriomedial edge of the biceps brachialis muscle), passing through HT-2. It descends medial to the Lung channel and Pericardium channel and passes through HT-3 at the medial border of the transverse cubital crease. It then descends through HT-4, HT-5, and HT-6 on the anterior aspect of the forearm and through HT-7 at the ulnar end of the transverse carpal crease. Then it enters HT-8 on the medial side of the palmar surface, runs along the lateral side of the little finger, and ends at HT-9 at the tip of the finger.

3.6.2 Connecting Vessel of the Heart *Shinkei no Betsuraku* 心経の別絡

The connecting vessel of the hand lesser yin Heart channel is called "Connecting Li" (HT-5). It starts one *cùn* superior to the wrist at HT-5 and diverges to ascend the Heart channel. It enters the Heart, connects to the root of the tongue, and then merges with the eyes.

3.6.3 Divergent Channel of the Heart *Shinkei no Keibetsu* 心経の経別

The divergent channel of the hand lesser yin Heart channel diverges from the primary channel deep within the axillary fossa and enters between the muscles to join with the Heart. It then ascends through the throat, emerges on the face, and gathers at the inner canthus of the eye.

3.6.4 Channel Sinews of the Heart *Shinkei no Keikin* 心経の経筋

The channel sinews of the hand lesser yin Heart channel start at the lateral edge of the little finger and

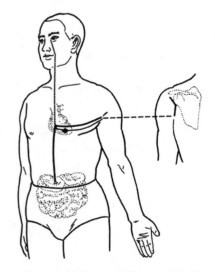

Figure 3–15: Divergent Channel of the Heart

gather at the pisiform bone at HT-7. They ascend to gather at the medial epicondyle of the elbow and then enter the axilla. After meeting with the Lung channcl thcy pass through the pectoral region and gather at the sternum. From there they descend through the cardiac orifice area and connect to the navel.

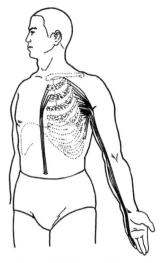

Figure 3–16: Channel Sinews of the Heart

3.6.5 Explanation

① According to the *Elaborations of the Fourteen Meridians* there are two network vessels of the Heart channel. One ascends to join the Lung and enters between the lobes of the lungs. The other one descends from the lungs, turns to run along both sides of the spinal column, and then joins with the grandchild vessel and the Kidney.

② Since the Heart channel is in a paired relationship with the Small Intestine channel , it joins with the Small Intestine two *cun* superior to the navel. The Heart channel circulates Heart ki, which prevents too much heat from collecting in the Heart organ. More will be explained about this later, but it should be understandable if you consider that the Heart channel is, like the Kidney channel, a lesser yin channel.

③ In Meridian Therapy the Pericardium channel is used as a substitute for the Heart channel, the reason for which will be explained later. However, it should be noted that the Heart channel does have its own unique effectiveness for treating certain conditions, which in many cases is the result of its being connected with the Kidney.

④ The divergent channel of the Heart runs all the way to the inner canthus of the eye. That is why HT-3 and HT-4 are effective treatment points when the patient has bloodshot eyes along with an great heat in the chest. Likewise, since the divergent channel also passes through the throat, HT-7 can be used to alleviate a sore throat.

⑤ Pain on pressure tends to be found between HT-4 and HT-3.

3.7.1 Flow of the Greater Yang Small Intestine Channel *Taiyō Shōchōkei no Ruchū* 太陽小腸経の流注

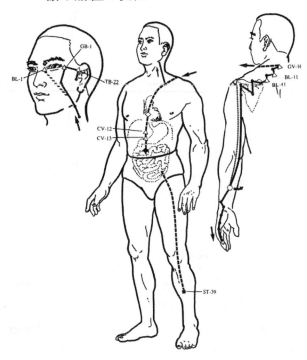

Figure 3–17: Main Channel and Connecting Vessel of the Small Intestine

The Small Intestine or hand greater yang channel starts at SI-1 on the tip of the little finger. It ascends through SI-2 and SI-3 along the ulnar edge of the hand through SI-4 and SI-5 at the wrist, passes through the styloid process of the ulna, and emerges at SI-6. It continues to directly ascend along the posterior aspect of the ulna, passing through SI-7 and through SI-8 at the medial side of the elbow. It then ascends the posterior aspect of the upper arm, where it connects to the Large Intestine and Triple Warmer channels. Then it emerges in the shoulder joint at SI-9 and SI-10 and passes through SI-11, SI-12, and SI-13 on the scapula and through SI-14, SI-15, and GV-14 on the upper back superior to the scapula. It enters at ST-12, and connects with the Heart at CV-17. It then passes through the throat, descends through the diaphragm, and through the Stomach at CV-13 and CV-12, and then joins with the Small Intestine in the area two *cùn* superior to the navel.

A branch ascends from ST-12 through SI-16 and SI-17 on the neck and through SI-18 on the cheek. It reaches to the outer canthus of the eye at GB-1 and then continues posteriorly to enter the ear at SI-19.

Another branch diverges from SI-18 on the cheek, ascends inferior to the eye, touches the nose, reaches BL-1 at the inner canthus of the eye, and then moves diagonally across the zygomatic arch.

3.7.2 Connecting Vessel of the Small Intestine *Shōchōkei no Betsuraku* 小腸経の別絡

The connecting vessel of the hand greater yang Small Intestine channel is called "Branch to the Correct" (SI-7). It diverges from the primary channel at SI-7, five *cùn* proximal to the wrist and penetrates to pour into the lesser yin channel. It ascends through the elbow and connects to LI-15 on the shoulder.

3.7.3 Divergent Channel of the Small Intestine
Shōchōkei no Keibetsu 小腸経の経別

The divergent channel of the hand greater yang Small Intestine channel follows the flow of the primary channel from SI-16. It also diverges and descends from the shoulder joint, entering the axilla, running though the Heart, and then connecting to the Small Intestine.

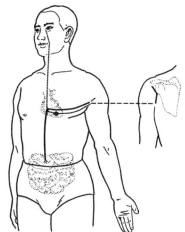

Figure 3–18: Divergent Channel of the Small Intestine

3.7.4 Channel Sinews of the Small Intestine
Shōchōkei no Keikin 小腸経の経筋

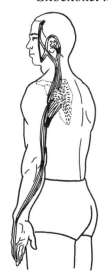

Figure3–19: Channel Sinews of the Small Intestine

The channel sinews of the hand greater yang Small Intestine channel start at the tip of the little finger and ascend to gather at the wrist. They then ascend along the medial aspect of the forearm to gather at the medial condyle of the humerus. If this area is bumped, the sensation will be felt all the way down to the tip of the little finger. These sinews continue to ascend, and gather in the axilla.

A branch that diverges from the axilla traverses upward posterior to the axilla, then ascends over the scapula and up the neck, where it flows anterior to the greater yang Bladder channel to gather at the mastoid process posterior to the ear.

A branch that derives from the mastoid process enters the ear.

The main path from the mastoid process ascends over the ear and descends to gather at the zygomatic bone. It ascends to gather at the outer canthus of the eye.

Another branch ascends from the lower jaw and gathers anterior to the ear. It connects to the outer canthus of the eye and ascends the forehead to gather at ST-8.

3.7.5 Explanation

① Acupuncture points belonging to the Small Intestine channel in the shoulder area are often used for treating stiff shoulders and pain in the shoulder joint. Indurations and pain on pressure are found especially at acupuncture points from SI-11 to SI-15. When moxibustion is used, points with indurations should be selected.

② Acupuncture points in the distal part of the arm are often used for rheumatism, arthritis, and stiff shoulders.

③ The Small Intestine channel can be used to treat acute febrile disease since it is a greater yang channel. It is effective for inflammation of the joints when there is urinary difficulty. The Heart and Small Intestine channels circulate through the ear, and hence they can be used for ear problems.

④ As it says in the *Ling Shu*, there are many times when it is convenient to think of the Small Intestine as a part of the Stomach. The Small Intestine channel should be treated after tonifying the Spleen when the tip of the tongue and face are red and when the accompanying symptom pattern includes a feeling of fullness and oppression below the Heart, borborygmus (i.e., rumbling intestines), belching, diarrhea, or constipation.

⑤ Chapter 4 of the *Ling Shu* says, "Illness of the Small Intestine causes pain in the lower abdomen that spreads to the lumbar vertebrae and testicles and that sometimes results in painful diarrhea. There can be signs such as heat in the area anterior to the ear, or extreme cold, or extreme heat on the top of one shoulder, or heat between the first and second fingers, or a sunken channel. These indicate illnesses of the hand greater yang channel." According to this passage, the Small Intestine channel is also related to the testes.

⑥ Pain on pressure also appears in the forearm, such as at SI-7. In the Sawada School, HT-7 is said to be effective for treating constipation, which is probably due to SI-4 being a traveling point (変動穴 *hendōketsu*).

3.8.1 Flow of the Greater Yang Bladder Channel *Taiyō Bōkōkei no Ruchu* 太陽膀胱経 の流注

The Bladder or foot greater yang channel starts at BL-1 at the inner canthus of the eye. It ascends the forehead, intersecting the Governing Vessel at GV-24, and travels up to the vertex where it again meets the Governing Vessel at GV-20.

A branch descends from GV-20 to the area above the ear and joins the Gallbladder channel at GB-8, GB-10, and GB-11.

The primary channel enters through the vertex to connect to the brain and reemerges to pass through BL-7, BL-8, and BL-9. It diverges at the nape of the neck (descending from BL-10 to GV-14 and GV-13) and descends medial to the scapula, alongside the spinal column, passing through BL-11, BL-12, BL-13, BL-14, BL-15, BL-16, BL-17, BL-18, BL-19, BL-20, BL-21, BL-22, BL-23, BL-24, BL-25, BL-26, BL-27, BL-28, BL-29, and BL-30. It enters at the lumbar region, passing through the vertebrae to intersect the Kidney and join with the Bladder.

A branch descends from the lumbar region, passing through BL-31, BL-32, BL-33, BL-34, and BL-35 along the sacrum, crosses the buttock through BL-36 and BL-37, and enters the popliteal fossa at BL-40.

A branch diverges and descends over the medial aspect of the scapula and then passes through BL-41, BL-42, BL-43, BL-44, BL-45, BL-46, BL-47, BL-48, BL-49, BL-50, BL-51, BL-52, BL-53, and BL-54 parallel to the vertebral column. It goes through the hip

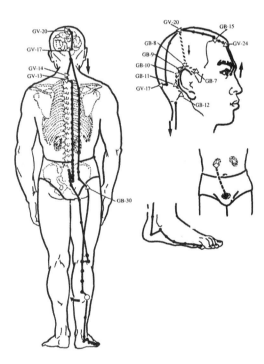

Figure 3–20: Main Channel and Connecting Vessel of the Bladder

joint then continues, descending the posterior aspect of the upper leg. It descends through BL-38 and BL-39 and merges at BL-40 in the popliteal fossa.

From BL-40 it continues to descend through BL-55, BL-56, BL-57, BL-58, and BL-59 on the gastrocnemius, then through BL-60 and BL-61 posterior to the lateral malleolus, and through BL-62 and BL-63 inferior to the lateral malleolus. It then passes through BL-64 and along the lateral aspect of the foot, passing through BL-65, BL-66, and BL-67 at the tip of the little toe.

3.8.2 Connecting Vessel of the Bladder *Bōkōkei no Betsuraku* 膀胱経の別絡

The connecting vessel of the foot greater yang Bladder channel is called "Taking Flight." It starts at BL-58 seven *cùn* superior to the lateral malleolus, and diverges to join the lesser yin channel.

3.8.3 Divergent Channel of the Bladder *Bōkōkei no Keibetsu* 膀胱経の経別

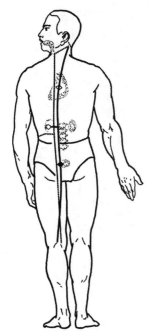

The divergent channel of the foot greater yang Bladder channel diverges and enters the popliteal fossa. It ascends to a point five *cùn* inferior to the buttock, where it diverges and enters the anus. It joins with the Bladder, then spreads and goes to the Kidney. It then ascends along the spine to the Heart, where it enters and disperses.

The primary channel ascends the spine to the nape of the neck and rejoins the greater yang channel.

3.8.4 Channel Sinews of the Bladder *Bōkōkei no Keikin* 膀胱経の経筋

The channel sinews of the foot greater yang Bladder channel start on the little toe and ascend to gather at the lateral malleolus. They then ascend diagonally to gather at the knee.

Figure 3–21: Divergent Channel of the Bladder

A branch travels along the lateral side of the foot to gather at the heel. It ascends and gathers at the popliteal fossa.

A branch that diverges from the path that ascends from the heel gathers at the medial side of the gastrocnemius. It then ascends to the medial aspect of the popliteal fossa and rejoins the path from which it diverged. They rejoin and ascend to gather at the buttock, and then ascend along the spine to the nape of the neck.

A branch separates from the nape of the neck to gather at the root of the tongue.

The primary path (from the nape of the neck) gathers at the occipital bone. It then ascends over the head and descends the face to gather at the nose.

A branch of the path that descends to the face goes to the area superior to the eyes and then gathers inferior to the eyes.

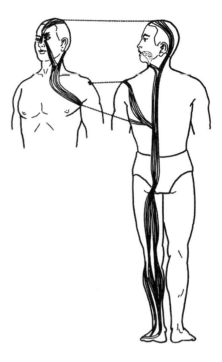

A branch separates from the path ascending along the spine and ascends from the lateral aspect of the back posterior to the axilla to gather at LI-15. A branch from LI-15 passes under the axilla, ascends

Figure 3–22: Channel Sinews of the Bladder

to ST-12, then continues to ascend to gather at GB-12. A branch from ST-12 ascends diagonally to the area inferior to the eye, where it meets the path that comes over the head.

3.8.5 Explanation

① The strong feature of the Bladder channel is its points on the back of the body. Abnormalities in the organs or meridians that are related to these points will be reflected at these points. At the same time they are used as treatment points. It is important to train the sensitivity of your fingertips to find the acupuncture points after you have studied their uses as explained in textbooks. Protuberances usually indicate excess, but there are times when there is deficiency even though the points have protuberances. These points can also show signs such as depressions, or they may be hot or cold to the touch. These are signs that appear when there is a cold or heat pattern due to deficiency of yin somewhere in the body. Moxibustion or needling should be used for these conditions. Tonification or dispersion must naturally be determined according to the deficiency or excess.

② Acupuncture points on the head can have pain on pressure when they show depressions or edema.

③ Acupuncture points that are between the bones of the scapula often have indurations when there are symptoms such as stiffness of the shoulders or disorders that appear above the neck. Indurations or pain on pressure can also appear when there are lung or heart problems.

④ Channel sinews branch off from the spinal column and go to LI-15 on the shoulder. This path most likely ascends along the scapula. The whole area around the scapula often has indurations in patients who complain of stiff shoulders.

⑤ BL-17 marks the border that separates the Upper Warmer from the Middle Warmer. In relatively new cases of illnesses of the Liver, Gallbladder, Stomach or Intestines, it is likely that there will be indurations or pain on pressure in the area of BL-17, BL-18, and BL-19. Deficient-type distention, depressions, indurations, and pain on pressure appear in the area of BL-20, BL-21, and BL-22 when there are chronic digestive tract problems.

⑥ Signs can be seen in acupuncture points below BL-22 when there are Kidney, Bladder, or uterine conditions, as well as when there is low back pain.

⑦ Acute illnesses with an aversion to cold, fever, and headaches are considered a symptom pattern relating to the greater yang Bladder channel. There is a tendency to develop a fever with the stagnation of yang ki in the greater yang channel that occurs along with an aversion to cold when there is a deficiency of Lung ki, which controls the external areas (the *hyō* areas of the body).

The Lower Warmer may become chilled and yang ki may stagnate in the Upper Warmer because the circulation of yang ki in the greater yang channel deteriorates during chronic illnesses. This condition can cause headaches, stiff shoulders, and hot flushes.

Stagnation of yang ki also causes stagnation of blood, which in turn causes tension and stiffness in the shoulder muscles. Stiffness in the Bladder channel most frequently appears at BL-10. Stiffness also tends to appear at BL-43 medial to the scapula.

⑧ Yang ki tends to be insufficient in the area centering on BL-22 in the Lower Warmer. Stiffness in the Upper Warmer is due to stagnation of yang ki, and stiffness in the Lower Warmer is due to insufficient yang ki. Stiffness in the Lower Warmer shows up not only in the lower back, but also tends to appear at BL-40, BL-58, or BL-60 in the lower limbs.

⑨ The Bladder channel points on the lower limbs are often used to treat sciatica, but are also effective for fatigue, weakness of the legs, cramps, and urinary difficulty.

3.9.1 Flow of the Lesser Yin Kidney Channel *Shōin Jinkei no Ruchū* 少陰腎経の流注

The Kidney or foot lesser yin channel starts at the inferior aspect of the little toe, where it receives the flow of the Bladder channel. It diagonally transverses the sole of the foot to KI-1, emerges inferior to KI-2, and then passes through KI-3 and KI-4 posterior to the medial malleolus. It diverges and enters KI-5 and KI-6 on the heel. It then continues, ascending through KI-7, KI-8, SP-6, and KI-9 on the medial aspect of the lower leg up to KI-10 at the medial edge of the popliteal crease. Then it ascends along the medial and posterior aspects of the upper leg,

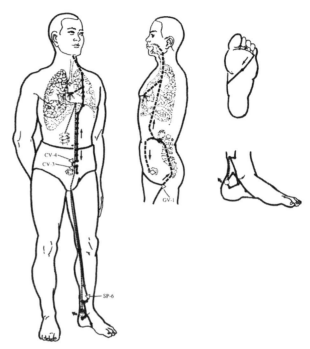

Figure 3–23: Main Channel and Connecting Vessel of the Kidney

penetrates the spinal column at GV-1, and emerges in the lower abdomen, where it passes through KI-11, KI-12, KI-13, KI-14, KI-15, and KI-16. It joins with the Kidney then connects to the Bladder at CV-4 and CV-3.

The primary channel (the channel that goes from KI-16 to the Kidney) ascends from the Kidney through KI-17, KI-18, KI-19, KI-20, and KI-21, then passes through the Liver and diaphragm at KI-22. It then enters the Lung, passing through KI-23, KI-24, KI-25, KI-26, and KI-27, passes through the throat, and terminates at the root of the tongue.

A branch leaves the Lung, encircles the Heart at CV-17, and then pours into the chest, connecting also to the Pericardium channel.

3.9.2 Connecting Vessel of the Kidney *Jinkei no Betsuraku* 腎経の別絡

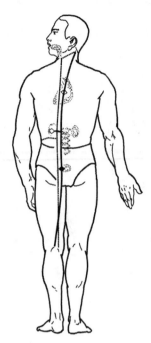

The connecting vessel of the foot lesser yin Kidney channel is called "Large Goblet" (KI-4). It starts at KI-4 posterior to the medial malleolus, passes through the heel, and then diverges to merge with the greater yang channel.

A branch ascends parallel with the primary channel, then runs through the Pericardium. It then descends to enter the lumbar vertebrae.

3.9.3 Divergent Channel of the Kidney *Jinkei no Keibetsu* 腎経の経別

The divergent channel of the foot lesser yin Kidney channel derives from the primary channel in the popliteal fossa and diverges to merge with the greater yang channel. From there it ascends through the Kidney, emerges from the second lumbar vertebra (L2) and merges with the girdling vessel. From there the primary channel connects to the root of the tongue and then emerges at the nape of the neck to meet the greater yang channel.

Figure 3–24: Divergent Channel of the Kidney

3.9.4 Channel Sinews of the Kidney *Jinkei no Keikin* 腎経の経筋

The channel sinews of the foot lesser yin Kidney channel start beneath the little toe. They align with the foot greater yin channel sinews and run diagonally to the area inferior to the medial malleolus, where they gather to the heel. They then ascend together with the greater yang channel sinews to gather at the medial aspect of the knee. From there, aligned with the greater yin channel sinews, they ascend the medial aspect of the thigh and gather at the genitalia. They pass through the spine and ascend alongside the spinal column, passing through the nape of the neck to gather at the occipital bone, where they join the foot greater yang channel sinews.

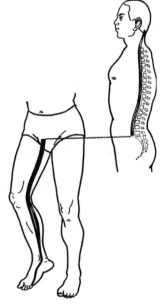

Figure 3–25: Channel Sinews of the Kidney

3.9.5 Explanation

① The Kidney channel picks up the flow of the Bladder channel and starts on the sole of the foot. It is difficult to needle KI-1 and KI-2, but they are very useful points for patients with yin deficiency with an abundance of deficient-type heat. It is also possible to apply pressure with a finger to these points instead of needling them. In that case, it best to press your finger until it feels like it sinks into the point.

② The acupuncture points from KI-3 to KI-7 are often deficient or cold. KI-3 is especially important as a diagnostic indicator, and can be used to examine the pulse of the lesser yin channel. Note that there is considerable blood stasis when the body is robust yet the lesser yin pulse is undetectable. A floating pulse that is easily detected is a sign of Kidney deficiency with abundant deficient-type heat.

③ Pain on pressure appears along the Kidney channel on the thigh when there are patterns of Kidney deficiency or Liver deficiency even though there are no acupuncture points belonging to the Kidney channel on the thigh above KI-10.

④ Acupuncture points in the abdominal area may be used as diagnostic points. Resistance and pain on pressure in the area around KI-11 superior to the pubic bone indicate Kidney deficiency. The Kidney channel above that point will often be deficient along with the Conception Vessel, and lateral to that the Stomach channel will be tense. This phenomenon occurs because deficient-type heat of the Kidney deficiency spreads to the Stomach channel. Conception Vessel deficiency appearing at the same time as a tense Stomach channel always indicates a Kidney deficiency heat pattern. Pain on pressure also commonly appears in the other acupuncture points in the abdominal area when there is diarrhea.

⑤ The Kidney channel in the thoracic area frequently has pain on pressure when there is Heart heat along with a Kidney deficiency heat pattern. Moreover, both the primary channel and divergent channel of the Kidney are connected to the throat and tongue, just as is the lesser yin Heart channel. Indeed, there are cases when throat pain immediately improves upon treating the Kidney channel (such as at KI-6).

⑥ The divergent channel of the Kidney is connected to the Girdling Vessel at the area of the second lumbar vertebra. The Girdling Vessel is also connected to the Gallbladder channel.

That is why low back pain often improves when the Gallbladder channel is tonified or dispersed after tonifying a deficient Kidney. However, it should also be noted that the Girdling Vessel seems to droop down along the inguinal fold along the abdomen.

⑦ The channel sinews of the Kidney ascend lateral to the spinal column and medial to the Bladder channel. Points here are also known as paravertebral points. Many patients have indurations in this area, especially the medial section between BL-23 and BL-25 in patients with low back pain.

3.10　Hand Reverting Yin Pericardium Channel　手の厥陰心包経

3.10.1　Flow of the Reverting Yin Pericardium Channel *Ketsuin Shinpōkei no Ruchū* 厥陰心包経の流注

The Pericardium or hand reverting yin channel starts in the chest. It emerges and joins with the Pericardium. It descends through the diaphragm and then links the Triple Warmer through CV-13, CV-12, and CV-7.

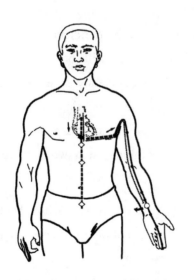

Figure 3–26: Main Channel and Connecting Vessel of the Pericardium

A branch traverses the chest toward the axilla, and emerges at PC-1, three *cùn* inferior to the axillary fold. It ascends up over the axilla, passes through PC-2 on the medial aspect of the upper arm, and descends between the greater yin (Lung) and lesser yin (Heart) channels. It then enters PC-3 on the cubital crease and descends between the muscles on the forearm, passing through PC-4, PC-5, PC-6, and PC-7. On the palm it enters PC-8 then continues along the middle finger to emerge at PC-9 on the tip of the finger.

A branch diverges from PC-8 on the palm and passes along the fourth finger (the ring finger) to emerge at the tip where it meets the Triple Warmer channel.

3.10.2 Connecting Vessel of the Pericardium *Shinpōkei no Betsuraku* 心包経の別絡

The connecting vessel of the hand reverting yin Pericardium channel is called "Inner Pass" (PC-6). It starts at PC-6, two *cùn* proximal to the wrist, and ascends the channel to connect to the Pericardium.

3.10.3 Divergent Channel of the Pericardium *Shinpōkei no Keibetsu* 心包経の経別

The divergent channel of the hand reverting yin Pericardium channel diverges from the primary channel of the Pericardium channel three *cùn* inferior to GB-22, where it enters the chest. It merges with the Triple Warmer and then emerges to ascend through the throat. Behind the ear it converges with the lesser yang channel inferior to the mastoid process.

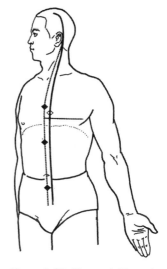

Figure 3–27: Divergent Channel of the Pericardium

3.10.4 Channel Sinews of the Pericardium *Shinpōkei no Keikin* 心包経の経筋

The channel sinews of the hand reverting yin Pericardium channel start on the middle finger. They align with the sinews of the greater yin (Lung) channel and ascend to gather at the medial epicondyle of the elbow. They continue to ascend the medial aspect of the upper arm to gather at the axilla and then descend from GB-22 to spread over the anterior and posterior aspects of the rib cage.

A branch enters through the axilla, spreads out in the chest, and gathers at the area of the cardiac orifice.

3.10.5 Explanation

① The Pericardium will be explained in the chapter on visceral manifestations, but it should be noted here that yang ki of the Heart flows through the Pericardium channel. This yang ki enters the Kidney after passing through the Bladder

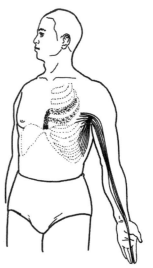

Figure 3–28: Channel Sinews of the Pericardium

---

channel, and then becomes yang ki of the life gate after combining with essence. That is why both the life gate and the Pericardium are examined at the proximal position of the pulse on the right wrist when doing pulse diagnosis. The Heart is the monarch and thus does not emerge to directly perform work. However, without the vital yang ki of the Heart the body cannot move. This is especially true for the Spleen, which has no yang ki, making yang ki of the Heart essential when there is Spleen deficiency. However, the Heart channel is a lesser yin channel and is thus is rich in cold ki, which is ki that is used to control heat in the Heart. Therefore, rather than tonify the Heart channel, which would strengthen cold ki, the Pericardium channel, in which the yang ki of the Heart flows, should be tonified when there is Spleen deficiency. (See the section on the Heart and the Small Intestine in Chapter 4, page 110.)

② The Pericardium channel should be tonified when there is Spleen deficiency. Many of the acupuncture points used for this are effective for treating heart disease. In such a case you should tonify when there is insufficient yang ki in the Heart and disperse when there is surplus heat in the Heart.

③ Along the Pericardium channel, pain on pressure and indurations most commonly appear at PC-4. Points from PC-5 through PC-7 do not get indurations, but rather often lose ki and become deficient.

3.11   Hand Lesser Yang Triple Warmer Channel   手の少陽三焦経

3.11.1 Flow of the Lesser Yang Triple Warmer Channel *Shōyō Sanshōkei no Ruchū* 少陽三焦経の流注

The Triple Warmer or hand lesser yang channel starts at TW-1 at the tip of the fourth finger (ring finger). It ascends between the fourth and fifth metacarpal bones, passing through TW-2 and TW-3, and then continues on through TW-4 on the dorsal aspect of the wrist. It ascends the posterior aspect of the forearm between the radius and ulna, passing through TW-5, TW-6, TW-7, TW-8, and TW-9 as well as TW-10 on the elbow. On the lateral posterior aspect of the upper arm it ascends through TW-11, TW-12, and TW-13 and continues to ascend through TW-14, SI-9, and SI-12 on the shoulder. It passes through

TW-15 posterior to the foot lesser yang (Gallbladder) channel and then crosses the Gallbladder channel at GB-21 to enter ST-12. It then descends to CV-17 and spreads to connect to the Pericardium. It continues to descend through the diaphragm and joins with the Triple Warmer at CV-13, CV-12, and CV-7.

A branch ascends from CV-17 to ST-12 and then ascends from GV-14 at the nape of the neck to the posterior border of the ear, where it connects TW-16, TW-17, TW-18, and TW-19. It then directly ascends to TW-20 at the superior border of the ear, and emerges through GB-6 and GB-4. It then continues, winding around the cheek to reach SI-18 on the zygomatic bone. A branch from GB-5 descends through GB-14 to BL-1.

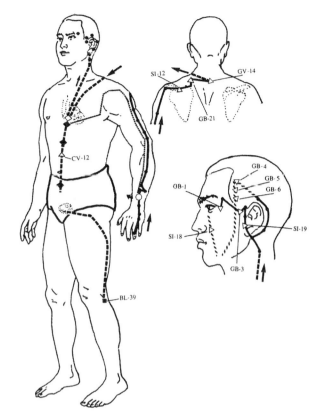

Figure 3–29: Main Channel and Connecting Vessel of the Triple Warmer

A branch enters the ear from TW-17 posterior to the ear and then emerges anterior to the ear to pass through SI-19, TW-21, and TW-22. After passing through GB-3 it continues transversing the cheek to GB-1 at the outer canthus of the eye.

3.11.2 Connecting Vessel of the Triple Warmer *Shanshōkei no Betsuraku* 三焦経の別絡

The connecting vessel of the hand lesser yang Triple Warmer channel is called "Outer Pass" (TW-5). It starts at TW-5, two *cùn* proximal to the wrist on the dorsal aspect. It travels up the posterior aspect of the arm and pours into the chest to meet the Pericardium.

3.11.3 Divergent Channel of the Triple Warmer *Sanshōkei no Keibetsu* 三焦経の経別

The divergent channel of the hand lesser yang Triple Warmer channel ascends along with the primary channel from TW-16. At the vertex it diverges and descends posterior to the ear on down to enter ST-12. It then runs through the Triple Warmer and spreads out in the chest.

3.11.4 Channel Sinews of the Triple Warmer *Sanshōkei no Keikin* 三焦経の経筋

The channel sinews of the hand lesser yang Triple Warmer channel start at the tip of the fourth finger and gather at the dorsum of the wrist. They ascend the forearm and gather at the elbow. They continue to ascend the posterior aspect of the upper arm, ascending over the shoulder and up the neck, where they join the hand greater yang (Small Intestine) channel.

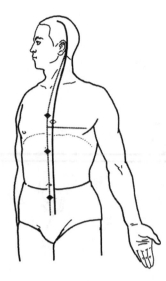

Figure 3–30: Divergent Channel of the Triple Warmer

A branch enters when it reaches the angle of the mandible and then connects to the root of the tongue.

Another branch ascends the ramus of the mandible, passes anterior to the ear, and connects to the outer canthus of the eye. It then ascends and gathers at the corner of the parietal bone.

3.11.5 Explanation

① According to the passage in *Ling Shu* Chapter 2 quoted below, the Triple Warmer channel runs between the Bladder channel and the Gallbladder channel. It is also known as the foot Triple Warmer channel, on which the most commonly used treatment point is BL-39. The Triple Warmer is related to heat and water, but the foot Triple Warmer channel is more important than the hand Triple Warmer channel in cases of illness with an abundance of water. Stiffness and pain on pressure is often found on the lower limbs between the Bladder and Gallbladder channels.

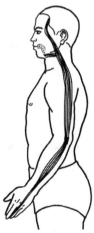

Figure 3–31:
Channel Sinews of the Triple Warmer

② There are important acupuncture points on the hand Triple Warmer channel, such as TW-5, TW-10, TW-13, and TW-17. These points are effective in all cases that involve surplus heat.

③ The character translated as "Warmer" in the phrase Triple Warmer means to burn or scorch. Thus, the Triple Warmer refers to the function of yang ki, of which there are various functions:

- Yang ki is essential for the production of ki, blood, and fluids in the Spleen and Stomach. This yang ki is called the yang ki of the Middle Warmer.

- Respiration begins when the Heart and Lung start to function due to the ancestral ki that was made in the Middle Warmer. This causes ki and blood to then be circulated throughout the body. The functioning of the ancestral ki is called the yang ki of the Upper Warmer.

- Yang ki of the life gate comes from the mixing of essence with yang ki of the Upper Warmer that descends into the Kidney. This yang ki is called the yang ki of the Lower Warmer.

- Digestion, absorption, and the excretion of wastes are all made possible by these yang ki functions.

④ The Triple Warmer should be used both when the body has become chilled due to insufficient yang ki and when there is too much heat due to insufficient yin ki. The fact that the Triple Warmer channel is a lesser yang channel makes it easier to understand why it is effective for treating heat patterns.

⑤ Pain on pressure on the Triple Warmer channel usually appears in acupuncture points on the upper arm. These points are effective for treating stiff shoulders.

> The lower *hé* [合 uniting] point of the Triple Warmer is located on the lateral posterior corner of the knee, lateral to the foot greater yang channel and posterior to the [foot] lesser yang channel. The point is BL-39, and it is a network point of the greater yang channel. The Triple Warmer channel influences the foot lesser yang and greater yang channels and is also a connecting vessel of the greater yang channel. It diverges five *cùn* superior to the lateral malleolus and passes through the calf, emerging at BL-39. It [ascends] parallel to the primary greater yang channel and then enters to spread around the Bladder and control the Lower Warmer. (*Ling Shu*, Chapter 2)

Illnesses of the Triple Warmer [tend to present with] abdominal distension, with the lower abdomen being especially firm [due to the distension]. [The patient] will have dysuria and will suffer from extreme [tension in the abdomen]. Water will stagnate [in the skin] causing edema. Signs [of this condition] appear along the great network vessel, anterior to the foot greater yang channel. The great network vessel is located in between the greater yang and lesser yang [channels]. When signs appear [in the great network] vessel, take BL-39 [as the treatment point]. (*Ling Shu*, Chapter 4)

3.12   The Foot Lesser Yang Gallbladder Channel   足の少陽胆経

3.12.1 Flow of the Lesser Yang Gallbladder Channel *Shōyō Tankei no Ruchū* 少陽胆経 の流注

The Gallbladder or foot lesser yang channel starts at GB-1, at the outer canthus of the eye. It passes through GB-2 and GB-3 and then ascends to the corner of the forehead and temporal region, where is passes through GB-4, GB-5, GB-6, GB-7, GB-8, and GB-9. It then passes through GB-10, GB-11, and GB-12 in the retroauricular region, through TW-20, GB-13, and GB-14, and then moves posteriorly through GB-15, GB-16, GB-17, GB-18, GB-19, and GB-20. It descends the neck, moving anterior to the Triple Warmer channel. From GB-21 on the superior aspect of the shoulder it crosses back over to the posterior side of the Triple Warmer channel to GV-14. It then passes through BL-11, TW-15, and SI-12 before entering ST-12.

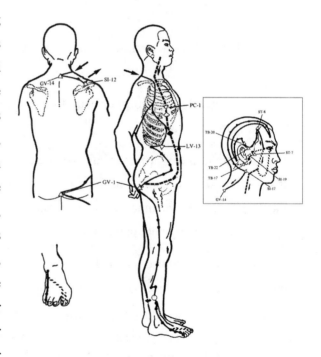

Figure 3–32: Main Channel and Connecting Vessel of the Gallbladder

From the retroauricular region a branch passes through TW-17 into the ear and emerges anterior to the ear to pass through SI-19 and GB-2 and then terminate posterior to GB-1 at the outer canthus of the eye.

A branch from the outer canthus of the eye descends to ST-5, meets the Triple Warmer channel inferior to the eye, descends through ST-6, and then descends the neck to ST-12. From there it continues to descend to the chest, crosses the diaphragm, connects to the Liver at LR-14, and then joins with the Gallbladder at GB-24. It then passes through LR-13 inferior to the rib cage on the flank, emerges at ST-30 in the inguinal region, traverses the border of the pubic region, and then moves laterally to the hip joint to enter GB-30.

The primary channel descends from ST-12 to the axilla; it passes through GB-22 and GB-23, then passes by the chest to the free ribs from where it descends through GB-25, GB-26, GB-27, GB-28, and GB-29. From GB-29 it joins BL-31, BL-33, and GV-1 and then proceeds to the hip joint. It continues through GB-32 and GB-33 on the lateral aspect of the thigh, then through GB-34 on the lateral side of the knee, and emerges to descend anterior to the fibula, passing through GB-35, GB-36, and GB-37. It then descends directly through GB-38 and GB-39 and on to GB-40, anterior to the lateral malleolus. It passes through GB-41 and GB-42 on the dorsum of the foot and enters between the fourth and fifth toes, passing through GB-43 and GB-44.

A branch diverges on the dorsum of the foot, enters between the first and second toes, and passes between the metatarsal bones to emerge at the tip of the big toe. It then turns back and passes through the nail to emerge at LR-1.

3.12.2 Connecting Vessel of the Gallbladder *Tankei no Betsuraku* 胆経の別絡

The connecting vessel of the foot lesser yang Gallbladder channel is called "Bright Light" (GB-37). It starts at GB-37, five *cùn* superior to the lateral malleolus, diverges to run with the reverting yin (Liver) channel, and then descends to connect to the dorsum of the foot.

3.12.3 Divergent Channel of the Gallbladder *Tankei no Keibetsu* 胆経の経別

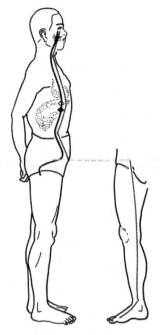

Figure 3–33: Divergent Channel of the Gallbladder

The divergent channel of the foot lesser yang Gallbladder channel runs through the thigh along with the primary channel and enters the pubic region to join the reverting yin (Liver) channel. It diverges and enters the area of the free ribs, and passes into the chest to join with the Gallbladder. It spreads and ascends to the Liver, passes through the Heart, and continues up alongside the throat. It then emerges from the jaw, spreads throughout the face, and joins the lesser yang (Gallbladder) primary channel at the outer canthus of the eye.

3.12.4 Channel Sinews of the Gallbladder *Tankei no Keikin* 胆経の経筋

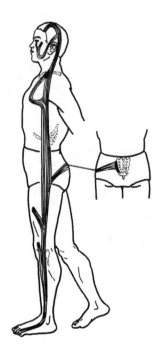

Figure 3–34: Channel Sinews of the Gallbladder

The channel sinews of the foot lesser yang Gallbladder hannel start on the fourth toe and ascend to gather at the lateral along the lateral edge of the tibia to gather at the lateral side of the knee.

Branches diverge from the fibula at the lateral side of the knee and ascend the thigh. The anterior branch gathers superior to ST-32, and the posterior branch gathers at the buttock.

The primary path ascends the lateral aspect of the rib cage, transverses anteriorly to connect to the pectoral area, and then gathers at ST-12.

A path ascends directly from the axilla up through ST-12. It then passes anterior to the greater yang (Bladder) channel, passes posterior to the ear, ascends the temporal region, passes through the vertex, and then descends around the jaw to ascend again to gather at the zygomatic bone.

A branch diverging from the zygomatic bone gathers at the outer canthus of the eye and becomes the connecting point of the eye.

3.12.5 Explanation

The strong feature of the Gallbladder channel is that it is connected to the Triple Warmer channel, which is also a lesser yang channel. The greater yang channel flows through the back area, the yang brightness channel through the abdominal area, and the lesser yang channel through the lateral aspects of the body.

Gallbladder points on the lateral aspect of the head can be used with Triple Warmer points to treat insomnia, headaches, and eye and ear problems. However, treating Gallbladder points on the lower leg (such as GB-41) often heals these conditions as well. Using a touching needle on the lateral aspect of the head is effective for treating insomnia and should always be used for the "irascibility bug" (*Kan no mushi* 疳の虫), a syndrome of children traditionally recognized in Japan, the general characteristics of which include crying at night, loss of appetite, and frequent irritability.

There are indispensable acupuncture points for stiff shoulders on the section of the Gallbladder channel that runs between the neck and the shoulders. It is best to alleviate tension in the whole meridian rather than aiming at just specific points when treating stiff shoulders.

The Gallbladder channel in the abdominal region is an important abdominal diagnostic area. Moreover, the acupuncture points in this area are related to abdominal conditions and to low back pain. (See the abdominal diagnosis section in Chapter 7, page 222.)

The Gallbladder channel on the thigh is often stiff and tense. For instance, this condition of stiffness and tension is always present during a Liver deficiency heat pattern, such as seen with hemiplegia. The Gallbladder channel on the lower leg is also often tense. However, tenseness does not always have to be a condition of excess.

Pain on pressure tends to appear at GB-41, GB-40, GB-38, and GB-31, regardless of whether there is Liver excess or Liver deficiency.

Signs of disharmony can appear on the Gallbladder channel in conjunction with any pattern of imbalance since cold and heat stagnation tend to manifest on the Gallbladder channel. Treating such conditions will improve the stability of internal organ function.

3.13.1 Flow of the Reverting Yin Liver Channel *Ketsuin Kankei no Ruchū* 厥陰肝経の 流注

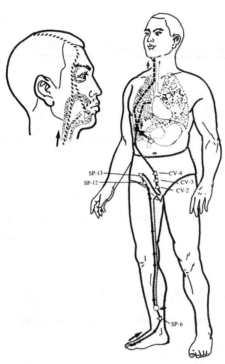

Figure 3–35: Main Channel and Connecting Vessel of the Liver

The Liver or reverting yin channel starts at LR-1 on the terminal phalanx of the big toe. It ascends the dorsum of the foot, passing through LR-2 and LR-3 and then through LR-4, one cùn anterior to the medial malleolus. It then ascends through SP-6, LR-5, and LR-6, and at eight *cùn* proximal to the medial malleolus it crosses to the posterior of the greater yin (Spleen) channel. Then it ascends through LR-7 and LR-8 on the medial aspect of the knee and through LR-9, LR-10, and LR-11 on the medial thigh and enters at SP-12 and SP-13 in the pubic region. After passing through the genitalia it goes through CV-2, CV-3, and CV-4 in the lower abdomen. It then passes by the Stomach at LR-13, joins with the Liver, connects to the Gallbladder, and crosses the diaphragm at LR-14. Then it spreads out in the costal region, ascends the posterior aspect of the throat, and ascends to enter the nasopharynx. It connects to the tissues around the eye and then ascends the forehead to meet the Governing Vessel channel at GV-20 at the vertex.

A branch descends from the tissues around the eye, goes through the inside of the cheek, and passes through the inner surface of the lips.

A branch diverges from the Liver, crosses the diaphragm, and ascends to pour into the Lung.

3.13.2 Connecting Vessel of the Liver *Kankei no Betsuraku* 肝経の別絡

The connecting vessel of the foot reverting yin Liver channel is called "Woodworm Canal" (LR-5). It starts at LR-5, five *cùn* proximal to the medial malleolus, diverges, and runs with the lesser yang (Gallbladder) channel.

In men a branch ascends through the leg then through the testes to connect to the penis.

3.13.3 Divergent Channel of the Liver *Kankei no Keibetsu* 肝経の経別

The divergent channel of the foot reverting yin Liver channel diverges on the dorsum of the foot and ascends to the pubic region. It meets the Gallbladder channel and runs along with the divergent channel of the Gallbladder channel.

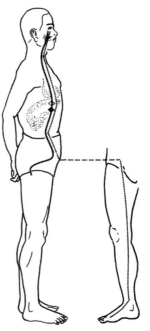

Figure 3–36: Divergent Channel of the Liver

3.13.4 Channel Sinews of the Liver *Kankei no Keikin* 肝経の経筋

The channel sinews of the foot reverting yin Liver channel start on the dorsal aspect of the big toe and ascend to gather at the medial malleolus. They then ascend along the tibia and gather at the inferior medial aspect of the knee. They continue to ascend, and gather at the genital area, where they connect with other channel sinews.

3.13.5 Explanation

The strong feature of the Liver channel is that unlike the other yin channels, part of it flows superior to the throat. Note especially that it goes to GV-20. This allows for moxibustion to be applied at GV-20 when there is high blood pressure due to a Liver deficiency pattern.

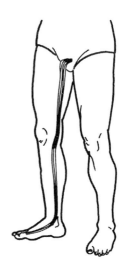

Figure 3–37: Channel Sinews of the Liver

The section of the Liver channel on the face flows through the same area as that of the yang brightness channel. It is likely that it flows deeper than the yang brightness channel. The yang brightness channel is often treated after tonifying Liver deficiency when treatment is being given for Bell's Palsy or trigeminal neuralgia. This treatment method was developed because the heat of a Liver deficiency heat pattern spreads to the yang brightness channel.

The Liver channel passes through the genitalia. Therefore, it is effective for treating priapism, pulling pains in the testes, and gynecological problems. Pulling pain the testes is an especially typical symptom pattern of the Liver channel.

There are many important Liver acupuncture points in the abdominal region. They are also used as diagnostic points. LR-14 especially shows resistance and pain on pressure when there is Liver heat, and it is used as a dispersion point in such conditions.

The points on the lower limbs each have their important uses, but LR-8 should always be used when there is a Liver deficiency heat pattern. LR-8 should be dispersed when there is blood stasis. Pain on pressure also tends to appear in LR-5 and LR-3, which are often used particularly for genital conditions such as prostatitis.

3.14   The Extraordinary Vessels   奇経

3.14.1 Flow of the Governing Vessel *Tokumyaku no Ruchū* 督脈の流注

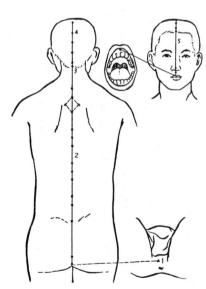

Figure 3–38: Governing Vessel Channel

The governing vessel begins at a point in the lower extremity [of the trunk], ascends the anterior aspect of the spine to GV-16, and then enters and joins with the brain. (*Nan Jing*, Chapter 28)

The governing vessel begins at a point in the lower extremity [of the trunk], ascends the anterior aspect of the spine to GV-16, and then enters the brain, ascends to the vertex of the head, and passes through the forehead to the bridge of the nose. It joins with the sea of yang vessels. *(Elaborations of the Fourteen Meridians)*

The governing vessel begins in the lower abdomen and descends to the center of the [pubic] bone. In women it enters and connects to the vagina, next to the urethral opening. The network vessel passes through the reproductive organs, [re]connecting [to the primary channel] in the perineum [CV-1]. [Together they] continue past the anus. [Another network vessel] diverges to pass through the buttocks to the lesser yin [Kidney channel]. It connects to the network vessel of the greater yang [Bladder channel], ascends along with the lesser yin [Kidney channel] through the posterior aspect of the inner crotch, and passes along the [visceral side] of the spine to join with the Kidney.

[Another network vessel] starts along with the greater yang [Bladder channel] at the inner canthus of the eye, ascends the forehead to mingle at the vertex of the head, and then enters to encircle the brain. It reemerges, splits, and descends the nape of the neck. It [descends] medial to the scapula and passes along the lateral edge of the spine to the lumbar region. It enters and passes through the buttocks to connect to the Kidney. In men it passes through the penis and then descends to the perineum, the same as in women. From the lower abdomen it ascends straight up through the center of the navel, passes through the Heart, enters the throat, ascends the chin, circles around the lips, and then ascends to the area beneath the eye. (*Su Wen*, Chapter 60)

The network vessel of the governing vessel is called Long Strong [GV-1]. It ascends parallel to the spine, ascends the nape of the neck, spreads out at the vertex of the head, and then descends to the scapular bones. It diverges and runs along the greater yang [Bladder channel], and passes through the back. (*Ling Shu*, Chapter 10)

3.14.2 Governing Vessel Explanation

The sub-section above presented passages from the classics that concern the governing vessel. The phrase "point in the lower extremity" from the *Nan Jing* and *Elaborations of the Fourteen Meridians* refers to CV-1. Whereas those texts give CV-1 as the starting point, the *Su Wen* says that the governing vessel "begins in the lower abdomen." The point in the lower abdomen from which it starts should be CV-3. From CV-3 it passes through the "center of the bone"—that is, through CV-2—to the perineum. From the anus it ascends along the midline of the back, but it also joins the Kidney and Bladder channels, entering at GV-1 and joining with the Kidney.

There is a branch that does not just travel along the midline of the back. From GV-20 it descends through the nape of the neck, passes between the scapular bones, and flows down along both sides of the spine to meet again at CV-1.

There is a network vessel that ascends from the lower abdomen along the path of the Conception Vessel. But, this vessel can be thought of as flowing deep to the Conception Vessel.

In short, the Governing Vessel is closely related to the Conception Vessel and the Bladder and Kidney channels; it is a highly important channel in terms of treatment.

Just as is implied by the governing vessel being called the sea of yang channels, it always manifests signs of a yang disease. Symptom patterns often improve just by treating the areas where those signs appear.

There are many important points on the Governing Vessel. Its points on the lower back are effective for treating illnesses related to the urinary tract, prostate, anus, and uterus. The mid-section of the Governing Vessel can be used for treating digestive tract disorders. In nervous diseases, such as insomnia, the section of the Governing Vessel on the upper back will often have pain on pressure.

3.14.3　Flow of the Conception Vessel *Ninmyaku no Ruchū* 任脈の流注

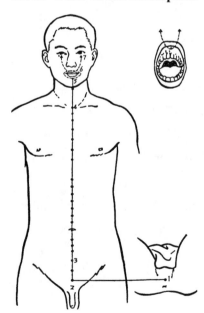

Figure 3–39: Conception Vessel Channel

The conception vessel starts below CV-3 and ascends toward the [pubic] hairline, passes through the inside of the abdomen, ascends through CV-4 and up to the throat. (*Nan Jing,* Chapter 28)

The connecting vessel of the conception vessel is called Tail Shadow [CV-15]. It starts at CV-15, descends, and disperses in the abdomen. (*Ling Shu,* Chapter 10)

The conception vessel starts below CV-3 and ascends toward the [pubic] hairline, passes through the inside of the abdomen, and ascends through CV-4 up to the throat. It ascends the chin, passes through the face, and enters the eyes. (*Su Wen*, Chapter 60)

The connecting vessel of the uterus is connected to the Kidney. (*Su Wen*, Chapter 47)

3.14.4 Conception Vessel Explanation

The Conception Vessel is a channel that ascends from the perineum up through the midline of the abdomen. Moxibustion should be used on its points in the lower abdomen when the Lower Warmer is deficient and there is a condition of cold. On the other hand, blood stasis is indicated when there is resistance and excess in these points.

Points on the Conception Vessel in the upper abdomen are fundamental points in relation to digestive tract disorders. It is absolutely essential to use CV-12 when the Spleen and Stomach are deficient. CV-14 often manifests resistance and pain on pressure when the patient has consumed too many liquids and foods with a high liquid content. Or, CV-14 can also manifest resistance and pain on pressure when there is Kidney deficiency.

CV-17 is a very important point in the thoracic region. Heat builds up in the chest when there is a heat pattern of Kidney deficiency or Liver deficiency. At that time the chest will feel hot to the touch and will manifest pain on pressure in an area centering on CV-17.

3.14.5 Flow of the Yang Heel Vessel *Yōkyōmyaku no Ruchū* 陽蹻脈の流注

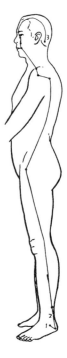

The yang heel vessel starts in the heel, passes through the lateral malleolus, and ascends to enter at GB-20. (*Nan Jing*, Chapter 28)

The yang heel vessel starts in the heel, passes through the lateral malleolus, and ascends to enter at GB-20. ... The heel vessels [*qiáo mài*] of both feet take as their root the connecting vessel of the greater yang [channel]. They merge with the greater yang [channels] and their ki flows upwards. If their ki circulates well together, the eyes will be moistened. If their ki does not nourish [the channel], the eyes cannot be used. Men count the yang [heel vessel], and women count the yin [heel vessel]. The channel that is counted is taken to be the [primary] channel, and the channel that is not counted is taken to be the network vessel.

The heel vessel is 8 *chǐ* long. It originates at BL-62 and takes BL-59 as its cleft [accumulation] point and BL-61 as its root. It merges with the foot lesser yang [channel][2] at GB-29, merges with the hand yang brightness [channel] at LI-15 and LI-16, merges with the hand and foot greater yang [channels] and the yang linking [vessel] at SI-10, merges

Figure 3–40: Yang Heel Vessel Channel

---

[2] The original text says lesser yin.

with the hand and foot yang brightness [channels] at ST-4, merges again with the hand and foot yang brightness [channels] at ST-3, and merges with the conception vessel and the foot yang brightness [channel] at ST-1. The above-mentioned points are the places where the yang heel vessel surfaces. This makes 20 points. *(Elaborations of the Fourteen Meridians)*

3.14.6 Yang Heel Vessel Explanation

According to the above arrangement, the yang heel vessel begins at BL-62 and reaches BL-61, BL-59, GB-29, SI-10, LI-15, LI-16, ST-4, ST-3, and ST-1. *Illustrations of the Three Powers in Japanese and Chinese*[3] says that the yang heel vessel also reaches to BL-1 and terminates at GB-20. This is most likely based on a consideration of passages from the *Nan Jing*.

In men, the yang heel vessel is the primary channel and the yin heel vessel is the network vessel. In women, the yin heel vessel is the primary channel and the yang heel vessel is the network vessel.

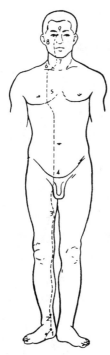

Figure 3–41: Yin Heel Vessel Channel

3.14.7 Flow of the Yin Heel Vessel *Inkyōmyaku no Ruchū* 陰蹻脈の流注

The yin heel vessel also starts in the heel and passes through the lateral malleolus. It ascends to the throat, merging with the penetrating vessel; [together they] pass [through the throat]. *(Nan Jing,* Chapter 28)

The heel vessel diverges at the connecting [vessel] of the lesser yin [channel] posterior to KI-2 and ascends above the medial malleolus. It ascends directly, passing through the inner thigh, and enters the groin. It ascends through the inside of the chest and emerges at ST-12. Then it ascends anterior to ST-9 and enters the nose. It connects to the inner canthus of the eye and merges with the greater yang [channel]. In women the [yin heel vessel] is the primary channel, and in men it is the network vessel. The *qiāo mài* [[heel vessel] of each foot is 8 *chǐ* long. However, the cleft (accumulation) point of the yin heel [vessel] is KI-8. *(Elaborations of the Fourteen Meridians)*

---

[3] The three powers are Heaven, Earth, and humankind.

3.14.8 Yin Heel Vessel Explanation

The yin heel vessel passes through KI-2, KI-6, KI-8, ST-12, and BL-1.

Based on the primary function of the extraordinary vessels, the yin heel vessel is effective in treating the symptom patterns that appear after a febrile disease. After the flow of the channels becomes hyperactive due to the stagnation of yang ki caused by the febrile disease, even though the original symptom pattern of the febrile disease may have disappeared, it is possible that the flow in the meridians that became hyperactive has not returned to normal. Consequently, ki and blood overflow in the extraordinary vessels, where they stagnate and manifest in specific symptoms.

3.14.9 Flow of the Penetrating Vessel *Shōmyaku no Ruchū* 衝脈の流注

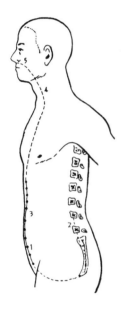

Figure 3–42: Penetrating Vessel Channel

The penetrating vessel starts at ST-30, [ascends] parallel to the foot yang brightness channel, ascends past the side of the navel, and continues up to the chest where it disperses. (*Nan Jing*, Chapter 28)

The penetrating vessel starts at CV-4 and ascends directly up along the abdomen. (*Su Wen*, Chapter 39)

The penetrating vessel is the sea of the [twelve] channels. It is in charge of permeating and irrigating every nook and cranny. It merges with the yang brightness [channel] in the ancestral sinews. The yin [penetrating vessel] and yang [brightness channel] preside over the convergence of the ancestral sinews. [They] converge at ST-30, and the yang brightness [channel] is the leader [in their work]. They join with the girdling vessel and connect to the governing vessel. (*Su Wen*, Chapter 44)

The penetrating vessel starts at ST-30, ascends parallel to the lesser yang channel past the sides of the navel, and continues up to the chest where it disperses. (*Su Wen*, Chapter 60)

The penetrating vessel is the sea of the five zang and six fu organs, which are all [moistened and nourished] by it. The ascending channel emerges at the upper mandible, spreads to the yang [areas on the face], and pours into the yin[4] [areas on the face]. The descending channel pours into the great network vessel [KI-4] of the lesser yin [channel]. [First] it emerges at ST-30 and passes along the medial thigh. It

---

[4] The original text says, "pours into the essences." The *Jiǎ Yǐ* says that "essences" is a mistake for "yin."

enters the popliteal crease and passes concealed through the posterior aspect of the tibia, then descends to reach the posterior aspect of the medial malleolus, where it joins [with the greater network vessel of the lesser yin channel] and then disperses. [This] descending channel runs parallel to the lesser yin channel and then spreads out to the three yin channels. The channel that continues along passes deep and then emerges at the ankle [at the superior aspect of the calcaneal tubercle], descends through the dorsum of the foot, enters between the big toes [the first and second toes], and spreads out to the connecting vessels [in the area] to warm the flesh. (*Su Wen*, Chapter 38)

The penetrating vessel is the sea of the twelve channels. It starts from the Kidney along with the great network vessel of the lesser yin [channel]. It descends to emerge at ST-30, passes through the inner thigh, enters the popliteal crease at an angle, passes along the medial posterior aspect of the tibia parallel to the lesser yin channel to enter [the area] posterior to the medial malleolus, and then enters the sole of the foot. A branch enters the inner malleolus at an angle, emerges and joins with the dorsum of the foot, enters between the big toes [the first and second toes], and pours into the network vessels, thereby warming the feet and lower legs. (*Ling Shu*, Chapter 62)

[In women] the penetrating vessel and conception vessel both start from the uterus and ascend along the visceral side of the spine, becoming the sea of the meridians. The [branches] that float up to the surface pass through the right side [and left side][5] of the abdomen, ascend to meet at the throat, and then diverge to encircle the mouth. (*Ling Shu*, Chapter 65)

The penetrating vessel and conception vessel both start from the uterus and ascend along the visceral side of the spine, becoming the sea of the meridians. The [branches] that float up to the surface pass through the abdomen, ascend and meet at the throat, and then diverge to encircle the mouth. Thus it is said, "The penetrating vessel starts at ST-30, parallels the foot lesser yin channel, passes along the side of the navel, and ascends to the chest, where it disperses. Diseases [of the penetrating vessel] cause people to have abdominal cramping with counterflowing ki." The *Nan Jing says*, "[The penetrating vessel] parallels the foot yang brightness channel. [However,] if one thinks about the [acupuncture] points, [it is like this]: The foot yang brightness [channels] ascend two *cùn* from both sides of the navel. The foot lesser yin [channels] ascend 5 *fēn* from both sides of the navel." According to the

---

[5] The original text gives the right side only. Most translations pass over this point since it is unclear.

acupuncture classic[6] the penetrating vessel starts along with the governing vessel at CV-1 and passes through the following 22 points[7] on the abdomen: KI-21, KI-20, KI-19, KI-18, KI-17, KI-16, KI-15, KI-14, KI-13, KI-12, and KI-11. These [points] all belong to the foot lesser yin [channel]. Therefore it is clear that the penetrating vessel parallels the foot lesser yin channel. *(Elaborations of the Fourteen Meridians)*

3.14.10   Explanation of the Penetrating Vessel

As can be seen from the above description, there are many different explanations concerning the Penetrating Vessel. The *Nan Jing* simply says that the Penetrating Vessel starts at ST-30 and ascends parallel to the yang brightness channel to the chest, where it disperses. A similar passage is given in Chapter 60 of the *Su Wen*. However, in this case the Penetrating Vessel ascends parallel to the lesser yin channel.

In the other explanations the penetrating vessel does not simply disperse in the chest, but rather reaches up to the throat and mouth. Some explanations say that the Penetrating Vessel starts at ST-30 while others say it starts at CV-4 or from the uterus. Thus, it must circulate through these areas as well.

The Penetrating Vessel also flows through the lower limbs. It passes through the same area as the Kidney channel and reaches all the way to SP-6, LR-3, and KI-1.

Cold feet and hot flushes, palpitations, and a clogged feeling in the throat indicate Kidney deficiency, but also indicate an abnormality of the Penetrating Vessel. Considering these symptom patterns it is easy to see how it can be said that the penetrating vessel ascends the lower limbs along with the Kidney channel, passes over the Stomach channel at ST-30, entwines itself in the perineum and at CV-4, touches the chest, and then reaches to the mouth from the throat.

On the one hand the Penetrating Vessel is called the sea of the twelve channels, and on the other hand it is called the sea of the five zang and six fu organs. Though this may seem like a contradiction, there are many such statements in the classics. This should be understood as an indication of the importance of the Penetrating Vessel.

---

[6] That is, the *Ling Shu*.

[7] Eleven points on each side of the abdomen.

3.14.11　Flow of the Girdling Vessel *Taimyaku no Ruchū* 帯脈の流注

> The girdling vessel starts at the free ribs and encircles the body. (*Nan Jing,* Chapter 28)

> The girdling vessel starts at the free ribs and encircles the body. [During] an illness of the girdling vessel the lumbar and abdominal [regions] become so slack as to resemble a water sack.[8] The area where the channel ki [of the girdling vessel] emerges is one *cùn* eight *fēn* inferior to the free ribs. It is aptly called the girdle vessel since it circles around the body like a girdle. Moreover, it meets the foot lesser yang [channel] at GB-28. The girdling vessel emerges at about four points. (*Elaborations of the Fourteen Meridians*)

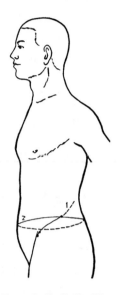

Figure 3–43: Girdling Vessel Channel

3.14.12　Explanation of the Girdling Vessel

The Girdling Vessel is undoubtedly connected with the Gallbladder channel, and among the other channels is mainly connected with the Kidney and Stomach channels. Almost all cases of low back pain are related to the Girdling Vessel. In cases of low back pain it is necessary to treat the Kidney and Stomach channels and not just the Gallbladder and Liver channels. Indeed, in the case of a Liver deficiency pattern all these channels are naturally chosen as treatment locations, so there is no need to worry much about channel selection.

The Girdling Vessel passes through the lower back at the level of the navel, but in the abdomen it is suspected that it dips down through the inguinal region. That is why pain on pressure appears in the inguinal region during most cases of a Liver deficiency pattern or a Kidney deficiency pattern. In those who have pain on pressure in the superior aspect of the inguinal region on the right side, most will have pain in the right side of their lower back. The same holds true for the left side. In considering various cases in terms of clinical practice, it seems that the Girdling Vessel is anything but formulaic.

---

[8] That is, they become bloated like a water sack that is full of water.

3.14.13 Flow of the Yang Linking Vessel *Yōimyaku no Ruchū* 陽維脈の流注

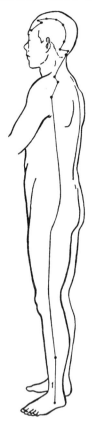

The yang linking [vessel] links the yang. It starts at the meeting [point][9] of the yang [channels]. Together with the yin linking [vessel], it links and connects the body. If [the yang linking vessel] cannot link yang with yang, then [one] becomes relaxed to the point that one cannot maintain one's posture. The channel ki emerges at BL-63 and diverges to GB-35, which is a cleft (accumulation) point. [The yang linking vessel] meets the hand and foot greater yang [channels] and the heel vessel at SI-10, and meets the hand and foot lesser yang [channels] at TW-15 and then again at GB-21. The part [of the channel] that goes to the head meets the foot lesser yang [channel] at GB-14, ascends [through] GB-13 and GB-15, ascends to reach GB-17, passes through GB-19, and then descends to reach GB-20. The places where [the yang linking vessel] meets with the governing vessel are GV-16 and GV-15. The *Nan Jing* says, "[During] a yang linking disease, [the patient] suffers from [alternating] chills and fever. The channel ki of the yang linking [vessel] emerges at about 24 points." (*Elaborations of the Fourteen Meridians*)

3.14.14 Explanation of the Yang Linking Vessel

Figure 33–44: Yang Linking Vessel Channel

Illustrations of the Three Powers in Japanese and Chinese says that the Yang Linking Vessel passes through BL-63, GB-35, GB-29, LI-14, SI-10, TW-15, GB-21, GV-15, GV-16, GB-20, and GB-13. However, there are different views on this. For instance, the *Book of Illustrations of the Transport Points on the Copper Man* says the Yang Linking Vessel also passes through GB-24.

There is no need to be overly concerned about the precise pathway of the acupuncture points. The Yang Linking Vessel is principally related to the lesser yang channel, and is used when there is an aggravation of heat during a lesser yang illness.

---

[9] BL-63.

3.14.15 Flow of the Yin Linking Vessel *In'imyaku no Ruchū* 陰維脈の流注

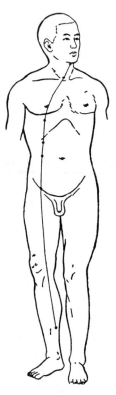

The yin linking [vessel] links the yin. The channel starts at the crossing [point][10] of the yin [channels]. If [the yin linking vessel] cannot link yin with yin, then [one] loses [his/her] will in a state of stupefaction. The place where the channel ki emerges is the cleft [accumulation] point of the yin linking [vessel]. It is called "Guest House" [KI-9]. [The yin linking vessel] meets the foot greater yin [channel] at SP-16 and SP-15. It again meets the foot greater yin [channel] and reverting yin [channel] at SP-13 and LR-14 and meets the conception vessel at CV-22 and CV-23. The *Nan Jing* says, "[During] a yin linking disease [the patient] suffers from heart pain. The channel ki of the yin linking [vessel] emerges at about 20 points." (*Elaborations of the Fourteen Meridians*)

3.14.16 Explanation of the Yin Linking Vessel

The Yin Linking Vessel starts at KI-9 and passes through the Spleen channel at SP-13 and SP-14. Therefore, considering this, one can see that the Yin Linking Vessel is inseparably connected to the Kidney and Spleen channels. Consideration of the symptom pattern also shows that the Yin Linking Vessel has its focal point on the Kidney channel.

Figure 3–45: Yin Linking Vessel Channel

---

[10] KI-9.

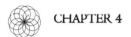 CHAPTER 4

Visceral Manifestations
蔵象

The organs and meridians are closely related. The functions of organs are exercised through the meridians. Likewise, if the circulation of ki and blood in the meridians is normal, the function of the organs is also kept normal. Therefore, tonifying and dispersing any deficiency or excess in the meridians will also immediately adjust the functioning of the organs. This is well indicated in the words of Takeyama Shin'ichirō, who said, "Approach the essence by way of the phenomena." That is the reason why we must understand visceral manifestations in detail.

The word *cáng xiàng* [蔵象 *zōshō*] comes from Chapter 9, Section 6 of the *Su Wen*, where the Yellow Emperor asks, "What is visceral manifestation?" and Qi Bo explains the function of the organs. The word *cáng xiàng* corresponds to physiology in the Western medical sense. However, the organs as such in Meridian Therapy are totally different from those recognized in Western medicine. It is important to avoid misunderstandings by keeping this in mind as you learn Meridian Therapy.

4.1   The Liver and Gallbladder   肝と胆

4.1.1 The Nature of the Liver

Chapter 8 of the *Ling Shu* says, "The Liver stores blood and blood houses the ethereal soul." The term "ethereal soul" describes the positive or active nature of the Liver, and the power to realize that nature is in the blood.

Chapter 8 of the *Su Wen*, says, "The Liver is a general and considers tactics." The phrase "considers tactics" describes the power to actively and completely achieve things according to plan. These qualities of the Liver can be made manifest if there is sufficient blood stored in the Liver. Chapter 5 of the *Su Wen* says, "The emotion of the Liver is anger." This does not mean that the Liver always has anger; again, it indicates the capability of the Liver to actively handle things.

These points are easy to understand when you consider the pathology and symptom pattern. In the case of Liver deficiency, even if one tries to do something according to plan, there is no progression, and in trying to be positive and active, people with Liver deficiency are halfhearted and impatient and make no actual progress. That makes the person irritated and angry. On the other hand, muscular pain, such as low back pain, tends to be brought on by completely overdoing something. Additionally, if the blood becomes any more insufficient, there will be a loss of the enthusiasm to do anything, leading to the tendency to fear.

4.1.2 Areas Controlled by the Liver

The eyes, nails, and sinews are areas controlled by the Liver. Blood stored by the Liver is appropriately distributed to these areas, enabling them to perform their various functions. If Liver blood becomes deficient, changes appear in the eyes, sinews, and nails.

The Liver controls the inside of the eyes. As seen in the flow of the meridians, the Bladder channel controls the upper eyelids and the Stomach channel controls the lower eyelids. The parts of the eyes that are specifically related to the Liver are the optic nerve, retina, cornea, and conjunctiva. Therefore, diseases such as cataracts, glaucoma, hemorrhaging of the eyegrounds, keratitis, and conjunctivitis can sometimes be cured by the treatment of the Liver transport (BL-18) point and the Liver channel.

Insomnia can also sometimes be cured by the treatment of Liver deficiency. Chapter 10 of the *Su Wen* says that the blood returns to the Liver at night and goes to work at the areas where it is needed during the day. It is the blood that makes it possible for you to walk and grasp things with your hands. However, insomnia will result if the blood does not return to the Liver at night.

The Liver also controls the sinews. Therefore, the diseases that affect areas composed of sinews are often caused by Liver deficiency. For example, gynecological problems sometimes present with a Liver deficiency pattern since the uterus has a lot of sinews. Also, low back pain and frozen shoulders (i.e., fifty-year-old's shoulder) are often caused by Liver deficiency. Likewise, nails that break easily can be considered a Liver deficiency problem since the Liver controls the nails.

4.1.3 The Liver and Sourness

Chapter 10 of the *Su Wen* says, "The Liver desires sourness." Sourness has the functional property of gathering. Therefore, it is thought that ki that has the power of gathering is always at work in the reverting yin Liver channel, and that the Liver tries to gather the blood to itself. This is a function of yin ki if you categorize the functional property by yin and yang.

From the clinical perspective, it is good to prescribe sour foods in order to reduce the heat of a Liver deficiency heat pattern. However, individuals who constitutionally tend to be Liver deficient like hot/spicy foods because they want to gain even the temporary power and energy to become lively. So, they tend to dislike sour foods, which have the functional properties of gathering and reducing.

4.1.4 The Liver and the Four Seasons

The springtime (or the morning within a single day) is the season when everything buds and comes alive. In the body, the ki of life in the springtime revitalizes the functioning of the Liver. Thus, if the Liver is normal, one can be positive and active in everything that one does. This is a function of the blood, which contains the power to grow and produce.

4.1.5 The Liver and Gallbladder

The Liver stores the blood and holds the power of generation or creation. This is a function of yang ki, which emerges into the Gallbladder and lesser yang Gallbladder channel. Chapter 8 of the *Su Wen* says, "The Gallbladder is the upright official who makes decisions." It is the blood that carries out this decision-making power of the Gallbladder.

This is easy to understand when thinking about the symptom pattern. If there is no blood, nothing can be generated or created, and yang ki of the Gallbladder and Gallbladder channel will diminish. The pulse will become sinking and thin, and the decision-making power will be lost, leading to a frequent sighing. On the other hand, if yin ki of the Liver becomes deficient and the Liver is not able to gather the blood, then the patient will present with a

Liver deficiency heat pattern. The heat created in this case spreads to other organs and meridians, but it is the Gallbladder and Gallbladder channel that sustain the most influence. If heat increases in the Gallbladder channel, it will rise to the Upper Warmer, causing the patient to become irritable. However, such patients are not able to do as many things as expected since there is insufficient blood.

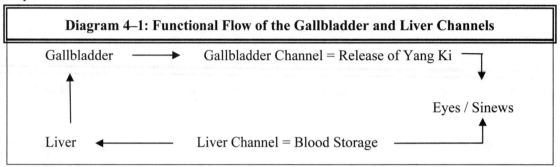

Diagram 4–1: Functional Flow of the Gallbladder and Liver Channels

Gallbladder ⟶ Gallbladder Channel = Release of Yang Ki

Eyes / Sinews

Liver ⟵ Liver Channel = Blood Storage

4.2   The Heart and Small Intestine   心と小腸

4.2.1 The Nature of the Heart

Chapter 62 of the *Su Wen* says, "The Heart houses the spirit," and Chapter 8 says, "The Heart is like a monarch; it eminates the spirit light." Spirit is the essential ki stored by the Heart. Therefore, the founders of Meridian Therapy said that there is no Heart deficiency pattern. The spirit is the most important thing, since if it is lost death will ensue.

Chapter 4 of the *Su Wen* says that the Heart is the "yang within yang" organ, and Chapter 5 says, "The emotion of the Heart is joy." The Heart is rich in yang ki because it is the yang within yang organ, and being rich in yang ki gives it all the more reason to manifest the emotion of joy.

But, what exactly is this yang ki of the Heart? Judging from the physiology of the other organs, it is considered to be a mixture of defensive ki and blood. This is called spirit. Thus, if there is no ki and no blood, death will follow. In the case that either the ki or blood of the Heart becomes deficient due to a deficiency in the other organs, symptom patterns related to the Heart may appear, but they will not lead to death.

On the other hand, if the yang ki of the Heart (i.e., the mixture of the blood and ki that equals spirit) becomes overbearing, heat increases and leads to excessive joy and laughter.

4.2.2 Areas Controlled by the Heart

The Heart is related to the tongue, complexion, and vessels.

The condition of the Heart tends to be revealed in the tongue. Usually, a red tongue can be considered an indication that there is an abundance of heat in the Heart. It is difficult to distinguish the tastes of food when there is an abundance of heat. Some patients cannot stick out their tongues as expected when asked to do so. This is caused by decreased yang ki in the Heart. A red face that is too lustrous is also an indication of heat in the Heart. On the other hand, death will occur if there is no luster, which is a sign that the spirit is gone.

The Heart also controls the blood vessels. Chapters 10 and 18 of the *Su Wen* say, "The Heart governs the vessels and stores the ki of the blood vessels." The terms "vessels" and "blood vessels" here mean the channels. The channels circulate ki and blood throughout the body. The driving force behind that circulation is yang ki, and that is why the Heart, which has an abundance of yang ki, controls the channels.

4.2.3 The Heart and Bitterness

Chapter 10 of the *Su Wen* says, "The Heart desires bitterness." Bitterness has the functional property of firming. Among the five zang organs, it is most proper that the Kidney be firmed up. Therefore, the Heart always desires Kidney ki.

The Heart is an organ rich in yang ki. But, if there is too much yang ki in the Heart, the patient will complain of palpitations and heart pain. In response, Kidney ki, in other words ki with the power to firm, is used in an attempt to reduce the Heart heat. This Kidney ki—ki that is tonified by bitterness—flows in the lesser yin channel.

Yin and yang theory explains that the balance between yin and yang is preserved since the Heart has yang ki and yin ki flows in the lesser yin channel, to which the Heart channel belongs.

Taking the logic to the next step, if yin ki (cold ki) in the lesser yin channel becomes very intense, yang ki in the Heart will be lost, which, as we have seen, results in death. So, it should now be clear why there is no Heart deficiency pattern. Likewise, it should now also be understood that the symptom pattern of the Heart is mainly related to heat in the Heart. At the same time, it can be said that heat in the Heart often points toward a Kidney deficiency pattern.

4.2.4 The Heart and the Four Seasons

Chapter 9 of the *Su Wen* says, "The Heart is the greater yang within yang and corresponds to the ki of summer." The Heart has an abundance of yang ki. It corresponds to the ki of summer (or daytime within a single day) since it is always active. Without yang ki the function of growth cannot take place.

4.2.5 The Heart and Small Intestine

The Heart and Small Intestine are paired organs. However, in the clinic it is convenient to consider the Large Intestine and the Small Intestine as both belonging to the Stomach, as stated in Chapter 2 of the *Ling Shu*. Actually, symptom patterns of the Small Intestine are mainly treated as a Spleen deficiency pattern.

Chapter 2 of the *Ling Shu* says, "The Small Intestine is the fu organ in charge of receiving," and Chapter 8 of the *Su Wen* says, "The Small Intestine is the official in charge of receiving and transforming." The Small Intestine also connects to the greater yang channel, to which the Bladder channel connects as well, and is thereby related to the function of urination. The ki coming down the greater yang channel must be abundant in order to urinate comfortably. That ki is yang ki of the Heart, and that is why the Heart and the Small Intestine are related as paired organs.

However, this particular yang ki is not spirit. Spirit does not perform work because it is the sovereign fire. The yang ki mentioned here is the ministerial fire—that is, the yang ki that flows in the Pericardium channel.

Explained another way, when the Small Intestine is considered as a part of the Stomach, the symptom patterns of the Small Intestine should be treated as cold or heat symptom patterns of the Small Intestine that are caused by Spleen deficiency. Rheumatism or arthritis tend to develop if one is affected by an external pathogenic factor at a time when there is poor circulation of ki in the greater yang channel and when urination is less than optimal. This is a channel disease, and in this case it is best to tonify the yang ki of the Heart (ministerial fire = yang ki of the Pericardium channel) in order to invigorate the yang ki of the greater yang channel. However, in order to invigorate the yang ki of the Heart, it is necessary to tonify the Spleen, which is in charge of producing ki and blood. That is why the Pericardium and Spleen channels are tonified in both fu organ diseases and channel diseases.

4.3   The Pericardium and the Triple Warmer   心包と三焦

4.3.1 The Nature of the Pericardium

As mentioned in the section on the Heart, yang ki of the Heart is called spirit and is a mixture of the yang ki of ki (i.e., defensive ki) and the yang ki of blood (i.e., the power of genesis or creation). It is the most important component in the body, and is therefore called the sovereign fire. The human body cannot function without yang ki, so the yang ki of the Heart moves to the outside to perform its function. That yang ki is called the ministerial fire. The ministerial fire functions through the Pericardium. Therefore, the Pericardium channel is used as the treatment area.

The nature of the ministerial fire is joy because it is yang ki of the Heart. That is why Chapter 8 of the *Su Wen* states, "The Pericardium is the ambassador and from it joy and happiness emanate." If the ministerial fire is vigorous, a person's character will be cheerful and relaxed. CV-17 is the diagnostic and treatment point that has an abundance of yang ki of the Pericardium. The term "ambassador" means a subject who serves the sovereign fire.

4.3.2 The Ministerial Fire of the Kidney

Yang ki of the Pericardium (the ministerial fire) travels to every organ, but it is the Kidney that requires the ministerial fire the most of all the organs because the Kidney itself does not have any yang ki.

Ministerial fire from the Pericardium spreads out to the five zang and six fu organs after going through the Bladder channel and entering the Kidney channel. At that time it unites with the essence of the Kidney and functions as the most fundamental and important yang ki. The *Nan Jing* calls this the "life gate," a name that indicates how important it is. It is also called source ki because it is the source of all the yang ki. It is further known as the source ki of the Triple Warmer. The term Triple Warmer refers to the three areas where yang ki functions. This will be discussed later.

The Spleen and Stomach, which are located above the Kidney and life gate, will function well if the essence of the Kidney and the ministerial fire (life gate) are vibrant. This relationship can be expressed metaphorically as a fire—the combination of essence and ministerial fire—glowing under the kettle—the Stomach and Spleen. There will be increased production of ki, blood, and fluids if the Spleen and Stomach function well. The fluids will be stored in the Kidney, the blood in the Liver, and the Lung ki will circulate, sending ki and blood to the Heart. Then the ministerial fire will come out from the Heart and again become the driving force to work the Triple Warmer.

4.3.3 Areas and Function of the Upper Warmer

The function of the Triple Warmer is divided into three parts: upper, middle, and lower. These areas each receive yang ki (the ministerial fire) and then play out their respective roles. However, the origin of this yang ki is yang ki of the life gate. That is why the life gate is called the original ki of the Triple Warmer—the source ki of three areas where yang ki functions.

The chest is the area of the Upper Warmer. The nutritive ki, defensive ki, and ancestral ki that are produced in the Stomach and Intestines rise to the Heart and Lung located in the chest. Ancestral ki becomes the motive power for breathing. Nutritive ki becomes blood and then the yang ki of the Heart. Defensive ki is circulated throughout the body by Lung ki. This is the function of the Upper Warmer.

4.3.4 Areas and Function of the Middle Warmer

The Spleen, Stomach, and Liver are contained in the area of the Middle Warmer. Fluids that come from the Kidney and yang ki of the life gate function within the Spleen and Stomach to produce ki and blood. The ki and blood rise up to the chest and become yang ki of the Upper Warmer. The Liver stores the blood and governs genesis/creation. These are the functions of the Middle Warmer.

4.3.5 Areas and Function of the Lower Warmer

The area below the navel is the Lower Warmer. The yang ki of the life gate is located here, and it is the source ki of all of the body's functions. Defensive ki is created in the Lower Warmer and rises to the Upper Warmer. The excretion of stool and urine also belongs to the function of the Lower Warmer.

For instance, if yang ki of the life gate decreases, the Lower Warmer becomes chilled, causing excessive urination and a tendency to have diarrhea. On the other hand, if heat increases due to a shortage of Kidney fluids, it will cause constipation or febrile diarrhea or else a decrease in urination.

4.4.1 The Nature of the Spleen

Chapter 8 of the *Ling Shu* says, "The Spleen stores the nutritive [ki] and the nutritive [ki] stores the intention." Intention is the essential ki stored by the Spleen. But, what is the nutritive ki that stores the intention? It is thought of as the Spleen's function in producing ki, blood, and fluids that nourish each part of the body, organs, and meridians. The Spleen uses intention to make the Stomach and Intestines produce ki, blood, and fluids.

The Spleen is called the most extreme yin within yin. Its nature is not forceful like the Liver and it does not circulate ki like the Lung. It is not always active like the Heart, and it does not crave the ministerial fire like the Kidney. The Spleen produces ki, blood, and fluids by intention, like a philosopher absorbed in quiet thought. In terms of human emotion, it could be expressed as "thought."

The Spleen does not have yang ki. Therefore, death will ensue if heat invades the Spleen due to some kind of illness. It is said that the essential ki of the Spleen usually works hard to send heat back to the Stomach. This is easy to understand if you think about what happens when there is no heat in the Stomach. For example, the appetite improves if the Pericardium channel is tonified when the Stomach is cold due to Spleen deficiency. This happens because the ministerial fire of the Pericardium does not go to the Spleen but rather to the Stomach.

4.4.2 Areas Controlled by the Spleen

The flesh, mouth, lips, and four limbs are the areas controlled by the Spleen.

The human body mainly consists of flesh. Even the internal organs are made of flesh. The Spleen, which produces the fluids and blood, governs the flesh since the fluids and blood are essential to the flesh. People whose flesh is flabby or flaccid tend to present with a Spleen deficiency pattern. People who have decreased functioning of their inner organs due to chronic illnesses also tend to present with a Spleen deficiency pattern. This indicates that the organs have become frail because of insufficient fluids and blood due to the Spleen deficiency.

The mouth is the starting point for the production of ki, blood, and fluids, and hence the Spleen also controls the mouth. If there is an abnormality in the mouth such as a canker sore, the condition tends to be Spleen deficiency.

The Spleen also controls the lips since they are made of flesh. In fact, the lips turn white in the case of a Spleen deficiency cold pattern and turn red in the case of a heat pattern. Also, individuals with big lips constitutionally tend to present with a Spleen deficiency heat pattern, and those with small lips tend to present with a Spleen deficiency cold pattern.

The four limbs contain an abundance of flesh. Therefore, complaints of lassitude, lack of strength, or emaciation of the four limbs indicate Spleen deficiency. The four limbs should be strong if there is plentiful production of ki and blood, and should also be strong in patients with an abundance of heat in the Stomach even if they have Spleen deficiency.

4.4.3 The Spleen and Sweetness

Chapter 10 of the *Su Wen* says, "The Spleen desires sweetness," and Chapter 56 of the *Ling Shu* says, "The sweetness of grain goes first to the Spleen." Sweetness has the functional property of relaxation and seems to encompass functions such as softening hardened things, relaxing tension, and moistening dry things. Blood and fluids are essential for performing such functions. The blood and fluids are produced in the Stomach and Intestines by order of the Spleen, and that is why sweetness goes to the Spleen.

Chapter 4 of the *Ling Shu* says, "If both the physical and energetic bodies are insufficient, do not use needles, but rather use sweet medicine to reestablish harmony." The term "physical body" refers to the hair/skin, blood vessels, flesh, sinews, bones, and organs. The term "energetic body" refers to yin ki and yang ki. Yin ki and yang ki should be tonified if there are symptom patterns due to their deficiency. However, if both the physical and energetic bodies are inadequate, it is best to stimulate the production of blood and fluids by using sweet herbs that activate the Spleen.

As mentioned above, sweetness tonifies the Spleen. However, in performing acupuncture treatment this can be considered as corresponding to the use of the earth points. For example, the earth point of the Liver channel can be used in the case of Liver deficiency with a cold pattern that shows a lack of the Liver blood.

Incidentally, in pulse diagnosis a soft pulse that has vibrant Stomach ki (a pulse quality) is considered a healthy pulse. A soft pulse appears when there is efficient production of ki, blood, and fluids, which moisten the channels.

4.4.4 The Spleen and the Four Seasons

The Spleen is very active during the *doyō*, which is a Japanese term that refers to the last 18 days of each season. It is also said that the Spleen corresponds to the ki of the doyō.

The ki of each organ becomes very active during the season to which it is related: spring, summer, autumn, or winter. Spring is the time when the Liver ki works to gather the blood and initiate generation or creation. During the summer, the Heart heat becomes vigorous, which greatly aids in growth. At the same time, the Heart heat is kept in check by the functioning of the lesser yin ki. In the autumn, the hair and skin shrivel because of the effects of the withering ki of autumn, the season of the lung. In the winter, the Kidney stores the fluids, and the yang ki of the life gate works to prevent the fluids from becoming overly plentiful.

However, all these functions are possible because of the ki, blood, and fluids that are produced in the Spleen and Stomach. Therefore, during the *doyō*, after each of the other four zang organs performs its role in its respective season, the Spleen becomes active and produces ki, blood, and fluids to distribute to the four zang organs. It is also said that the Spleen is located in the center because of its central importance.

4.4.5 The Spleen and the Stomach

In Chapter 45 of *Su Wen* it says that the Spleen circulates the fluids produced in the Stomach (see quote on page 116). However, the Spleen cannot function without the fluids stored in the Kidney. That is why the Spleen controls the Kidney.

The Stomach contains yang ki, which, as previously mentioned, is the ministerial fire that comes from the Pericardium. Ki, blood, and fluids are produced from the fluids that come from the Kidney and the ministerial fire that comes from the Pericardium.

The relationship between the Spleen and the fu organs also deserves a few words.

As mentioned in the discussion on the Small Intestine, it is more convenient in the clinical setting to regard both the Large Intestine and the Small Intestine as belonging to the

Stomach. Moreover, Chapter 11 of the *Su Wen* says, "The Stomach is the sea of food and drink and the great source of the six fu organs," and Chapter 9 says, "The Spleen/Stomach, Large Intestine, Small Intestine, Triple Warmer, and Bladder are the original storehouses." Thus, it seems acceptable to think that each of the six fu organs is related to the production of the ki and blood in the Stomach. Therefore, it can be said that the Spleen controls all the fu organs. There are many cases where symptom patterns appear in the fu organs due to Spleen deficiency.

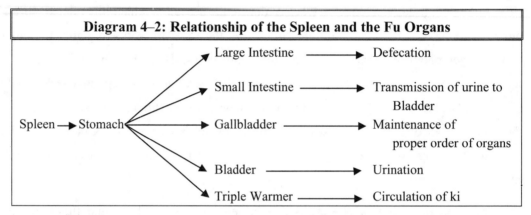

Diagram 4–2: Relationship of the Spleen and the Fu Organs

If the Spleen is diseased, it cannot bring the fluids to the Stomach. There is only a membrane between the Spleen and the Stomach, and thus the fluids are easily brought to the Stomach. (*Su Wen,* Chapter 29)

The Spleen governs circulation of the fluids for the Stomach. (*Su Wen,* Chapter 45)

The five tastes go into the Stomach from the mouth. The Stomach produces the essential ki, and the Spleen distributes it. (*Su Wen,* Chapter 47)

4.5 The Lung and Large Intestine 肺と大腸

4.5.1 The Nature of the Lung

Chapter 8 of the *Ling Shu* says, "The Lung stores ki and ki houses the corporeal soul." This passage indicates that the Lung is related to ki. Further, Chapter 18 of the *Su Wen* says, "The Lung circulates the nutritive ki, defensive ki, and yin and yang." Thus, the Lung governs the circulation of ki throughout the whole body. The corporeal soul is the essential ki stored by the Lung, and it is the driving force for the Lung to circulate ki. So, what kind of entity is the ki that the Lung circulates?

As was previously mentioned, the skin and hair have pores that protect the body from the changes in the exterior temperature, humidity, and pressure. When it is cold the pores close, and when it is hot the pores open to release sweat. It is Lung ki and yang ki that activate the opening and closing of the pores. That is why the Lung governs the skin and hair.

Chapter 8 of the *Su Wen* says, "The Lung is like a minister from whom policies are issued." This means that the Lung aids something. The Heart contains the sovereign fire, which goes to the Pericardium and becomes the ministerial fire. However, the ministerial fire cannot circulate around the body by itself, and thus the Lung ki distributes it throughout the body. Therefore, it is the Heart that the Lung aids. In the five elements theory, the Heart controls the Lung since the Heart always requires the Lung ki.

Chapter 5 of the *Su Wen* says, "Grief is the emotion that injures the Lung." It is said that grief is the emotion of the Lung. When the Lung is diseased the emotions that manifest are grief and sadness or idle complaints. However, when the Lung is normal the emotions that manifest infer a quiet and alone condition.

The Lung desires the functional property of gathering, which is opposite to the functional property of releasing. Therefore, the Lung craves the condition that is opposite to releasing. That is the concept described by the word "grief."

4.5.2 Areas Controlled by the Lung

The skin and hair and the nose are the areas controlled by the Lung. Chapter 44 of the *Su Wen* says, "The Lung governs the skin and hair," and Chapter 37 of the *Nan Jing* says, "The Lung ki goes to the nose." Moreover, Chapter 40 of the *Nan Jing* says, "The Lung governs the voice." The skin and hair are the most superficial part of the body and serve to wrap up the body. Since the Lung governs the skin and hair, the Lung itself can be regarded as having the function of wrapping up the body. That is why "the Lung desires gathering." (*Su Wen*, Chapter 22)

As previously mentioned, there are pores in the skin and hair. The body is protected from external pathogens by the opening and closing of the pores, which harmonizes yin and yang ki. The Lung also controls body hair. For example, individuals who have constitutionally weak Lung and who tend to be cold have an abundance of body hair.

Some internal areas of the body are continuous with the skin. One area is the internal surface of the nose, trachea, and lungs. This is the relationship that leads to the Lung governing the voice. The area along the inside of the mouth, esophagus, stomach, intestines, and anus is also continuous with the skin. The inside of the Bladder and uterus are likewise continuous with the skin. These areas should be considered as being related to the Lung. Since they are related to the Lung, if yang ki does not circulate due to Lung ki deficiency, then yang ki does not circulate inside these areas either, which leads to them becoming chilled. On the other hand, if the heat in the Lung increases, heat stagnates in these areas as well.

For instance, warming the skin and hair causes hunger because it improves the circulation of the Lung ki, which invigorates the yang ki inside the Stomach. On the other hand, overeating when one has a cold causes a stuffy nose and more fever.

4.5.3 The Lung and Pungency/Spiciness

The Lung itself desires the functional property of gathering. Thus, in terms of the functioning of the pores, it works more toward the closing of the pores. However, if the pores close and the Lung ki is not diffused, yang ki will not circulate throughout the body, or it will stagnate in one place, creating heat. That is why Chapter 10 of the *Su Wen* says, "The Lung desires pungency/spiciness." This means that eating pungent or spicy food improves the circulation and release of ki.

In terms of yin and yang, the Lung should be considered as having an abundance of yin ki and the function of gathering, and the Lung channel should be considered as circulating ki and releasing it. These two functions are the visceral manifestation of the Lung.

4.5.4 The Lung and the Four Seasons

The autumn (or evening within a single day) is the time when everything gathers. Leaves fall and fruits ripen. Animals prepare for hibernation. If this principle is applied to the zang organs, it corresponds to the functioning of the Lung. That is why Chapter 22 of the *Su Wen* says, "The Lung governs autumn," and "The Lung desires gathering."

4.5.5 The Lung and Large Intestine

The Lung and the Large Intestine are paired organs. The Large Intestine is located in the Lower Warmer and is influenced by the yang ki of the life gate. Moreover, the Large Intestine is a part of the Stomach. Thus if heat in the Stomach increases with Spleen deficiency, the heat also goes to the Large Intestine. Thus, it may seem like the Lung and the Large Intestine do not have any relationship, but there is one. For example, those who tend to have Lung deficiency also tend to have diarrhea as soon as they drink cold beer or milk. This results because the inside of the stomach and intestines, which are continuous with the skin, becomes chilled. As mentioned above, the skin and hair of a Lung deficient individual tends to be cold.

On the other hand, if heat stagnates in the Lung, the heat also appears in the Large Intestine and in the Large Intestine channel.

4.6   The Kidney and Bladder   腎と膀胱

4.6.1 The Nature of the Kidney

Chapter 8 of the *Ling Shu* says, "The Kidney stores the essence, and the essence houses the will." Will is the power to continuously do something. Young babies cannot concentrate on a single matter even when playing since their Kidneys are not yet physiologically firm. Adults who are constitutionally Kidney deficient seldom complete goals even though they may dabble in various activities. It is said that this power to persist and persevere is found in the Kidney essence. In terms of yin and yang, this functioning belongs to yin. Yin ki by nature firms things. That is why Chapter 22 of the *Su Wen* says, "The Kidney desires firmness."

Chapter 44 of the *Su Wen* says, "The Kidney is the water organ," and Chapter 34 says, "The Kidney is the water organ and governs the fluids." The Kidney has an abundance of fluids. Since the Kidney desires firmness, essential ki and fluids firm it. Essential ki and fluids have a yin function.

It is said that the emotion possessed by the Kidney is fear. People who are easily scared and frightened tend to be Kidney deficient. Infants are easily scared and frightened. Fear is a passive feeling that connotes non-activity and stillness. The Kidney is yin within yin. As mentioned before, Kidney essence is yin ki. The fluids also belong to the yin aspect. Thus, not being active is good for the Kidney, which should be thought of as an organ that tries to prevent the depletion of the body fluids.

However, if a person is always passive and quiet, nothing is accomplished. Therefore, as mentioned in the section on the Triple Warmer, the ministerial fire of the Pericardium descends and becomes the yang ki of the life gate, thereby allowing the body to become active. However, the Kidney essence and fluids are essential in order for the ministerial fire of the Pericardium to descend to the Lower Warmer.

In terms of yin and yang theory, the Kidney essence and the fluids are yin, and the ministerial fire of the Pericardium is yang. Thus, health is maintained when these yin and yang aspects intermingle in the Upper and Lower Warmers. That is also why the Kidney controls the Heart.

4.6.2 The Areas Controlled by the Kidney

The Kidney controls the bones, ears, two lower orifices, and hair on the head.

The ears are also related to the Heart since the Heart and the Kidney are connected in the Upper and Lower Warmer through the lesser yin channel. If there is an outbreak of heat due to a deficiency of Kidney fluids, this heat rises up to the Heart through the lesser yin channel. This is called yin deficiency fire moving. If there is an abundance of heat in the Heart, the excess heat will rise up to the head, causing deafness. That is why the ears are related to both the Kidney and the Heart.

The two lower orifices are the openings through which stool and urine are excreted. As mentioned in the section on the Triple Warmer, defecation and urination will cease or will exceed normal if there is no yang ki of the life gate. That is why it is said that the Kidney is related to the two orifices.

The Kidney controls the hair on the head. However, balding and having white hair have different meanings. Balding is caused by hair falling out due to the vigorous release of yang ki from the head. That is why it is said that people who are bald are full of vitality. However, losing hair with age results from the heat caused by deficiency of Kidney fluids rising up to the head. On the other hand, white hair is a phenomenon caused by decreasing yang ki of the life gate in those who tend to be deficient in Kidney fluids.

The Kidney also controls the bones and bone marrow. The marrow is connected to the brain, so the brain should also be thought of as being controlled by the Kidney. Fluids are essential for the bones and bone marrow to properly function. The bones dry up and are easily fractured if there are insufficient fluids. Osteoporosis is said to be a result of a lack of calcium, but from the standpoint of Meridian Therapy it is caused by Kidney deficiency. Likewise, cases of hernia with low back pain always involve Kidney deficiency.

The water inside the bones is heated up when there is an outbreak of heat due to deficiency of fluids. If this condition becomes severe the brain is also heated up, which tends to result in dementia.

4.6.3 The Kidney and Saltiness

Chapter 10 of the *Su Wen* says, "The Kidney desires saltiness." Saltiness has the functional property of softening. For example, if salt is sprinkled on a fresh radish or Chinese cabbage, water will be drawn out and it will shrivel. The term softening here is meant to describe that kind of function—that is, the release of stiffness from something that is firm due to having been solidified by water in the East Asian medical sense. Therefore, the Kidney requires saltiness so that it does not become too firm with fluids.

From the viewpoint of yin and yang, the fluids are yin. If they increase more than necessary the body becomes chilled. Therefore, the saltiness works to maintain proper levels of fluids. This function is the same as that of the yang ki of the life gate. On the other hand, the lesser yin channel, which is connected to the Kidney, tries to control heat and increase yin ki and the fluids, which firm the Kidney. This is the opposite function of the yang ki of the life gate. When the functions of yin ki and yang ki harmonize, the Kidney performs its proper physiological role.

4.6.4 The Kidney and the Four Seasons

The Kidney works hard during the winter (and during the nighttime within a single day). The winter is the time to store—as in storing up for the winter. It is the time when everything is concealed, under cover. Since the Kidney is the organ that by nature has abundant yin ki, it is best for it to remain in hiding, quietly fearing. Because this is the same function as that of the fluids, the Kidney is said to be robust in the winter.

4.6.5 The Kidney and Bladder

The Kidney and the Bladder are paired organs. Clearly, urination abnormalities appear whether the fluids become insufficient or overly plentiful due to Kidney deficiency. This is related to the yang ki of the life gate.

As previously mentioned, yang ki is able to descend from the Pericardium to the Lower Warmer because of the essence and fluids of the Kidney. Urine is secreted by the power of this yang ki as it descends to the Kidney. However, urination becomes uncomfortable when there is a heat pattern caused by a fluid deficiency of the Kidney, which makes it difficult for the yang ki to descend to the Lower Warmer.

On the other hand, large quantities of urine are excreted if the contracting power of the Kidney is weakened due to an insufficiency of yang ki caused by a deficiency of both the essence and the fluids of the Kidney. Also, as was mentioned in the section on the Lung, the Bladder is continuous with the skin. If the skin becomes chilled, the Bladder itself also becomes chilled, leading to frequent urination.

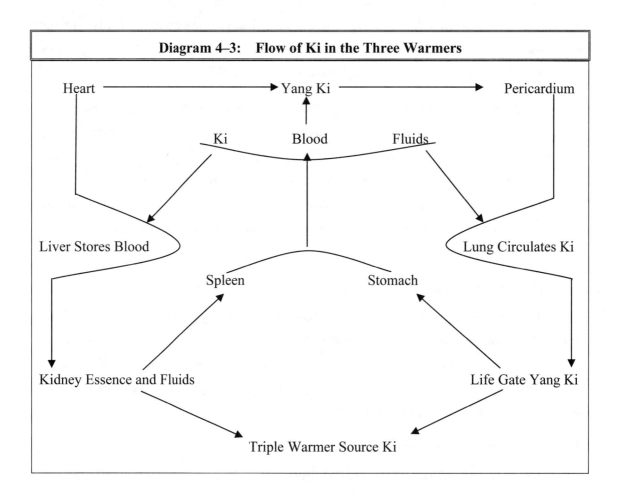

Diagram 4–3:   Flow of Ki in the Three Warmers

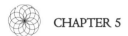 CHAPTER 5

Etiology

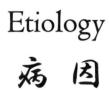

Etiology is divided into three categories: endogenous factors, exogenous factors, and non-endogenous/non-exogenous factors.

The term "endogenous factors" refers to the concept that illness can result from emotional inclinations. These include anger, joy, pensiveness, sorrow, grief, fear, and fright and are together called the seven affects.

The term "exogenous factors" refers to changes in external temperature, pressure, or humidity, the effects of which can cause illness. These include wind, cold, summerheat, dampness, dryness, and fire and are together called the six factors (six excesses) or external pathogenic influences (external evils).

Causes that are neither endogenous nor exogenous are those things that do not fit into the above categories, and they include food and fatigue.

The concept of food as an etiological factor includes overeating, starvation, and food poisoning. In the classics it said that overindulgence or inadequate consumption of the five tastes, the ingestion of cold foods or drinks, or the drinking of alcohol could cause disease. Also included nowadays are iatrogenic disorders caused by modern medications.

The term fatigue refers to the causation of infirmities by overexertion, the concept of which also includes trauma and overindulgence in sex. The aftereffects of surgery are also included in this category.

Weeding through etiology is not done simply in order to find the reason that someone came down with an illness. Understanding etiology allows one to understand the pathology of disease and makes it easier to determine the pattern of imbalance.

5.1　Constitutional Factors　　　　　　　素因

It may seem strange to include one's physical constitution within the parameters of etiology. But, from the viewpoint of Meridian Therapy there are no perfectly healthy people. Everyone lives with some kind of irregularity. The term physical constitution is a phrase that is used to help explain a pattern of imbalance. That is, a person with a certain physical constitution is always living with a certain pattern of imbalance, or in other words, certain patterns of imbalance will easily manifest with only a slight disruption of one's health.

Among the patients who come for acupuncture treatment, there are many who are essentially healthy but who have slightly deviated from their physical constitution. It is an easy matter to treat such people, but just because it is easy does not mean that their treatment should be taken lightly. Having such patients means that even those with indefinite complaints can be treated with acupuncture, which in turn points to the breadth of acupuncture's range of applicability. Moreover, continual treatment can prevent illness by maintaining health. Clinicians should have some experience with this. Chapter 2 of the *Su Wen* says, "Cure the illness before it appears!"

There are many ways to classify constitutional factors, which are also known as predisposing factors. In Chapters 2, 64, and 72 of the *Ling Shu*, among others, they are given as features of everything from personality to physical characteristics. Here we will categorize them by the pattern of imbalance so that they will be of immediate usefulness in the clinic. For more detailed explanations, please consult the classical texts.

5.1.1　Constitutional Liver Excess Pattern *Kan-Jitsu-Shō Taishitsu* 肝実証体質

Observational Signs: The size of the eyes is proportional to the amount of blood stored in the Liver. Therefore, individuals with large eyes naturally tend towards having Liver excess. Because this physical constitution also tends to cause blood stasis, these individuals will have relatively dark, rough skin with patches of discoloration. They tend to have sturdy, muscular physiques.

Personality: Persons of this type tend to be broad-minded, and they like to look out for the welfare of others. They do not get shaken up over trifles, quickly finish their work, and have loud, deep voices. In the case of women they tend to be simple and innocent, and also tend to be athletic.

Symptom Pattern: Persons of this type often complain of stiff shoulders and muscle soreness. They have hearty appetites and like to drink alcohol. Their stools are firm and dark in color, or they tend to have constipation. They do not often get angry, but when they do, their anger is so intense that they cannot be approached.

5.1.2 Constitutional Liver Deficiency Heat Pattern *Kan-Kyo Nesshō Taishitsu* 肝虚熱証 体質

Observational Signs: People with a constitutional Liver deficiency heat pattern tend to have long and slender eyes and chiseled facial features. Moreover, in these people the antihelix tends to protrude out past the helix. This can be clearly seen from behind. Persons of this type also tend to have slender yet muscular physiques.

Personality: Persons of this type tend to be fanatical about cleanliness and methodical. They cannot feel at ease unless everything is done just right, and they feel they must carry through to the end everything that they begin. However, they cannot do everything just as they would like, since they naturally tend to be deficient in blood. That makes them irritable. Even so, since they are also concerned about the activities of others, they tend to take on more than their bodies can handle.

Symptom Pattern: Persons of this constitution are irritable and tend to get insomnia from thinking too much. They often have dreams. They easily get Gallbladder channel related headaches and stiff shoulders, and also tend to become constipated.

5.1.3 Constitutional Liver Deficiency Cold Pattern *Kan-Kyo Kanshō Taishitsu* 肝虚寒 証体質

Observational Signs: Small eyes characterize persons of this type. Their ears have the same shape as people with a constitutional Liver deficiency heat pattern. They tend to be slender, but with feeble muscles. In the case of women, they tend to be anemic and easily get cold.

Personality: Persons of this type tend to lack both drive and physical strength, and thus are often timid. Or, due to a persecution complex there are times when they tend to dislike being with people. However, when they are in good health they tend to get irritable while they work, just like someone with a constitutional Liver deficiency heat pattern. They tend to switch back and forth between times of timidity and aggressiveness. They can show consideration for others.

Symptom Pattern: Persons with this constitution tend to have cold hands and feet since they lack sufficient blood, and also easily get frostbite. Many are infertile. They tend to get stomachaches when they are cold. Women tend to have diarrhea when they have their menses. They do not have strong appetites, though they eat a normal amount. They tend to sigh a lot.

5.1.4 Constitutional Spleen Deficiency Heat Pattern *Hi-Kyo Nesshō Taishitsu* 脾虚熱証体質

Observational Signs: People with a constitutional Spleen deficiency heat pattern naturally tend to have an abundance of heat in their Stomach and Intestines, and thus have well-defined jaws or large mouths and lips.

Personality: At their best they are magnanimous. At their worst they exaggerate and talk boastfully.

Symptom Pattern: The symptoms are divided into two categories, Stomach excess heat and Stomach deficiency heat.

Those with constitutional Stomach excess heat have large appetites and tend to overeat. They may even eat glass! They sweat when they eat (even in the winter), and when they drink alcohol they tend to want to take their clothes off. They suffer when they have constipation, and feel relieved by having diarrhea. When there is abundant heat in the Stomach and Intestines there is also heat in the four limbs, so they tend to be very active. They also tend to enjoy singing. If this condition of Stomach excess heat continues too long they will become manic.

Those with constitutional Stomach deficiency heat are healthy when they have a good appetite. But, when they eat too much they tend to lose their appetite, get diarrhea, have stomachaches, and complain of weariness in their hands and feet or even throughout their whole bodies.

5.1.5 Constitutional Spleen Deficiency Cold Pattern *Hi-Kyo Kanshō Taishitsu* 脾虚寒証体質

Observational Signs: Persons of this type tend to have small mouths that are often left open, and their lips tend to be pale. The area around their mouths tends to be yellowish. They tend to have weak flesh and be lanky.

Personality: Persons of this type tend to be passive in all that they do, and they lack power and perseverance. They tend to be lost in thought. They do not have good memories. Since they have difficulty getting energy into their limbs they tend to be lazy.

Symptom Pattern: Persons of this type tend to have small appetites and cold bodies because they naturally have insufficient yang ki in the Stomach. If they overeat even a little they tend to get worn-out from diarrhea. They tend to have stomachaches and weariness throughout their bodies. They also tend to accumulate saliva and to pass large quantities of slightly cloudy urine.

5.1.6 Constitutional Lung Deficiency Heat Pattern *Hai-Kyo Nesshō Taishitsu* 肺虚熱証体質

Observational Signs: Persons of this type tend to have light complexions and lots of body hair. In fact, chest hair and heavy beards tend to characterize these people. They tend to have surprisingly muscular physiques. Women tend to have very fair skin and a lot of peach fuzz.

Personality: Persons of this type tend to have low toned, powerful voices. Many are full of self-confidence. There are also many who are self-righteous and poor at showing consideration for others.

Symptom Pattern: People with constitutional Lung deficiency easily release yang ki. However, if they release too much yang ki they will become cold. Thus, to defend against that happening, they tend to have an abundance of body hair.

When they are healthy, they feel refreshed when they expel sweat, stool, urine, or semen because it improves the circulation of ki. When yang ki cannot be released, heat tends to stagnate in the Large Intestine channel anterior to the Lung, which tends to cause stiff shoulders.

People with this physical constitution tend to get diarrhea from drinking beer or milk. Also, they tend to get swollen tonsils.

5.1.7 Constitutional Lung Deficiency Cold Pattern *Hai-Kyo Kanshō Taishitsu* 肺虚寒証体質

Observational Signs: Like people with a constitutional Lung deficiency heat pattern, people with a constitutional Lung deficiency cold pattern have fair skin and an abundance of body hair, but their body hair is very fine. Children often have peach fuzz on their backs if they are constitutionally Lung deficient. Such children are prone to catching colds.

Personality: Persons of this type have weak voices and are not active. They tend to worry over the most minor problems and are full of idle complaints.

Symptom Pattern: People with a constitutional Lung deficiency cold pattern tend to get cold easily. They expel large quantities of slightly cloudy urine when they are cold and regularly sneeze and have runny noses. They also have a tendency to be depressed.

5.1.8 Constitutional Kidney Deficiency Heat Pattern *Jin-Kyo Nesshō Taishitsu* 腎虚熱証体質

Observational Signs: The condition of the Kidney is revealed in the ears. People with large ears and slightly dark and lustrous skin are not likely to become Kidney deficient, and thus tend to live long lives.

However, people with a healthy Kidney are likely to become Kidney deficient due to overindulgence in sex. To make matters worse, naturally there is nothing that can be done about slipping towards Kidney deficiency with increased age. When people become Kidney deficient, even large ears will darken and curl forward, and because of the decreased firming ability of the Kidney, these people tend to become overweight from middle age on.

Personality: People with a constitutional Kidney deficiency heat pattern tend to have a humble demeanor, which is a manifestation of the emotion of fear that is related to the Kidney. Becoming mild mannered with age is also a condition of becoming Kidney deficient.

Symptom Pattern: The feet of these people tend to become uncomfortably hot because of the tendency to have insufficient Kidney fluids. Or, the bottoms of their feet may hurt. They also tend to urinate during the nighttime, be short of breath, and get palpitations. They usually have a hearty appetite, but tend to get diarrhea when they have decreased urination or constipation when they have increased frequency and volume of urination.

5.1.9 Constitutional Kidney Deficiency Cold Pattern *Jin-Kyo Kanshō Taishitsu* 腎虚寒証体質

Observational Signs: The size of the ear is proportional to the size of the Kidney. Even though the constitutional Kidney deficiency heat pattern and the constitutional Kidney deficiency cold pattern are both Kidney deficiency patterns, those who have the cold pattern have small ears or ears that seem to have shrunk into the head. Recently, this condition has become more common in children. These children tend to have enuresis (bedwetting) at night and are unusually squeamish.

Personality: Persons of this type tend to lack perseverance and the drive to carry through with anything. They are timid and passive by nature. Many are not ambitious in life, and hence may not have successful careers or marriages.

Symptom Pattern: These individuals have hands and feet that tend to be cold, and they are always prone to catching colds. They do not sweat even in the summer. They have poor appetites and tend to get diarrhea. Also, they usually have weak sexual desire and low energy. They have a low ability to resist disease and tend to become inflicted with serious illnesses when they lose their health even just a little.

Table 5–1: Characteristics of Constitutional Factors	
Liver	Size of the eyes and shape of the ear
Spleen	Color and size of the mouth and lips
Lung	Body hair and the color of the skin
Kidney	Size of the ears

5.2 Endogenous Factors 内因

Endogenous factors are also referred to as the seven affects. These include anger, joy, pensiveness, grief, sorrow, fear, and fright. Experiencing these emotions in the extreme leads to the appearance of particular patterns of imbalance. For example, extreme anger leads to

Liver deficiency, and extreme joy leads to Heart heat. Pensive worrying leads to Spleen deficiency, and extreme grief and sorrow lead to Lung deficiency or Lung heat. Extreme fear leads to Kidney deficiency, which causes increased heat in the Heart, resulting in people becoming easily frightened.

Nonetheless, there are those who get angry and those who do not get angry no matter what conditions they encounter, since everyone has a unique personality. For example, imagine someone getting into a car accident. There are those who will get angry at this, and those who will become sad thinking about the future consequences. There are also those who will worry over the problems of taking care of everything related to the accident. Each individual's emotional nature—the fluctuations and tendencies that arise from their physical constitution—is different, even though they find themselves in similar situations. Therefore, it can be said that endogenous factors enhance a person's constitutional factors.

Constitutional factors are closely related to endogenous factors. Be that as it may, suppose that while you are conducting the questioning part of an examination, the patient says that he became unwell because of something irritating that happened. Even if you do not have confidence in your pulse diagnosis abilities, based on this information you can treat the patient as having a Liver deficiency pattern. On the other hand, even if the symptom pattern presents as a condition of anger, there are times when it is not possible to determine in questioning whether the symptom pattern actually resulted from extreme anger. It is only natural that the Liver deficiency could have resulted from another cause and then produced the condition of anger. The same holds true for the other endogenous factors as well.

Besides the consideration of endogenous factors there are many circumstances when the etiology cannot be ascertained by questioning. In these cases it is necessary to determine the pattern of imbalance without relation to the etiology. You may think that it is not necessary to learn the etiology theory if there are times when it is not possible to ascertain the etiological factors, but it is important to do so for the following reasons.

Learning the etiology gives you clues for determining the pattern of imbalance, and it also teaches the important skill of knowing what kind of changes to ki, blood, and fluids are brought about by each of the etiological factors. From this you can imagine the pathology, and work backwards to the etiological factors through questioning about the current conditions. By pursuing this method it becomes easy to grasp the pathological condition and determine the pattern of imbalance.

5.2.1 Anger = Liver Deficiency *Do = Kan-Kyo* 怒＝肝虚

Anger is the natural emotion of the Liver. It is displayed in emotional states such as activeness, deliberateness, thoroughness, and being fanatical about cleanliness. However, these can turn into the cause of illness and lead to Liver deficiency.

There are people who cannot feel at ease unless they deliberately engage in activities and thoroughly carry out all that they do. Such people are constitutionally Liver deficient and tend to develop abnormal Liver deficiency patterns. Regardless of physical constitution, people tend to develop Liver deficiency patterns when they find themselves in positions where they need to think carefully or do very detailed work. Likewise, people tend to become Liver deficient when they get angry at home or at work. The pattern of imbalance should be determined as Liver deficiency if the above conditions can be ascertained through questioning during the examination.

Blood is essential for minute planning and carrying things out in a thorough manner. Thus, anger consumes blood. Chapter 5 of the *Su Wen* says, "Violent anger injures yin." If blood is consumed, people with constitutional Liver deficiency easily develop an abnormal Liver deficiency, and even those with other constitutional types develop a Liver deficiency pattern when blood is consumed. Naturally, even if blood becomes insufficient due to other causes the same kind of emotional states will appear.

The discussions above describe people who have developed Liver deficiency. Conversely, come people develop Liver excess. They may bear their anger in silence, such as those who want to get angry at home, but who do not allow themselves to do so. People who hold in their anger develop a state of emotional depression. Liver excess results from the stagnation of blood along the Liver reverting yin channel caused by this state of depression. Just as in Liver deficiency, there will be symptom patterns such as stiffness medial to the scapula, tension in the neck muscles, headaches, and insomnia. Nonetheless, Liver excess and Liver deficiency can be distinguished because the emotional states and signs in the pulse and abdomen will be different.

5.2.2 Joy = Heart Heat *Ki = Shin-Netsu* 喜＝心熱

Joy is the normal emotion of the Heart. Normal means that the yang ki of the Heart has emerged as and is functioning as the ministerial fire of the Pericardium. Chapter 39 of the *Su*

Wen says, "Laughing causes the ki to relax … when one laughs, the ki harmonizes, the will is realized, nutritive and defensive ki efficiently circulate; in other words, the ki is relaxed." Therefore, it can be said that people with a sunny disposition have normal yang ki of the Heart. However, heat will increase in the Heart if one becomes too cheery. In such cases, joy becomes an etiological factor.

Chapter 5 of the *Su Wen* says, "Wild joy injures yang." This means that the Heart, which is stimulated by heat, overworks because ki rises to the Upper Warmer due to the extreme joy. Too much yang ki could also be released when the Heart overworks. This is expressed in Chapter 8 of the *Ling Shu* as, "Exceeding joy causes the spirit to lose its inhibition, and hence it can no longer be stored." This is a Kidney deficiency Heart heat pattern since it is caused by the inadequate ability of the Kidney to perform its functional property of firming and tightening. There are actual cases of people becoming ill from excessive joy.

Conversely, excessive joy can result from too much heat in the Heart due to some other factor. For example, it should be considered that there is too much heat in the Heart when the patient is overly cheerful when giving answers to questions during an examination or laughs while giving answers to questions about a serious illness. In such cases, it is best to pay attention to the left distal position on the pulse and also check their blood pressure and confirm any past illnesses. Chapter 62 of the *Su Wen* says, "Laughter doesn't cease when there is a surplus of spirit."

5.2.3 Pensiveness = Spleen Deficiency *Shi = Hi-Kyo* 思＝脾虚

Chapter 5 of the *Su Wen* says that "pensiveness" is the natural emotion of the Spleen. Pensiveness has connotations of thoughtful prudence and contemplativeness. People have good memories and the ability to deliberate and think things through in a calm manner when the Spleen is healthy. However, when one is overly pensive, making one wrong step can lead to illness. Chapter 5 of the *Su Wen* says, "Pensiveness injures the Spleen."

People who tend to develop Spleen deficiency have a constitutional tendency to think too much about everything. Similarly, those who think too much or worry a lot tend to develop Spleen deficiency, regardless of their physical constitution. When conducting the questioning examination, if the patient claims to have become ill due to having so many things to worry about, she likely has a Spleen deficiency pattern.

The circulation of ki deteriorates when one ruminates too much. Chapter 39 of the *Su Wen* says, "Pensiveness causes the ki to get all tangled up. ... When one thinks too much the mind becomes fixated and the spirit becomes attached, the healthy (right/true) ki stagnates and does not circulate; in other words, the ki gets all tangled up." The functioning of the yang ki of the Heart deteriorates when the ki becomes tangled. This does not mean that the Heart stops functioning, but rather that there is a reduction in the ministerial fire that emerges into the Pericardium. Chapter 49 of the *Nan Jing* says, "Anxious worrying injures the Heart." This has the same meaning. As was mentioned in the chapter on visceral manifestations, yang ki of the Stomach decreases when there is a lack of ministerial fire of the Pericardium. That is why people lose their appetite when they think too much.

5.2.4 Grief and Sorrow = Lung Deficiency *Yūhi = Hai-Kyo* 憂悲＝肺虚

Chapter 5 of the *Su Wen* describes "grief" as the natural emotion of the Lung. Grief includes the connotation of a state of quiet solitude. However, sinking too deeply into grief will injure the Lung. Sorrow deepens the more one grieves.

Those with constitutional Lung deficiency are likely to fall into grief and sorrow because of the poor diffusion and circulation of ki. However, the Lung can also be weakened when there are woeful or sorrowful happenings, regardless of one's physical constitution. It is good to treat Lung deficiency for those who claim to have lost their health due to sad events.

Chapter 39 of the *Su Wen* says, "Being sorrow-stricken extinguishes the ki. ... When one is sorrow-stricken, the Heart and surrounding tissues are stressed, the lobes of the Lungs swell up and obstruct the Upper Warmer, nutritive and defensive ki are not diffused, and heat accumulates inside; thus, being sorrow-stricken extinguishes the ki." The circulation of Lung ki deteriorates when there is deep grief or sorrow. Also, one's drive slackens off, and the voice becomes diminutive. Or, there are also cases when there will be an appearance of flu-like symptoms.

If the grief and sorrow deepen any further, heat will stagnate in the Lung, which normally tends to result in asthma or coughing. In people who continuously cough like they are trying to clear their throats, the circulation and release of Lung ki has been weakened by the activation of the gathering function of the Lung.

When this kind of stagnation of the Lung ki occurs, people usually try to release ki by grumbling about things. Such behavior can often be seen in people with constitutional Lung deficiency, since they tend to develop Lung heat because they do not release the stagnated ki even though they gripe a lot. Conversely, there are people who harbor grief and sorrow and have many complaints even if they develop Lung deficiency or Lung heat from other causes.

5.2.5 Fear/Fright = Kidney Deficiency Heart Heat *Kyō • Kyō = Jin-Kyo Shin-Netsu* 恐・驚＝腎虚心熱

Chapter 5 of the *Su Wen* says that fear is the natural emotion of the Kidney. The meaning of fear implies a passiveness and a state of quiet restraint, and it also corresponds to the Kidney's functional property of tightening and firming. This can be expressed another way as remaining in a state of perfect calm, or as a state of humbleness. In actuality, people who have a firm and strong Kidney have a tendency to great or distinguished people with a dignified bearing. They do not fight with others and do not become abnormally angry or sorrowful.

However, even these great people can become Kidney deficient if they have too much fear. Chapter 5 of the *Su Wen* says, "Fear injures the Kidney." Chapter 39 says, "Fear causes the ki to descend. … When one is terror-stricken, the essence recedes; when the essence recedes, it closes off the Upper Warmer; when the Upper Warmer is closed off, the ki returns [to the Lower Warmer]; when the ki returns, the Lower Warmer becomes distended; thus, the ki does not circulate."

Kidney deficiency results from the reduction of essence that is caused by fear. This type of Kidney deficiency is accompanied by heat. The Upper Warmer is closed off if one develops Kidney deficiency. In other words, the ministerial fire of the Pericardium has a difficult time developing into the yang ki of the life gate. This will cause heat to stagnate in the chest, which will cause one to be easily frightened.

There are not many cases of people becoming Kidney deficient due to fear. But, they do exist, such as people who have accidents at sea or adventurers with frightening close-call experiences. It is said that once construction workers who work high up on scaffolding experience the feeling of fear while on the job, they will not be able to ascend the scaffolding again. Also, there are cases of people becoming Kidney deficient after witnessing a fatal accident or a fire. The patient should be treated without hesitation as Kidney deficient if any of the above–mentioned extraordinary experiences are revealed during the examination.

It is normal for fright or surprise to accompany fear brought on by Kidney deficiency. Fright is related to the Heart, but it is not the natural emotion of the Heart. Fright is both the cause of illness and a symptom pattern. Chapter 39 of the *Su Wen* says, "Fright throws the ki into chaos—when one sustains a great fright the mind has no place to rest, the spirit loses that which it depends upon, and there is no place to stabilize one's anxiety. Thus, the ki is thrown into confusion." Being easily frightened is a result of increased heat in the Heart due to Kidney deficiency. In saying that the spirit loses that which it depends upon, it means that the spirit cannot be quieted within the Heart, which results because of the increased heat in the Heart.

Further, symptomatic fear appears in cases of a Liver deficiency cold pattern, as well as in cases of a Kidney deficiency heat or cold pattern. However, these patterns have different characteristics. The fear that accompanies a Liver deficiency cold pattern is passive. Persons of this type dislike meeting others. The fear that comes with Kidney deficiency can manifest as either true terror or as tendency to be overly modest and reserved.

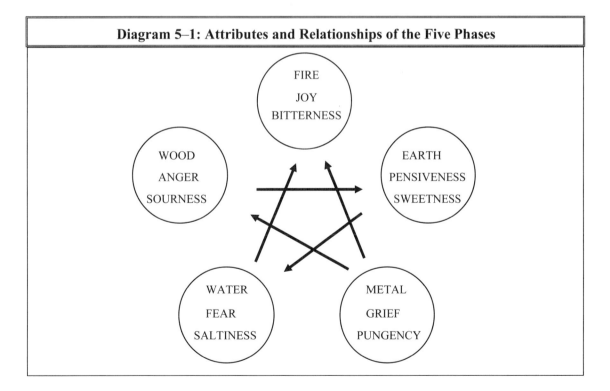

Diagram 5–1: Attributes and Relationships of the Five Phases

5.2.6 Other Emotions

In addition to the seven affects mentioned above, people have other emotions such as envy, jealously, and bitter feelings. These are not given separate attention because they are purely abnormal emotions that do not correspond with the visceral manifestations. In actuality there are many people who become ill due to feelings such as jealousy. However, this is most likely related to the personalities they have that relate to their physical constitutions. In other words, envy will transform into depression or grief, and bitter feelings will transform into sorrow or anger. Please take these points into consideration as references for determining the patterns of imbalance.

5.3   Food and Drink   飲食

Such things as excessive or insufficient intake of the five tastes, overeating, starvation, or food poisoning can be suspected in cases where illness results from food or drink.

Excessive or insufficient intake of the five tastes is, in the modern sense, the same as unbalanced nutrition, but in Meridian Therapy the categories are set by the flavor of the foods. These flavors are: sourness, bitterness, sweetness, pungency/spiciness, and saltiness. Eating balanced quantities will help maintain health, while eating unbalanced quantities will lead to illness. However, illness will not manifest quickly even if one's diet is unbalanced, and it is often difficult to determine which flavor was the culprit that caused the illness, since people eat so many different foods. Knowing the functions of each flavor allows one to understand the pathologies and symptom patterns that are caused by deficiency or excess of each of the organs. This knowledge will also allow you to give the patient dietary instructions.

Overeating and starvation are problems of quantity, and both can lead to illness.

Food poisoning clearly results in a symptom pattern.

Additionally, there were many cases of illness due to roundworm in ancient China. Today such cases are rare, but in their place we now have illness caused by the side effects of medication and artificial food additives.

5.3.1 Excessive/Deficient Intake of the Five Flavors

① **Sourness**

Sour foods have the functional property of gathering. Gathering can be thought of as the function of collecting together things that are scattered or of sinking things that are floating. Applying this, it follows that sourness is necessary when there is an increase of ki in the yang aspect due to a deficiency of yin. For example, people who have a red face due to high blood pressure, or people who like to drink alcohol, should eat sour foods. Conversely, sourness is bad for the person who is cold due to insufficient yang ki.

Chapter 56 of the *Ling Shu* says, "Each of the five tastes proceeds to the place where it is most preferred. Sourness goes first to the Liver." The Liver prefers sourness because the blood is gathered to the Liver by the functional property of gathering that is inherent in sourness. Therefore, as a rule, people with Liver deficiency should be given sour foods to eat.

Most people who are Liver deficient will say that they do not like sour foods. They say this because they enjoy the good feeling brought on by the diffusion of yang ki from Liver blood, and eating sour foods slows this diffusion. Most of these people like spicy foods, which allow for quick diffusion of yang ki.

Sour foods include such things as vinegar, Japanese pickled plums (*umeboshi*), and lemons. Chapter 22 of the *Su Wen* says that green foods, sesame, dog meat, *sumomo* (Chn: *lǐ*) (a kind of plum), and leeks are sour. It is thought that this grouping is based more on the medicinal properties than on the actual taste of the foods.

② **Bitterness**

Bitterness has the functional property of firming. This functionality should be thought of as soothing things that are flaring up, and, even more actively than sourness, pacifying things that are floating. Firming also increases yin ki. Heat is reduced by the increase of yin ki. Thus, bitterness is thought of as having the ability to reduce heat.

Applying this principle, it is appropriate for people with too much yang ki to ingest bitter foods. This would include those who overeat, have heat in the Heart, are sensitive to heat, or have constipation due to excess heat in the Intestines. Conversely, eating bitter foods is especially bad for people who have a tendency to get chills, have cold-induced diarrhea, or those who lose their appetites due to coldness of the Stomach.

Chapter 56 of the *Ling Shu* says, "Bitterness goes first to the Heart." This is because bitterness serves to check the heat in the Heart, of which there is always a lot. In other words, bitterness not only tonifies the lesser yin channel, it also stimulates the firming function of the Kidney. Heat in the Heart decreases relative to the firming of the Kidney by fluids, which also soothes other parts of the body that have heat. That is also why Chapter 63 of the *Ling Shu* also says, "Bitterness goes to the bones."

General bitter foods include such things as green peppers, garland chrysanthemums, green vegetable juice, and *maccha* (Japanese powdered green tea). Green vegetable juice is especially good for the body, and there are people who drink it excessively. However, eating a food that does not match one's pattern of imbalance will have the opposite effect. For example, it is said that a person who has a tendency to get a chilled stomach and has no appetite will have a "green vegetable juice burp" all day long if they drink green vegetable juice. The *Su Wen* says that wheat, mutton, apricots, and shallots are bitter.

③ Sweetness

Sweetness has the functional property of relaxing. Relaxing means to enrich and soften each part of the body with increased ki and blood and with fluids. Therefore, people who are feeling weak, yet who do not have any particular ailments, should first of all eat something sweet. That is why it is said to be good to eat something sweet when one is tired from physical exertion.

Chapter 56 of the *Ling Shu* says, "Sweetness goes first to the Spleen." Sweetness goes to the Spleen because when the Spleen is made robust there will be active production of ki, blood, and body fluids. Also, Chapter 23 of the *Su Wen* says, "Sweetness goes to the muscles," which means sweetness first of all nourishes the flesh. That is why it is better to make weak children eat a larger portion grains, and a lesser portion of animal protein. Conversely, people who are overweight and "generously-proportioned" should most likely refrain from eating sweet foods.

Sweet foods include such things as sweet potatoes, rice, white potatoes, pumpkin, and honey. In the *Su Wen* it says that beef, jujube, and hollyhock are sweet. Although they are called sweet in everyday language, refined sugar and artificial sweeteners do *not* belong in this category.

④ Pungency/Spiciness

Pungency/spiciness has the functional property of warming by increasing yang ki. Therefore, people who have modest amounts of yang ki and a tendency to be cold should eat pungent/spicy foods. However, it is also possible to become chilled from eating spicy foods because it causes sweating.

Chapter 56 of the *Su Wen* says, "Pungency/spiciness goes first to the Lung." Pungency/spiciness acts to tonify the Lung and stimulate the release and circulation of ki. For example, warming the body with something pungent/spicy—ginger, garlic, *tamagozake* (Japanese eggnog)—will cure a light case of the flu. However, as was previously mentioned, spicy foods in the proper amount are fine, but too much or too little can, in opposite fashion, cause heat to be trapped inside or yang ki to be lost.

In the *Su Wen* it says that such foods as millet, chicken, peaches, and scallions are spicy. Other spicy foods include chillies, *wasabi* (Japanese horseradish), garlic, curry, and ginger.

⑤ Saltiness

Saltiness has the functional property of softening and loosening things that are tight or firm with water. Thus, saltiness is thought of as tonifying yang ki even though it is passive. Or, it can be thought of as decreasing water. Accordingly, salty foods should be strictly prohibited for people who are yin deficient with an abundance of heat. For example, salty foods are not good for people with high blood pressure.

Chapter 56 of the *Su Wen* says, "Saltiness goes first to the Kidney." It goes to the Kidney because it is needed there to prevent fluids from becoming excessive in the Kidney, which has the most body fluids in the body. Therefore, salty foods are the worst foods for people with a Kidney deficiency heat pattern.

Heat in the Heart increases relative to development of deficient-type heat caused by insufficient fluids in the Kidney. Consequently, salty foods should also be prohibited for people with abundant heat in the Heart. Conversely, it is advisable for people with an overabundance of fluids to consume an appropriate amount of salty foods in order to expel the fluids through the urine.

In the *Su Wen* it says that soybeans, pork, and chestnuts are salty. Therefore, these should be eaten when there is an increase of fluids in the Kidney.

Saltiness is not a problem as it comes in particular foods, but it is a problem as a spice. Adding a lot of salt to food causes the blood to become viscous, which increases the blood pressure and makes it difficult for the body to cool down. That is why people who live in cold climates like salty foods.

5.3.2 Overeating and Starvation

① Overeating and Overdrinking

Alcohol is the biggest problem when it comes to overconsumption. Alcohol belongs to the category of spicy among the five tastes. Spicy foods warm the body, but overingesting spicy foods will cause cooling, which is due to the resultant exceeding loss of yang ki. Many people who like alcohol are also thin because they lose fluids along with yang ki.

Moreover, alcohol causes heat to be trapped somewhere in the body, especially in the Liver, Gallbladder, and Stomach. The patterns of imbalance that tend to be seen in this condition are Spleen deficiency with Liver, Gallbladder, or Stomach heat patterns. Also, the Gallbladder channel tends to manifest pain on pressure in people who like alcohol.

Chapter 49 of the *Nan Jing* says, "Cold drinks injure the Lung." Drinking too many cold drinks also leads to a tendency to catch colds as a result of the deterioration in production of yang ki that results from coldness of the Stomach. The onset of coldness of the Stomach can also lead to yang ki being pushed to another part of the body, where it will stagnate and cause heat. The repetition of this pattern tends to result in stomach cancer.

Excessive fruit consumption also falls within the category of cold food and drinks. Eating a lot of fruit tends to cause the skin to become rough. Young people have the tendency to eat a lot of fruit in the name of going on a diet, but they get rough skin. To achieve smooth skin, it is best to eat sweet grains. Moreover, contrary to their dietary intent, people can put on water eating fruit because it is rich in sweetness and water.

Generally, overeating is caused by excess heat in the Stomach. However, Stomach heat can be caused by either Spleen deficiency or Kidney deficiency. In the case of Stomach heat caused by Spleen deficiency, people tend to not gain weight. They can even lose weight despite the fact that they eat, since there is an insufficiency of fluids due to the Stomach heat. At the same time though, they can turn maniacal on the emotional level.

People who overeat as the result of heat in the Stomach caused by Kidney deficiency will become overweight without fail. The shortage of fluids caused by the Kidney deficiency produces deficient-type heat, which in turn creates heat in the Stomach, resulting in a hearty appetite. At the same time, weight is put on due to the weakening of the tightening/firming power of the Kidney. Therefore, people who wish to lose weight should refrain from eating too many sweet foods, eat more bitter foods, and also tonify the Kidney.

② Starvation

Naturally, starvation is also not good for the body. Recently there has been quite an increase in cases of anorexia, an emotional problem which it may be conjectured involves a subconscious desire to not become an adult which triggers the refusal to eat.

While it is natural for anorexics to lose weight, the characteristic of the disease is that they remain lively and are able to do anything they wish. However, in the case of women, a continuation of this condition for a number of months results in a loss of the menses. This is quite difficult to cure, but counseling is the best approach. If you are not familiar with counseling methods, it is fine just to be a good listener. Giving sermons or trying to be persuasive is not effective. Concurrently, restoring some of the balance of the body and inducing relaxation through acupuncture treatment will help the return of the appetite.

5.3.3 Roundworm, Food Poisoning, and Harmful Effects of Medicines

① Roundworm

There are not as many cases of roundworm now as there used to be, but occasionally a patient who is emaciated from roundworms comes for treatment. Mostly these patients are treated with antiparasitic Chinese herbs.

② Food Poisoning

Food poisoning can be life threatening. If you detect serious cases you should direct them to medical specialists. The levels of cases appropriate for acupuncture treatment are normally ones that subside after vomiting once or twice and having diarrhea. However, the patient can become dehydrated if diarrhea continues and nausea persists even though the stomach has been emptied. The patient should immediately be sent to the hospital if his or her consciousness becomes hazy. However, if it is not a life threatening case of food poisoning, it can usually be treated with moxibustion on the famous *uranaitei* (裏内庭) point (a point that corresponds to ST-44 on the plantar aspect of the foot).

③ Harmful Effects of Medicines

It is no wonder that medicines sometimes have harmful effects since modern medicines inherently have side effects in addition to the primary effect. However, the reality is that people must take medicines despite some minor side effects because to not do so could be life-threatening.

Some patients who come to acupuncture clinics will be taking modern medicines. Sometimes they ask for advice as to whether they should be taking the medicines, but in principle you should not interfere with the doctor's instructions, and you should not on your own advise them to quit taking medications. To suddenly stop taking medicines can be life threatening. For example, you should not tell people to stop taking anticancer drugs, hormone drugs, hypertension drugs, or medications for emotional or nervous system disorders. If you are consulted about medicines, it is appropriate to tell the patient that their doctor would most likely reduce the quantity of medication if their condition improves as a result of acupuncture treatment.

In reality, it is best not to take medications. All modern medicines bring heat to the chest, where the Heart and Lung carry the burden of the increased heat. A strain is also placed on the Spleen and Stomach, which leads to numerous cases of Spleen deficiency that normally would have been Liver deficiency. That only makes it very difficult to cure. You should readjust the body as much as possible through acupuncture, but if you find there is not much you can do, you should recommend taking medications as a last resort. If you can judge before then that acupuncture treatment is not appropriate, you should introduce the patient to a medical specialist.

It is not a problem to stop the patient from taking over-the-counter painkillers or medicines for the stomach and bowels. However, it is meaningless to have them stop taking the medicines if you do not relieve their suffering through acupuncture treatment.

Additionally, even though problems such as environmental pollution and artificial food additives have become a social dilemma, there is nothing we can do about it from where we stand. Even if you do not choose to eat chemically laden products, there is probably no way around it. The only thing that we can say for sure is that acupuncture is a natural therapeutic method that does not cause harmful medicinal side-effects. Such harmful effects of medicines should be preventable to some degree if the body's balance is being properly adjusted through acupuncture.

5.4 Fatigue 劳倦

Fatigue refers to weariness of the mind and body. In the *Essential Prescriptions of the Golden Coffer* (*Jīn Guì Yào Lüè*), it is called "deficiency taxation illness," which means an illness that occurs as a result of becoming fatigued from working while having a deficiency. Overindulgence in sex is also included in the category of fatigue (deficiency taxation). Childbirth, miscarriages, trauma related to traffic accidents, and the aftereffects of surgery are also included in this section.

In all cases of fatigue the patient will complain of being tired, but it is important to determine the pattern of imbalance by questioning to find out what caused the fatigue. However, simple connections should not be drawn between the etiology and the pattern of imbalance. The patterns of imbalance should be thought of in light of what pathological conditions are brought about by the etiology. Fatigue is easy to identify and should most certainly be checked during the questioning examination.

In the following subsections, explanations will be given for each organ, with each division beginning with a quote from Chapter 23 of the *Su Wen*.

5.4.1 Fatigue

① Liver

"Remaining active for a long time injures the sinews."

It should be considered that Liver deficiency would result from the consumption of blood that occurs when someone undertakes a task with unremitting perseverance, since the sinews are nourished by the blood and thus are controlled by the Liver. Examples include things like spending the whole night checking up on something or knitting. More than anything, emotionally related activities or activities with little movement are the activities that cause Liver deficiency. Office workers tend to get Liver deficiency. Also, housewives and those who doggedly pursue a hobby tend to become Liver deficient. These points should be considered and relevant questions should be asked about them during the examination.

People who steadfastly work on things tend to be constitutionally Liver deficient because they just cannot feel at ease until things have been brought to an end. Therefore, when they start something, they will keep at it all night long without even giving a thought to the consequences. That is why fatigue is closely related to the constitutional factors, or rather, tirelessly working on something often enhances the constitutional factors.

② Heart

"Staring at something for a long time injures the blood."

This quote means that if one overuses the eyes it will cause a shortage of blood. The Heart is connected to this because it produces the blood. Thus, you might imagine that someone could develop Heart deficiency, but that is not the case. The yang ki of the Heart will become insufficient if the blood is depleted. Therefore, tonification should be given as if for Spleen deficiency in order to increase the blood. Or, there are cases of people getting a Liver deficiency cold pattern when there is a lack of blood. In the end, it is a matter of constitutional factors that determines which pattern of imbalance will affect different individuals.

During the examination you should ask your patients if they overuse their eyes. Recently, there has been a definite decrease in average eyesight due to the increase in the use of computers. The patient will recover from it if they are treated for a Liver deficiency pattern from false nearsightedness.

③ Spleen

"Sitting for a long time injures the muscles."

This quote indicates that the Spleen will become deficient if one only sits around, since the Spleen controls the muscles. More specifically, this probably means that the muscles will atrophy if one remains sedentary. It is a fact that the functioning of the Stomach and Intestines declines when one sits for prolonged periods. Taxi drivers tend to have Spleen deficiency. We said that office workers tend to have Liver deficiency, but depending on their constitutional factors, there are also those who get Spleen deficiency.

Chapter 49 of the *Nan Jing* says, "Fatigue injures the Spleen." Overuse of the limbs tends to result in Spleen deficiency, and the yang brightness channel actually becomes drawn with tension. However, this is also related to the constitutional factors. Those who have a tendency to be Spleen deficient are generally not dynamic because they have weak limbs. Lazy people usually sit around and thereby weaken the Spleen all the more.

④ **Lung**

"Sleeping for a long time injures the ki."

It may seem strange to include doing nothing but sleeping in the category of fatigue, but it belongs there since sleeping for prolonged periods impairs the circulation and release of ki. Thus, sleeping for prolonged periods injures the ki—specifically the yang ki that is controlled by the Lung. Yang ki becomes insufficient due to both extreme activity and too little activity. It is best to circulate and release ki by maintaining an appropriate level of activity.

It is difficult to ascertain whether inactivity is a cause since everyone becomes less active when they are not feeling well. But some people become sluggish even when they have no real ailments, and others go to bed when they have the slightest problem. In these cases, you should suggest exercise if the person has constitutional Lung deficiency. People with constitutional Lung deficiency will recover their health by improving circulation and releasing ki through exercising. Their health tends to deteriorate when they stop exercising.

In other words, in cases of ailing ki, you should recommend exercise if you can judge that healing would follow with just an improvement in the circulation of ki. If you are incorrect in your judgment though, for example by recommending exercise to someone who has Spleen deficiency, they could become exhausted from overuse of their limbs. People with constitutional Liver deficiency become attached to exercise, and so a hobby becomes much more than simply a hobby, which is detrimental to health.

⑤ **Kidney**

"Standing for a long time injures the bones."

Standing for prolonged periods puts stress on the bones and also tends to lead to a decrease in the yang ki of the life gate because of a cooling from the feet upwards. Chills in the lower half of the body result in an increase in the frequency of urination and can also cause irregularities in the menstrual cycle, as well as low back pain.

Kidney deficiency can also result from doing manual labor such as lifting heavy bundles. As was previously mentioned, the pattern of imbalance that will manifest with fatigue depends on the constitutional factors of each individual. Manual labor that puts an undue burden on the bones tends to result in Kidney deficiency.

5.4.2 Overindulgence in Sex

There are statements throughout the classics that overindulgence in sex causes illness. This can be a difficult matter to ask about during the examination. Therefore, this information is usually gathered from the pulse and abdominal diagnoses. As you gain experience and proficiency you will gain the respect of your patients, and they may reveal such information to you without you having to ask.

Chapter 66 of the *Ling Shu* says, "Jumping into bed while drunk and then standing in the wind after perspiring injures the Spleen." Alcohol tends to induce sweating because it invigorates the yang ki. Sexual intercourse at that time tends to cause profuse sweating. Attempting to cool off by standing in front of a fan or an air-conditioner can cause Spleen deficiency, which is probably a result of extreme excess heat collecting in the limbs, which makes it difficult to move them. Conversely, it could be due to cooling resulting from the expending of yang ki.

However, these cases are also related to the constitutional factors. For example, when people with Liver deficiency stand in the wind in order to cool off after engaging in sexual intercourse, they are likely to get hemiplegia or paralysis. Or, their blood pressure could suddenly shoot up. People who tend to have hot bodies are likely to develop heat patterns when they overindulge in sex, and those who tend to be cold are likely to develop cold patterns.

People with constitutional Lung deficiency enjoy the expulsion of stool, urine, sweat, and semen, since the expulsion invigorates the circulation of ki. Therefore, people with constitutional Lung deficiency are very energetic and do not often become ill due to overindulgence in sex. However, really overdoing it can lead to changing over to Kidney deficiency.

Overindulgence in sex manifests as different patterns of imbalance in men and women. Women "sweat" a lot during sex because vaginal lubricating fluid is a transformation of sweat. Thus, they tend to get a Liver deficiency cold pattern. In men, semen, which in Japanese is literally "essence fluid," is a bodily fluid. Therefore, men who overindulge in sex tend first of all to develop a Kidney deficiency heat pattern.

In contrast to overindulgence in sex, one's health can also deteriorate in the absence of a lover, still resulting in Kidney deficiency or Liver deficiency. Heat is produced because yang ki cannot be released while one is feeling gloomy or depressed in this situation. The heat causes deficiency of the fluids of the Kidney and the blood of the Liver, which appear the same as the conditions resulting from overindulgence in sex. (See the quotation on the following page from *Bìngyīn Zhǐnán*, Fire Pattern Chapter.)

5.4.3 Trauma

Traffic accidents and other forms of trauma damage the blood, usually either by causing blood stasis or blood deficiency that results in Liver deficiency. There are also many cases of Liver deficiency and Spleen deficiency resulting from blood deficiency after surgery.

Chapter 4 of the *Ling Shu* says, "Falling down causes an internal stagnation of bad (i.e., unhealthy) blood ... which collects in the subcostal area, causing injury to the Liver." There are many such passages in the classics. This refers to the formation of blood stasis in the subcostal area caused by internal bleeding due to bruises and strains that, for example, are sustained in an accident if some nature. Since the Liver stores the blood, blood stasis is always more frequent in areas that are controlled by the Liver or Liver channel (subcostal area and lower abdomen) when there is a stagnation of blood. In terms of the pattern of imbalance, blood stasis corresponds to Liver excess.

5.4.4 Antepartum and Postpartum

Pregnancy, childbirth, miscarriage, and abortion are such important concerns that they require their own section.

Women tend to become blood deficient or get blood stasis after giving birth. Blood deficiency corresponds to a Liver deficiency heat pattern, and blood stasis corresponds to a Spleen deficiency Liver excess pattern. Miscarriage and abortion often result in a Liver deficiency cold pattern. Repeated abortions can also cause Kidney deficiency.

A number of women's illnesses are related to childbirth. During the questioning examination you should inquire as to whether the woman has experienced childbirth, and if so whether or not it was a normal delivery. However, this questioning is used only when it is difficult to determine the pattern of imbalance and should not be used up front as a standard part of the examination.

In the old days people used to warn women to not strain their eyes after giving birth because it could cause postpartum blood deficiency. These days, many young women ignore that admonition and watch TV or read the newspaper after giving birth, which will make them prone to getting cataracts or other eye diseases in the future.

> In court ladies, women who protect their chastity, and older women who have never married, the ki of sexual desire becomes clogged in the lower warmer, causing an arousal of the ministerial fire. The burning of the ministerial fire causes an eventual wasting away of kidney yin. This produces the same symptom pattern as in one who overindulges in sex, which results in yin deficiency and an arousal of fire.
>
> Due to unfulfilled five minds and seven affects, ki of the heart and liver accumulates, causing an intensification of heart fire and liver fire, which eventually results in blood deficiency of the heart and weakening of liver blood. ... Such conditions are very common. (*Bìngyīn Zhǐnán*, Fire Pattern Chapter)

5.5 Exogenous Factors   外因

The term "exogenous factors" refers to the idea that illness can result from changes in the natural environment, namely wind, cold, summerheat (fire), dampness, and dryness. These are known as external pathogenic influences or the six factors. Generally, fire is included within the category of summerheat.

Illness does not arise solely due to these exogenous factors. Illness can result from the combination of an exogenous factor with a deficiency of essential ki, or from the combination of an exogenous factor with a deficiency of ki, blood, or fluids that resulted in turn from the combination of an endogenous factor with a deficiency of essential ki.

In some cases the pattern of imbalance can be determined even without having a detailed understanding of the pathology simply by asking about the etiology, such as endogenous factors or fatigue. For example, if the patient's illness was brought on by anger, treatment can be given for Liver deficiency without knowing the fine details of the pathology. However, this is not the case with exogenous factors. Simply knowing the exogenous factors does not lead directly to ascertaining the pattern of imbalance. For example, just because someone came down with an illness upon being "struck by wind," does not mean they simply have wind stroke disease and can be treated for Liver deficiency.

Certainly wind is related to the Liver, and Chapter 49 of the *Nan Jing* says that wind stroke is a pathogenic influence that affects the Liver. But, wind can also affect other zang organs. Therefore, it is essential to know the fundamental visceral manifestations—that is, in what ways the ki, blood, and fluids of each zang organ change—in order to know what pathogenic influence caused a certain condition of illness. In other words, the pathological condition is more important than the actual cause. When the classics talk about the etiology, it has the same meaning as the modern usage of the term pathology. Therefore, you should remember that the words used to describe the etiology are also describing the pathology.

As previously mentioned, the classics described which zang organs tend to be invaded by which etiological factors, as well as the effects produced on other zang organs by an invasion of those factors. It follows that 25 types of pathological conditions can be considered, since each of the five pathogenic influences (wind, cold, summerheat fire, dampness, and dryness) can invade each of the five zang organs (Liver, Heart, Spleen, Lung, and Kidney).

Figure 5–2: Five Zang Organs in Multiple Configuration with External Pathogenic Influences			
Wood		Wind	
Fire		Cold	
Earth	X	Summerheat	= 25 types of pathological conditions
Metal		Dampness	
Water		Dryness	

The *Nan Jing* points out wind stroke, summerheat damage, food and fatigue, cold damage, and dampness stroke as the five pathogenic influences, and indicates that they respectively affect the Liver, Heart, Spleen, Lung, and Kidney. This was done in an attempt to connect etiology with treatment points. For example, if the Lung is suffering from wind stroke, the wood point (which corresponds to the Liver) on the Lung channel should be used as a treatment point since the Liver is the organ that is injured by wind. More will be given about this in the chapter on treatment.

Alternatively, Chapter 23 of the *Su Wen* says that the Liver has an aversion to wind, the Heart has an aversion to heat, the Spleen has an aversion to dampness, the Lung has an aversion to cold, and the Kidney has an aversion to dryness. It should be noted that it is *excessive exposure* that turns these exogenous factors into pathogenic influences.

The rest of this section summarizes the pathological conditions that result when each of the exogenous factors influence the five zang organs.

5.5.1 Wind

Wind corresponds to the ki of spring and is a power that promotes generation. However, when Heaven is deficient—in other words, when there is disorder and confusion in the rhythm of nature—wind becomes a pathogenic ki and attacks the body. Illness will result if the body is suffering from a deficiency at that time. This is called wind stroke disease.

The pathological condition that results from wind is a generation of heat due to the wind drying up the fluids, just as happens when one is whipped by a strong wind. The heat that is generated by wind is called deficient-type heat.

① Wind and the Liver

Being struck by wind while one has Liver deficiency produces heat because the wind dries up the fluids in the blood that are stored by the Liver. The manifestations of this heat mainly appear in the sinews. Chapter 5 of the *Su Wen* says, "Wind injures the sinews." For example, muscle ache, neuralgia, numbness, and various kinds of paralysis are often caused by wind stroke.

The generation of deficient-type heat tends to produce heat vexation (煩熱 *hannetsu*) in the extremities and also perspiration. The person becomes sinewy as they lose weight due to further depletion of fluids in the form of perspiration. There is a tendency to have constipation as fluids become insufficient. The heat rises and causes headache, hot flushes, insomnia, and sometimes a rise in blood pressure.

The pulse is floating and large. It has power, but is deficient underneath.

According to the *Nan Jing*, wind is the primary pathogenic influence for the Liver. It causes light swelling and pain in the subcostal area, a blue coloration somewhere on the face, and a wiry pulse.

② Wind and the Heart

The Heart by nature has an abundance of heat. But, the addition of wind further increases Heart heat.

Some individuals have red faces and high blood pressure, and are emotionally unstable, perspire a lot, and have red tongues. The pulse at the left distal position is strong, showing that there is heat in the Heart. This is a condition of wind stroke of the Heart.

According to the *Nan Jing*, wind is the deficient-type pathogenic influence for the Heart. It causes light swelling and pain in the subcostal area, body fever (i.e., deep fever), a red face and tongue, and a floating, large, and wiry pulse.

③ Wind and the Spleen and Stomach

The Spleen requires fluids. Deficient-type heat is produced when there are insufficient fluids due to being struck by wind when the Spleen is deficient.

The newly generated deficient-type heat spreads to many parts of the body, particularly the Stomach and Stomach channel. The extremities could feel heavy and sluggish because of stagnant heat in the flesh, as it says in the chapter on greater yin diseases in the *Shāng Hán Lùn*: "Wind stroke of the greater yin [channel causes] vexing soreness in the four limbs." General symptom patterns include a bitter taste in the mouth, a dry throat, and abdominal distension. The pulse is wiry, floating, large, and powerful.

According to the *Nan Jing*, wind is the bandit pathogenic influence for the Spleen. The symptom patterns include light swelling and pain in the subcostal area, heaviness in the body, fondness for sleep, and lassitude in the limbs. The pulse is wiry and moderate, and the body is yellowish.

④ Wind and the Lung

Being struck by wind while there is some difficulty in the circulation of Lung ki will cause a malfunction in the opening and closing of the pores of the skin and hair. This will cause symptom patterns to appear in the greater yang channel. This kind of condition is recorded in the *Shāng Hán Lùn*, which in the chapter on greater yang diseases gives representative symptoms: "Greater yang diseases [in which there is] fever, perspiration, aversion to wind, and a moderate pulse are called wind stroke." Thus, the pathology and symptom pattern of the illnesses caused by wind stroke of the Lung are different from wind stroke disease of the other organs.

According to the *Nan Jing*, wind has a weak pathogenic influence on the Lung, which means that it only produces mild symptoms, including an aversion to cold, gasping for breath, coughing, and light swelling and pain in the subcostal area. The pulse is choppy and wiry.

⑤ **Wind and the Kidney**

Being struck by wind while there is Kidney deficiency causes further depletion of fluids and generation of heat. This is called wind stroke disease of the Kidney.

When there is abundant deficient-type heat in the Kidney there is a tendency to perspire and to have heat vexation in the feet and hands. Or possibly, the heat vexation and soreness could be felt only in the plantar aspect of the foot. Symptoms include low back pain and both urinary difficulty and copious urination. The pulse tends to be floating and large or slippery, or sinking and slippery, and in all cases will be deficient underneath.

According to the *Nan Jing*, wind is the excess-type pathogenic influence for the Kidney, and thus is rather difficult to treat. Symptoms include light swelling and pain in the subcostal area, coldness in the lower abdomen, and cold feet. The pulse is sinking, soggy, and wiry. The body has a blackish tint, which is caused by heat in the blood due to a lack of fluids. The cold feet result from the chronic lack of fluids, which causes a loss of the heat that could cause heat vexation.

5.5.2 Summerheat (Fire)

Summerheat is the ki of the summer, which is the power that causes all things to grow. However, if Heaven is deficient and the summerheat goes to extremes, it can become a pathogenic ki and cause illness. But, the body will not be affected by that pathogenic ki unless there is a deficiency in the body.

The *Nan Jing* says that summerheat is the pathogenic influence that injures the Heart, but it also affects the other organs as well. It injures the Heart because the Heart relates to the ki of summer, and when summerheat becomes a pathogenic ki, the Heart, which always has an abundance of heat, suffers the brunt of the burden. Summerheat as a pathogenic influence affects the other organs because summerheat is equivalent to pathogenic heat, and pathogenic heat affects all the organs. Thus, the term summerheat as a pathogenic influence indicates pathology with an abundance of heat.

Furthermore, the heat that results from pathogenic summerheat is more intense than the heat that results from insufficient fluids due to wind, and tends to manifest as a condition of excess.

① Summerheat and the Liver

People tend to develop Liver excess heat when heat increases in the blood, because the Liver stores the blood. In the *Nan Jing* it says that summerheat is the excess-type pathogenic influence for the Liver, which means that when heat invades the Liver, the Liver becomes excess.

When summerheat invades the body, there is a change in body odor, because the heat consumes fluids. When summerheat invades the Liver the body smells rancid, and one also agonizes from body heat. The urine is a reddish yellow color, and there is abdominal pain. The pulse is floating, large, and wiry.

② Summerheat and the Heart

The Heart is rich in yang ki, and thus it has an aversion to things with an abundance of heat. The *Nan Jing* says that summerheat is the primary pathogenic influence for the Heart. Even just a little increase in heat has an effect on the Heart.

When heat increases in the Heart the body odor smells burnt, body heat is generated causing irritableness and distraction, and the chest hurts. The pulse is floating, large, and scattered. Increased heat in the Heart organ can also cause palpitations, shortness of breath, hot flushes, and nausea. There could be heat vexation in the feet and hands and possibly weight loss.

③ Summerheat and the Spleen

Summerheat as a pathogenic influence acting on the Spleen while there is Spleen deficiency causes the condition of being worn out by the heat of summer. Even though the cause is the high temperature of summer, this can still result in a Spleen deficiency cold pattern, since no heat will be trapped inside such as occurs when summerheat invades the

Liver. Of course, when there is a Spleen deficiency heat pattern there will be complaints of heat vexation in the hands and feet, general fatigue, loss of appetite, and a dry mouth.

According to the *Nan Jing*, summerheat is the deficient-type pathogenic influence for the Spleen, which means that it causes only minor symptoms. When summerheat enters the Spleen the body smells of a fragrant odor, and body heat is generated. These symptom patterns indicate that the fluids of the Spleen have become dried up by heat.

④ Summerheat and the Lung

The *Nan Jing* says that summerheat is the bandit pathogenic influence for the Lung because it can be life-threatening if the Lung becomes filled with heat. The body odor smells of flesh when there is an abundance of heat in the Lung. The patient could also bring up fleshy-smelling sputum.

When the Lung becomes filled with heat the patient will present with symptom patterns of internal heat such as a yellow coating on the tongue, body heat, wheezing and coughing, and chest pain. At the same time, the surface of the body becomes chilled because of perspiration due to the internal heat.

Conditions such as those mentioned above are usually treated as a Kidney deficiency heat pattern or a Liver deficiency heat pattern, and not as Lung deficiency. This is because heat in the Lung itself indicates Lung excess.

⑤ Summerheat and the Kidney

The *Nan Jing* says that summerheat is the weak pathogenic influence for the Kidney. The Kidney is not particularly fond of heat, but it is rather resistant to heat as long as endogenous factors do not deplete the fluids. However, summerheat, as well as heat due to other causes, can invade the Kidney if there is a lack of fluids for some reason. Increased heat in the Kidney always results in the same pathological conditions regardless of the etiology, because the heat promotes the depletion of fluids. Therefore, the result is a Kidney deficiency heat pattern. If the Kidney's fluids reach their limit of insufficiency, there will be a striking pulse, followed by death.

The *Nan Jing* says that the body odor will smell rotten if summerheat enters the Kidney. This is because the heat will make the fluids putrid, just like water can become putrid.

Additional symptom patterns include numbness in the lower limbs, heat vexation in the soles of the feet, a dry mouth, and body heat.

⑥ Fire as a Pathogenic Influence

Fire as a pathogenic influence is a side effect of moxibustion. For example, using a lot of moxibustion on the back of someone with hypertension could cause headache, dizziness, palpitations, insomnia, and even higher blood pressure. Even if there is no hypertension, it can cause the same conditions as excess heat in the Upper Warmer. Moreover, the same symptom patterns can appear if moxibustion is used on women who tend to get hot flushes, such as women with menopausal syndromes or those who recently gave birth.

There are very few patients with critical conditions like those described in the passage below from the *Shāng Hán Lùn* chapter on greater yang, but there are people with conditions similar to these. For example, some patients become irritable and restless and cannot sit still or sleep when they have had extensive moxibustion.

Even with *kyūtōshin* (灸頭鍼 moxa-on-the-handle needles) the same conditions can result. Side effects of moxibustion should be treated as a Kidney deficiency heat pattern or a Liver deficiency heat pattern.

> [When in a condition of] wind stroke [within] a greater yang disease, fire is used to induce sweating, pathogenic wind is exacerbated by fire-heat, [causing] blood and ki to overflow, [thereby] disrupting their normal [function]. The two yang(s) [pathogenic wind and fire-heat] will fumigate and scorch each other, [resulting in] yellowing of the body. [Due to] the exuberance of yang, a nosebleed is on the verge of occurring. [Due to] yin deficiency, urination is difficult. [Due to] the exhaustion of both yin and yang, the body becomes desiccated, there is sweating on the head only above the neck, abdominal distension, a light asthmatic [condition], a dry mouth, inflammatory erosion of the throat, or constipation. [If this condition] endures, [the patient] will have delirious speech, [and when] severe there will be dry heaving, kicking and struggling with the four limbs, and unconscious gripping of the clothes and groping in bed. If urination is uninhibited the patient can be treated. (*Shāng Hán Lùn*, Chapter on Greater Yang Diseases)

5.5.3 Dampness

Water is the foundation of all life in the natural world. In the human body as well, without fluids the body becomes dried out and heat is generated. Conversely, too much fluid causes various symptom patterns.

Illnesses that worsen when there is high humidity, or those that manifest certain pathological conditions due to stagnation of excess fluids, are classified into three categories: dampness disease, phlegm retention disease, and water-ki disease. The names accord to the area where there is excess water or to the apparent symptom pattern.

Dampness diseases are illnesses in which the muscles and joints become swollen and painful with water. Such illnesses occur in people who tend to naturally retain a lot of water and then suffer exposure to wind or cold.

Phlegm retention diseases are illnesses in which water gets trapped, especially in the stomach, and causes coughing, dizziness, shortness of breath, and vomiting.

Water-ki diseases are illnesses in which poor circulation and release of ki causes water to accumulate in the skin, resulting in edema and painful joints.

① Dampness and the Liver

The Liver is not very susceptible to the influence of dampness. However, the Liver stores the blood, which is made from water. Therefore, water will accumulate if there is a stagnation of blood.

The stagnation of blood causes blood stasis (i.e., Liver excess). Some people with a lot of blood stasis will have so-called water retention obesity. In the case of women, questioning usually reveals that they started to gain weight after menopause. Normally when there is little urination, defecation becomes easier, but in these people there is a tendency to have constipation.

The *Nan Jing* says that dampness is the deficient-type pathogenic influence for the Liver. It causes a tendency to cry, a sinking, soggy, and wiry pulse, cold feet, light swelling and soreness in the subcostal area, and pain in the lower abdomen.

② Dampness and the Heart

The Heart has an aversion to water since it is a yang organ among the zang organs—that is, since it will lose yang ki if water increases in blood vessels, which are controlled by the Heart. If there is a decrease in yang ki, water will also increase in the Small Intestine and Small Intestine channel, which are paired with the Heart. Excess water in the meridians causes painful joints and edema, and excess water in the Small Intestine causes a decrease in urination. Concurrently, the decrease in yang ki causes shortness of breath, an aversion to cold, and leaking sweat. Such symptom patterns are often seen in patients with polyarticular rheumatism and should be treated as a Spleen deficiency cold pattern.

The *Nan Jing* says that dampness is the bandit pathogenic influence for the Heart, and that it tends to cause perspiration. Because there is a decrease in yang ki as dampness encroaches upon the Heart, it is a very serious illness.

③ **Dampness and the Spleen**

The Spleen sets the Stomach and Intestines into work producing ki, blood, and fluids, and concurrently causes them to absorb and expel any excess water. An increase in water while there is Spleen deficiency will cause either a dampness disease with swelling due to accumulation of water in the muscles and joints or a phlegm retention disease in which there is an increase of water in the Stomach and Intestines.

The term "dampness disease" corresponds to the modern classifications of articular rheumatism and arthritis. However, in Spleen deficiency, as was just mentioned, the Small Intestine channel can deteriorate or the yang brightness channel can deteriorate. A dampness disease of the Small Intestine is a cold pattern and is common with rheumatism. A dampness disease of the yang brightness channel is a heat pattern and seems to be common with arthritis. In either case there is little urination and defecation feels comfortable.

Phlegm retention disease refers to illnesses in which there is an increase of water in the Stomach and Intestines due to Spleen deficiency. Phlegm retention disease is caused mainly by food and drink. In other words, it is not directly related to the humidity of the external environment. However, the term "dampness stroke" as used in the *Nan Jing* has the same meaning as phlegm retention, and therefore dampness, in the sense of a pathogenic influence, is used to refer to illnesses with water-related symptom patterns and not only to cases where the cause is actually humidity.

The Spleen has an aversion to dampness. Water tends to accumulate in the muscles, Stomach, and Intestines when there is Spleen deficiency. Therefore Chapter 68 of the *Nan Jing* says Earth points are the primary treatment points for a "heavy body and joint pain." A heavy feeling in the body and pain in the joints are both caused by accumulation of water in the muscles and joints due to a deficiency of the essential ki of the Spleen. To be more exact, joint pain is a symptom pattern related to external dampness, and heaviness in the body is related to internal water accumulation.

The *Nan Jing* says dampness is the weak pathogenic influence for the Spleen. It causes an increase in drool and a sinking, soggy, and moderate pulse. Naturally, the limbs become heavy. The increase in drool results from a lot of extra water in the Stomach and Intestines due to phlegm retention. The classification of weak pathogenic influence means that there will not be an acute and severe presentation of symptom patterns. Or one could think that there will be no symptom patterns like those seen when there is excess in the pulse. An excess pulse can result from a stagnation of blood, but not from an accumulation of water.

④ Dampness and the Lung

Water will accumulate in the Lung when the Lung is deficient, because the Lung circulates ki. Water will accumulate near the surface of the body if there is Lung deficiency alongside Kidney deficiency. Such conditions are referred to as water-ki diseases.

The circulation of yang ki deteriorates as water increases in the Lung itself. However, it is more likely that symptom patterns said to be caused by water in the Lung actually result from the influence upon the Lung of increased water in the Stomach due to Spleen deficiency. This is because such cases commonly get better when treated as Spleen deficiency. An actual increase of water in the Lung would be considered a very serious illness.

The *Nan Jing* says dampness is the excess-type pathogenic influence for the Lung and an excess of nasal mucus is a sign of such a condition. Of course, the patient will also tend to present with coughing and with panting and puffing.

⑤ Dampness and the Kidney

The Kidney is firmed to the appropriate degree by fluids. However, an excess of fluids will cause the Kidney to become chilled. Water is necessary for the Kidney, but at the same time, the Kidney has an aversion to water. That is why the *Nan Jing* calls dampness the primary pathogenic influence for the Kidney. The *Nan Jing* also says the amount of saliva increases with an increase of water in the Kidney. Copious of saliva indicates a Spleen deficiency cold pattern. So, the question is: How is that related to the Kidney?

When water increases in the Kidney it causes a lack of yang ki in the life gate, which then causes a lack of yang ki in the Stomach above it. Thus, excess saliva is related to the Kidney. But, it should be treated as a Spleen deficiency cold pattern.

Some people with Kidney deficiency have water retention obesity, which is caused by deficient-type heat produced by the deficiency of fluids in the Kidney. Heat naturally radiates outward. The more heat causes a release of sweat, the more one loses weight. But, longstanding deficient-type heat only pushes water to the surface. The water will accumulate at the surface if at this time there is poor circulation of Lung ki. Such a condition is referred to as a water-ki disease.

Sensitivity to heat and cold, as well as deteriorated joints, usually accompanies water-ki diseases. However, care must be taken to not mistake this condition for the arthritis or edema caused by Spleen deficiency. To that end, pulse diagnosis is critical. Speaking of symptom patterns, Kidney deficiency is often indicated by general water retention throughout the body and edema in the lower limbs. Additionally, it is also good to take note of fatigue in the limbs and the state of appetite and the stool when differentiating Kidney deficiency from Spleen deficiency.

5.5.4 Cold

Cold corresponds to yin ki and the ki of winter. Cold is the ki of the natural world that causes all things to hide away and conceal themselves. However, this too can become a pathogenic ki and a cause of disease when it is in excess.

Cold is possibly the strongest external pathogenic influence since it has a great ability to rob yang ki, and because damage due to cold often produces heat. That heat becomes a pathogenic ki and strikes inwards, causing all kinds of illnesses.

① Cold and the Liver

When the Liver is affected by pathological cold it is referred to as cold stroke. Pathological changes tend to occur in the muscles or uterus, which are controlled by the Liver, if the body becomes chilled when there is a lack of blood in the Liver due to fatigue, overindulgence in sex, or childbirth. Such conditions are referred to as blood deficiency resultant cold patterns or, in other words, as Liver deficiency cold patterns.

The *Nan Jing* says if the Liver is damaged by cold, it will cause light swelling and soreness in the subcostal area, an aversion to cold, and a wiry, choppy pulse. These symptom patterns appear in both Liver deficiency heat patterns and Liver excess heat patterns.

The light swelling and soreness in the subcostal area caused by Liver deficiency will either objectively show resistance with no pain on pressure, or it will show little resistance but will mainly exhibit pain on pressure. The light swelling and soreness in the subcostal area caused by a Liver excess heat pattern refers to a condition in which there is pain on pressure, resistance, and water stagnation. The patient may also complain of spontaneous pain.

In the case of an aversion to cold caused by Liver deficiency, there is only an aversion to cold and no subjective awareness of fever, since this is an aversion to cold caused by an insufficiency of blood. Cases of an aversion to cold caused by Liver excess will present with a condition of alternating chills and fever in which there is a recurring cycle of an outbreak of fever after an aversion to cold. Such a condition manifests when heat invades the lesser yang channel channel and indicates that the condition of pathogenic cold has already passed.

The *Nan Jing* says cold is the bandit pathogenic influence for the Liver. Therefore, it is harmful for the blood to become chilled at the deep level.

② Cold and the Heart

It is difficult for the Heart to become chilled since it is a yang organ among the zang organs and has an abundance of yang ki. That is why the *Nan Jing* says that cold is the weak pathogenic influence for the Heart. However, it is possible for the Heart to suddenly suffer a chill, which will result in death.

③ Cold and the Spleen

When it is said that the Spleen has been damaged by cold it is normally not the Spleen itself but rather the Stomach that has sustained the injury. The Stomach has a tendency to hold heat, but conversely it also easily becomes chilled. This is also referred to as cold stroke.

People yawn after eating when there is a decrease in yang ki in the Stomach. Or, they become sleepy. They could also have watery nasal mucous and accumulation of saliva in the mouth. There will be a loss of appetite and a loss of strength in the extremities when they have diarrhea.

The *Nan Jing* says cold is the excess-type pathogenic influence for the Spleen, and that it will cause one to sing with an altered voice. However, it is more likely that this is a result of excess-type heat in the Stomach and Intestines caused by cold that creates heat.

④ **Cold and the Lung**

Conditions that exhibit certain pathologies and symptom patterns that result from an invasion of pathological cold are referred to as "cold stroke" or as "cold damage." Cold stroke refers to cases in which the areas of the body that are deeper than the external areas (skin and hair) become cold due to a lack of yang ki; there is neither an aversion to cold nor fever but there is a lack of yang ki due to a very slow onset of coldness of the body; or there is no presentation of acute and severe symptoms and no influence upon other areas of the body even though there is an aversion to cold and fever.

In comparison, cold damage indicates injury sustained by cold and is seen mainly as a pathological change in the meridians. Pathological cold will invade the body when there is poor circulation and release of Lung ki, which is controlled by the skin. This always causes an aversion to cold because of the sudden loss of yang ki from the skin. The illness could then pass, or there could be an outbreak of fever after an aversion to cold. If the illness progresses with only an aversion to cold, it will eventually lead to the onset of coldness of the innards that will cause diarrhea and cold hands and feet. Sometimes this progression will reverse itself and cause a very high fever.

If the illness progresses mainly with a fever, that heat will become a pathogenic ki and spread to other areas. Ultimately it will develop into heat in the Stomach and Intestines and become an illness for which the use of a purgative is efficacious.

The *Nan Jing* says cold is the primary pathogenic influence for the Lung and that the symptom is wailing (in the sense of mourning). Wailing implies weeping, but in the case of Lung deficiency it carries the sense of sorrowfully weeping. This symptom is generally seen in people with Lung deficiency. But, it is often not apparent in Lung deficient people who also have been struck by cold damage.

⑤ **Cold and the Kidney**

It would be a rather serious problem for the Kidney to become chilled since it has an abundance of water. Therefore, it also has yang ki that protects it from coldness. This is known as the yang ki of the life gate.

The yang ki of the life gate passes from the chest through the greater yang channel and enters the Kidney. It follows that in cases where the Kidney has been invaded by pathogenic cold, this means that there has been a loss of yang ki from the greater yang channel. Acute conditions caused by this situation are referred to as lesser yin diseases, and chronic conditions are referred to as cold stroke of the Kidney. Either case should be treated as a Kidney deficiency cold pattern.

Low back pain is the first result when there is cold stroke of the Kidney. Additional symptoms include copious urination, constipation due to excessive urination, cold feet, slightly cloudy urine, and loss of spirits and vitality.

The *Nan Jing* says cold is the deficient-type pathogenic influence for the Kidney and that the symptom is groaning or moaning.

5.5.5 Dryness

Dryness as a pathogenic influence refers to dryness as the cause of illness. However, the pathology that results from dryness is the same as that for wind, since there is a resemblance to the lack of fluids caused by wind.

① Dryness and the Liver

The sinews become tense if the Liver is invaded by dryness when there is Liver deficiency. However, the symptom patterns are generally lighter than when there is wind stroke.

② Dryness and the Heart

It would be rather problematic for the Heart to have heat caused by dryness. However, the Heart most likely is not directly affected by dryness. If there is heat in the Heart, it should be treated as either due to wind or as Heart heat resulting from a heat disease striking inwards.

③ Dryness and the Spleen

It is best for the Spleen to be moderately moist since it draws upon fluids from the Kidney. In other words, it is not fond of dryness. If the fluids in the Spleen dry up, the symptom pattern appears as a Spleen deficiency heat pattern. However, this condition does not easily arise due to external pathogenic influences, since the Spleen is a deep organ. Generally, it is caused by lack of fluids as a side effect of such things as purgatives.

It is best for the Stomach to be slightly dry. A lot of water in the Stomach causes diarrhea and a loss of appetite. But a dry Stomach produces an abundance of heat, and thus makes the appetite hearty. Of course, if the Stomach becomes too dry it creates too much heat and causes constipation.

④ Dryness and the Lung

Dryness most easily enters the Lung. There are many people who have a cough due to the Lungs actually becoming dry. This condition has particular characteristics. You should ask patients who have a cough what happens to the cough when they are warm. If they say that their throats become scratchy and they begin to cough when they are warm, that is a cough resulting from a dry Lung. If this progresses to a severe case it can result in pneumonia, so it is important to ascertain whether heat is present or not when there is a dry Lung cough. Some patients with asthma also have dry Lungs. They tend to have an easier time during the rainy season when there is high humidity and a worse time in the winter. Conversely, those whose asthma worsens during the rainy season have a dampness disease.

⑤ Dryness and the Kidney

The Kidney has the strongest aversion to dryness since it is the water organ. However, pathogenic dryness does not enter all the way to the Kidney. Nevertheless, the Kidney can show a dryness-like condition if the fluids are consumed through such things as overindulgence in sex. In the final analysis, dryness diseases of the Kidney tend to have the same pathology as would be seen with pathogenic wind. The patient will have a blackish complexion when the Kidney starts to dry out, and the face will shine like it has oil on it. Of course, there will be heat vexation in the hands and feet. Such a condition should be treated as a Kidney deficiency heat pattern.

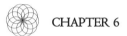

CHAPTER 6 # Pathology and Symptom Patterns
病 理 と 病 証

In previous chapters, descriptions of pathology and symptom patterns have already been given in sections dealing with deficiency and excess, visceral manifestations, and etiology because it would have been meaningless to not make reference to the determination of the patterns of imbalance. Even so, symptoms patterns and pathology are so important that they deserve their own chapter.

Concerning the arrangement of symptom patterns, we wanted to be able to connect it with the determination of the pattern of imbalance in such a way that a certain symptom would correspond to, say, Liver deficiency or Spleen deficiency. But, when we actually tried to organize symptom patterns, it was found that we could make very few definite statements as to certain symptoms always appearing with certain patterns of imbalance. For example, stiff shoulders or headache appear along with many patterns of imbalance. Actually, that type of differentiation has many inherent problems. Therefore, in order to overcome these difficulties we have decided to arrange symptom patterns in relation to pathology.

First we will give categories of patterns of imbalance based on deficiency and excess of yin and yang and on the presence of cold or heat. This will be useful for gaining a broad understanding of pathology and will make determining the pattern of imbalance easier. More than anything it is supposed to help you gain an understanding of the proper degree of tonification and dispersion, since it is important to neither insert needles deeper than necessary nor to insert too shallowly and fail to illicit a beneficial effect.

Next we will give pathologies that typically appear in certain organs or meridians in relation to symptom patterns. Then we will organize the symptom patterns, differentiating them according to symptom patterns in relation to organs and symptom patterns in relation to meridians.

When introducing certain symptom patterns we will also give the modern names of diseases and syndromes, since in our times many patients complain about specific illnesses. Of course, it is natural that certain illnesses will not always correspond to certain patterns of imbalance. But, knowing the modern medical names of some types of illnesses can be a useful reference for determining the pattern of imbalance.

Finally, we will include summary tables of symptom patterns of the internal, internal and external, and external areas, of pathology and symptom patterns of ki, blood, and fluids, and symptom patterns of the extraordinary vessels.

6.1 Yin and Yang: Deficiency/Excess and Cold/Heat

陰陽の虚実と寒熱

6.1.1 Pathology of Yang

① Yang Excess Patterns *Yō-Jitsu-Shō* 陽実証

Yang excess is a condition in which there is a repletion and stagnation of yang ki and the resultant profusion of heat in yang areas of the body such as the greater yang channel, yang brightness channel, fu organs, and Lung.

The Lung is hollow and as such is comparable to the fu organs. That is why a condition of heat stagnation in the Lung is also referred to as yang excess. Heat in the lesser yang channel is treated as yin excess since its influence reaches all the way to the reverting yin Liver channel.

An excess yang channel can result from Liver deficiency, Kidney deficiency, or Spleen deficiency, which are caused mainly by blood deficiency or a lack of fluids. But, these conditions are not referred to as yang excess since the primary factor is yin deficiency. These distinctions are made because the treatment methods vary depending on such distinctions.

Table 6–1: Yang Excess Patterns	
Yang Excess Symptom Patterns of the Yang Channel	Acute cases may present with an aversion to cold, fever, stiffness and pain in the nape of the neck, headache, lack of perspiration, and arthralgia. As a rule the organs due not show symptoms.
	Chronic cases may present with empyema, rhinitis, certain types of dermatosis, and neuralgia in the upper half of the body.
	Cases of heat in the yang brightness channel may present with inflammation and pain in the joints, a dry mouth, and dermatosis.
Yang Excess Symptom Patterns of the Fu Organs	Acute cases will present with heat and no aversion to cold, perspiration from the hands and feet with irritable restlessness, and delirious speech. There may be constipation with high fever in the afternoon.
	In chronic cases the patient may eat nonfood items, as well as eat huge amounts of food.
	There may be asthma, coughing, breathing trouble, and constipation in cases of yang excess of the Lung.
Pulse Condition	In cases of yang excess of the greater yang channel: floating, rapid, tight, and excess.
	In cases of heat in the yang brightness channel: floating and excess, or excess at the deep level.
	In cases of yang excess of the fu organs or Lung: slippery, excess, and rapid, all at the deep level.
Treatment Principles	After tonifying the deficient channel, do a general dispersion by shallowly needling with rapid insertion and removal.
Patterns of Imbalance	Lung deficiency greater yang channel excess heat pattern
	Lung deficiency yang brightness channel excess heat pattern
	Spleen deficiency yang brightness channel excess heat pattern
	Spleen deficiency Stomach excess heat pattern (including a Lung excess heat pattern)

② Yang Deficiency Patterns *Yō-Kyo-Shō* 陽虚証

Yang deficiency is a condition in which there is a relatively large amount of cold in the yang areas of the body due to a deficiency of yang ki. This condition is one in which deficiency of the yang ki of the organs and of the blood (which is the embodiment of the functioning of yang ki), manifests as cold in the yang areas of the body. It is not simply a deficiency of the yang ki of the yang channels but rather amounts to a condition of both yin and yang deficiency.

The progression of yang deficiency typically leads to yin exuberance (which is different from yin excess). The yin exuberance then causes cold to increase internally as well. The *Su Wen* expressed this as "yin exuberance internal cold."

Table 6–2: Yang Deficiency Patterns	
Symptom Patterns of Yang Deficiency	Acute cases may present with an aversion to cold, fever, headache, perspiration with an aversion to wind, frequent urination, loss of spirits, poor facial complexion, and cold feet. Chronic cases may present with a loss of appetite, diarrhea, sensitivity to cold, and cold hands and feet.
From Yang Deficiency to Yin Exuberance	The patient may only be aware of an aversion to cold, but taking their temperature will show a fever. There is no more perspiration. There is copious clear, whitish urine. There will be lientery (diarrhea containing incompletely digested material). The face may become reddish with an outbreak of fever if the cold becomes overly intense. This condition is called *true cold false heat* (真寒仮熱 *shinkan kanetsu*). The patient will by no means get out from the covers of his or her bed even though they have a fever, and will not drink even though they complain of thirst. When chronic cases go from yang deficiency to yin exuberance there may be diarrhea with a loss of appetite, a complete loss of spirits, and either copious urination or urinary difficulty.
Pulse Condition	In acute cases: floating, large, rapid, and deficient. In chronic cases: floating, large, and deficient (hollow). When the condition turns to yin exuberance these qualities will be seen together: soft, weak, thin, choppy, minute, and rapid or slow. A true cold false heat condition may present with the addition of a tight quality.
Treatment Principles	Use touch needling. Even only slightly deep needling can cause palpitations and irritable restlessness. As likely as not it would cause a greater aversion to wind and an increased temperature. Moxibustion is not appropriate for acute cases and must be used only with caution in chronic cases as it could cause an even greater loss of yang ki. Retention of needles must be applied with great caution.
Patterns of Imbalance	Lung deficiency cold pattern Spleen deficiency cold pattern Liver deficiency cold pattern Kidney deficiency cold pattern

6.1.2 Pathology of Yin

① Yin Excess Patterns *In-Jitsu-Shō* 陰実証

Chapter 62 of the *Su Wen* says, "What causes yin excess? Qibo answered, 'Unrestrained emotions cause yin ki to reverse and rise, which causes a deficiency in the Lower Warmer. Yang ki then rushes to the deficient Lower Warmer, and hence it is called excess'." This passage shows that yin excess is a stagnation and repletion of yang ki in the yin areas of the body, and is thus the opposite of yin exuberance internal cold. The yang ki of this passage actually refers to heat and blood. As was previously mentioned, blood also belongs to the yang aspect (yang within yin).

Table 6–3: Yin Excess Patterns	
Symptom Patterns of Liver Excess Heat	Alternating chills and fever, loss of appetite, constipation, a dry mouth, vomiting, and spontaneous pain in the thoracic rib cage area.
Symptom Patterns of Liver Excess	There could be stiffness from the area medial to the scapula up to the neck, pain in the upper abdomen, melancholia, spontaneous pain in the thoracic rib cage area, irregular menstruation, menstrual cramps, various gynecological diseases, and low back pain. The skin could be cold with a lot of heat in the organs, which can cause a hearty appetite, constipation, a dry mouth, and coldness in the lower half of the body with heat in the upper half.
Pulse Condition	Liver heat pulse wiry, rapid, and excess; or, rapid, choppy, and excess at the deep level. Liver excess pulse choppy, thin, and excess at the deep level.
Treatment Principles	Needles that are inserted shallowly and retained for long duration and deep needling are both effective. Moxa-on-the-handle needle and bloodletting can also be used. When using moxibustion use a lot on selected indurations.
Patterns of Imbalance	Spleen deficiency Liver excess heat pattern Spleen deficiency Liver excess pattern Lung deficiency Liver excess pattern

The Liver is responsible for causing the stagnation and repletion of blood and heat in the yin parts of the body. The fu organs and the Lung and Heart among the zang organs are yang areas, so heat in them would not be called yin excess. The Spleen does not take up heat and thus does not have the ability to cause stagnation of heat and blood. The Kidney stores the fluids, so adding heat to it only causes it to dry out but not to become excess. Therefore, the Liver is the only possibility for causing yin excess.

The Liver causes stagnation of blood because it stores the blood and because the functional property of gathering is at work in the reverting yin channel. Heat often accompanies the stagnation of blood.

② Yin Deficiency Patterns *In-Kyo-Shō* 陰虚証

Yin deficiency is a condition in which there is a deficiency of ki, blood, and fluids, which belong to the yin aspect, and an outbreak of heat. This heat is called deficient-type heat since it is produced from deficiency.

The heat that is produced internally tries to escape to the outside. The heat that goes to the outside spreads to other organs and meridians where it becomes heat in those areas and obstructs the circulation of ki and blood.

Table 6–4: Symptom Patterns of Yin Deficiency	
Symptom Patterns of Yin Deficiency	Red face, hot flushes, heat vexation in the hands and feet, tendency to perspire, hearty appetite with a tendency to constipation, abdominal pain, muscle aches, copious urination, lassitude, a dry mouth, edema.
Pulse Condition	The pulse could be floating or slightly floating. When it is floating the pulse could be large and powerful, or it could be large and slippery. It could also be tight at the deep level.
Treatment Principles	Retain needles at a general depth of 1–2 mm. Moxibustion can be used on areas with pain on pressure or indurations.
Patterns of Imbalance	Liver deficiency heat pattern Kidney deficiency heat pattern Spleen deficiency Stomach deficiency heat pattern

What causes yin excess? Qibo answered, "Unrestrained emotions cause yin ki to reverse and rise, which causes a deficiency in the Lower Warmer. Yang ki then rushes to the deficient Lower Warmer, and hence it is called excess. … Yang deficiency causes external cold. … Yin deficiency causes internal heat. … Abundant yang causes external heat. … Abundant yin causes internal cold." (*Su Wen*, Chapter 62)

6.1.3 Summary of Deficiency and Excess of Yin and Yang

Table 6–5 below summarizes yang excess, yang deficiency, yin excess, and yin deficiency. What is being shown here is a categorization of pathology based on passages from the *Su Wen*. It is not a grouping according to pulse qualities or symptom patterns.

To illustrate the difference, imagine for instance a pulse that is sinking and deficient. The sinking pulse represents yin and the deficient pulse indicates deficiency, so this would have been expressed as yin deficiency. Such a pulse would be seen with symptom patterns such as low spirits and general chills. In other words there would be a yin-type, deficient condition, and from that perspective it would be correct to label the condition as yin deficiency.

However, in classifying by pathology this condition would clearly be correctly labeled yang deficiency, which would be in accord with the *Su Wen*, because the pulse is sinking and deficient due to the relative increase of yin ki caused by the lack of yang ki and because of the presence of chills. Please keep this in mind as you look over the table.

Table 6–5: Deficiency and Excess of Yin and Yang		
	Deficiency	**Excess**
Yang (Heat)	Pulse: soft, weak, minute, thin, choppy, tight, slow, hollow, deficient, scattered, rapid, hasty	Pulse: floating, large, excess, flooding, rapid
	Acute heat conditions present with an aversion to cold but no fever, sensation of internal and external onset of coldness with low spirits, diarrhea, and loss of appetite	Acute heat conditions present either fever and an aversion to cold with no change in appetite, urination or defecation; or, fever, constipation, and delirious speech
	Tonify both yin and yang channels	Tonify the yin channel and disperse the yang channel
Yin (Cold)	Pulse: floating, large, slippery, deficient, wiry, moderate, hasty, rapid, leathery	Pulse: sinking, wiry, slippery, excess, slow, choppy, knotted, hidden
	Internal and external heat vexation, or cold lower limbs and hot flushes in the upper body; tendency toward constipation; good appetite	Acute heat conditions present with alternating chills and fever with no appetite, cold body surface but abundant internal heat, or tendency toward constipation, hearty appetite
	Tonify the yin channel, and sometimes disperse the yang channel	Tonify the yin channel and disperse the yin channel

6.2.1 Pathologies of the Liver and Gallbladder

A Liver deficiency pattern refers to a condition in which there is a deficiency of the essential ki of the Liver as well as a deficiency of the blood stored by the Liver due to any of a number of etiologies. Within a Liver deficiency pattern there could be a heat pattern or a cold pattern.

A Liver excess pattern refers to a condition in which there is heat due to stagnation of the blood of the Liver. Within a Liver excess pattern there could be a Liver excess heat pattern or a Liver excess pattern that developed along with blood stasis. Spleen deficiency causes the Liver excess heat pattern. The Liver excess due to blood stasis can be caused by either Spleen deficiency or Lung deficiency.

① Liver Deficiency Heat Pattern

A Liver deficiency heat pattern refers to a condition in which heat is generated when there is a deficiency of fluids of the Kidney at the same time as a deficiency of fluids in the Liver blood. This condition is also called yin deficiency or blood deficiency. The heat that is generated is called deficient-type heat because it results from the deficiency of fluids.

Because heat naturally radiates to the outside and to the Upper Warmer, deficient-type heat, apart from affecting the Kidney and Liver channels, can spread to all the organs and other channels with the possibility of bringing about a whole array of symptom patterns.

There will be heat vexation in the soles of the feet and the pulse will be sinking and hard when there is an excess of deficient-type heat in the Kidney channel due to a lack of fluids.

Insomnia, excessive dreaming, and irritability result from an abundance of deficient-type heat in the Liver channel due to blood deficiency.

The Gallbladder channel is the meridian most easily affected by heat. When there is an abundance of heat in the Gallbladder channel the patient may have cramping tension in the channel and complain of migraine headaches or stiffness in the neck. The pulse will be distinctly felt at the superficial level and may sometimes be excessive. That is why a Liver deficiency heat pattern is also expressed as a Liver deficiency Gallbladder excess pattern.

There is a sudden rush of overcoming warmth when heat appears in the Gallbladder channel. But since it is deficient-type heat, cooling will follow upon the release of some of this heat. This cooling triggers a shivering tremor through the body. Such symptom patterns represent the subjective feeling of alternating chills and heat.

The same alternation of chills and heat will appear in an acute case of Liver excess heat. However, the fever will be detectable by thermometer as well as being a subjective symptom.

Palpitations, chest pain, heat vexation in the palms, as well as increased blood pressure can occur when heat spreads to the Heart. In this case the pulse will be strong at the left distal position.

Coughing and asthma may result from the spread of heat to the Lung. The coughing will be especially bad during the middle of the night. The pulse will be strong at the right distal position.

Abnormalities associated with urination, such as cystitis, urethritis, or prostatomegaly, may develop if heat increases in the Bladder.

A large appetite with constipation may result from the spread of heat to the Stomach and Intestines.

Additionally, the spreading of heat to the meridians will impair the circulation of ki and blood in those channels and may cause the formation of indurations, muscle aches, and neuralgia. The exact locations affected by heat are identified through palpatory pulse and abdominal diagnoses in addition to symptom differentiation. The location should be simple to determine if the individual pulse qualities of the six pulse positions are carefully examined.

② Liver Deficiency Cold Pattern

This pattern of imbalance is one in which cold is produced by deficiency of fluids of the Kidney and yang ki of the life gate along with an actual depletion of the blood of the Liver. The overall pulse is weak. This pattern can alternatively be referred to as a deficiency of both yin and yang, yang deficiency, or as blood collapse (i.e., severe blood loss).

The cold that is produced will predominately affect the areas controlled by the Kidney and Liver channels, but symptoms will also appear with the spread of cold to the other meridians and organs.

If the entire body gets chilled, that is, should the yang ki of the body entirely vanish, death will follow. Therefore, in actuality some heat will be retained in the Upper Warmer (i.e., the Pericardium and Lung). This heat will bring about symptoms, but it should not be removed by dispersion since it was pushed up to the Upper Warmer by the cold.

The condition given above is one in which the body is cold from the Middle Warmer down and hot in the Upper Warmer, and as such could alternatively be described as an absence of exchange between the yin and yang of the upper and lower portions of the body. An abrupt cessation of exchange between the yin and yang of the upper and lower portions of the body may result in fever and an aversion to cold with vomiting and diarrhea.

If the Kidney becomes chilled the Bladder will also become chilled. This may cause low back pain and copious urination, and possibly a loss of the ability to forcefully expel urine.

The menstrual period will be accompanied by diarrhea if the Liver becomes chilled. At this time the yang ki of the Gallbladder will also be depleted, resulting in poor decision making ability, jumpiness, and a tendency to frequently sigh.

If cold spreads to the Stomach and Intestines the patient will be able to eat despite having a poor appetite. There is also the possibility of developing such disorders as chronic diarrhea, ulcerative colitis, or Crohn's disease.

If a lot of heat is forced up to the Heart and Pericardium by cold, it may cause chest pain, palpitations, arrhythmia, or similar problems.

It is also possible for heat to build up in the Lung, which may cause a sore throat, hot flushes, and coughing.

③ Spleen Deficiency Liver Excess Heat Pattern

Heat that occurs due to an acute febrile disease is not serious as long as it remains in the greater yang and yang brightness channels, but if not appropriately treated the heat may invade the lesser yang channels, the Gallbladder, the reverting yin Liver channel, and even the Liver itself. Such a condition is known as a lesser yang disease.

Since the lesser yang channel is close to the fu organs, if heat enters that channel it readily becomes Gallbladder heat. A bitter taste in the mouth and nausea develop when the heat in the Gallbladder increases. There is also the possibility of developing such problems as tympanitis, cholecystitis (inflammation of the gallbladder), or cholelithiasis (gallstones).

When there is an increase of heat in the Gallbladder the neighboring Stomach and Intestines will take on heat, which occurs because of a deficiency in the essential ki of the Spleen. At the same time, the heat from the Stomach and Intestines will dry up the fluids of the Spleen. An abnormal increase of heat in the Stomach and Intestines causes a loss of appetite, constipation, and a dry mouth. Furthermore, the fever will go up from the afternoon onward. Such a pattern of imbalance should be treated as a Spleen deficiency Liver excess heat pattern.

The reason the heat can penetrate all the way to the Liver is because the heat will be gathered towards the Liver in the same manner that the Liver gathers the blood in performing its natural function of storing the blood, and because the functional property of gathering is at work within the Liver channel. Heat that has invaded the Liver will at times show up in the lesser yang channel. At that time fever goes up, and as heat increases in the reverting yin channel heat, it decreases in the lesser yang channel, causing an aversion to cold. This is referred to as alternating chills and fever. Such a condition can be seen in those with an acute liver problem.

Moreover, the menstrual period may suddenly begin if heat goes all the way to the Liver. Conversely, if a fever develops during the menstrual period it should be considered as Liver excess heat. If the fever is temporarily alleviated with an antipyretic, menstrual cramps could develop from the next menstrual period onward.

It is possible for the Liver heat to enter the Lung, in which case there will be a cough which could worsen to become asthma, pneumonia, or pleurisy.

Liver heat may also spread to the Kidney or Bladder, in which case the fever will be accompanied by urinary difficulty. Acute cystitis, pyelitis, or acute nephritis may result.

Apart from the above there is a possibility of heat spreading to all the channels. It is likely that there will be cramping pain along the meridians in which an abundance of heat has gathered. The pulses of the meridians and organs that contain an abundance of heat will be strong.

④ **Liver Excess Patterns**

There are three types of Liver excess patterns.

One is a pattern in which there is a lot of blood stasis in the subcostal area, which can be caused by factors including bruises sustained in traffic accidents or falls, visceral problems such as hepatitis, and as well surgical operations, recurrent febrile disease (old Liver excess heat), or holding in one's anger.

There is a tendency to become gloomy when there is blood stasis in the subcostal area, which can cause a loss of vitality and a likelihood of getting stiff muscles between the neck and medial aspect of the scapula. There is also a strong possibility of getting stomach or duodenal ulcers. This pattern of imbalance is also apparent in cases of chronic hepatitis.

Because blood stasis is the primary pathology in this pattern of imbalance, with little influence from heat or cold, there is a concern that it will obstruct the circulation of ki and blood in all the organs and channels. This pattern should be treated as a Spleen deficiency Liver excess pattern.

In the second type of Liver excess pattern there is a lot of blood stasis in the lower abdomen. This is often seen in young women. Blood stasis in the lower abdomen can be caused by menstrual irregularities and an unbalanced diet.

This pattern is classified as a Spleen deficiency Liver excess pattern since that is the pattern that the pulse quality shows. However, even though it is called Spleen deficiency, there is no symptom pattern of the Stomach. However, there are gynecological abnormalities due to blood stasis, skin problems, and also constipation and hemorrhoids.

In this pattern as well there is little effect due to cold and heat since the primary pathology is blood stasis, but there is the possibility of a disruption of the circulation of ki and blood in all the organs and meridians.

The other type of Liver excess pattern is one that is common in people who have a lot of old blood stasis. This condition is treated not as Spleen deficiency, but rather as a Lung deficiency Liver excess pattern.

This pattern is one in which there is a deterioration in the circulation of Lung ki and a loss of moisture from the Liver blood due to a deficiency of fluids of the Kidney, which causes a stagnation of blood and then blood stasis. There will be a lot of blood stasis in the subcostal area and the lower abdomen, and the patient could have a chronic disorder.

Characteristic symptom patterns include such things as stiffness from the area medial to the scapula up to the neck, melancholy, constipation, cold lower limbs and hot flushes in the upper body, unstable neurosis, and palpitations. Additionally, this pattern could be apparent in people with hypertension, diabetes, heart disease, chronic hepatitis, trigeminal neuralgia, various tumors, various eye problems, atopic dermatitis, various women's diseases, and obesity. Because this pattern of imbalance is a blood stasis pattern there is the possibility of influence on all the organs and meridians.

The conditions given above are for chronic patterns of imbalance, but there are also patterns for acute cases of Lung deficiency Liver excess, in which the patient could complain of such things as an aversion to cold, fever, night sweats, diarrhea, or cold feet. Some people will have hepatitis, tuberculosis, or abnormalities of the thyroid gland.

6.2.2 Symptom Patterns of the Liver and Liver Channel

① Meridian-Associated Symptom Patterns

Headache; dizziness on standing up; vertigo; hardness of hearing; epilepsy; difficulty moving the tongue; low back pain; cramps or pain in the thoracic rib cage area, flanks, and inguinal region; pain upon bending the knees; muscle cramps; paralysis; shakes (hemiparalysis, Parkinson's disease); cramps along the inner thigh; swelling or a twitch in or swelling of the testes (inguinal hernia); distension of the lower abdomen (including conditions such as menstrual cramps and irregular menstruation in women); cold feet; a discolored patch on the face; itchiness in the groin.

② Organ-Associated Symptom Patterns

Anger; fear; hives; nosebleeds; body fever; frequent desire to lie down; enuresis (bed wetting); anuria (prostatomegaly or urethritis); loss of vitality; yellowish urination; diabetes; a dry mouth; diarrhea; abdominal distension; dry heaving; a feeling of oppression in the chest; nausea with a congested feeling in the epigastric area; a bitter taste in the mouth; vomiting.

6.2.3 Symptom Patterns of the Gallbladder and Gallbladder Channel

① Meridian-Associated Symptom Patterns

Headache; hardness of hearing; pain in the outer canthus of the eye; pain in the jaw; swelling and pain in ST-12; lymphadenitis of the cervical lymph nodes; swelling in the subcostal area; pain in the lateral sides of the chest that prevents one from rolling over while in bed; low back pain; pain in the lateral side of the hip joint; pain in the lateral side of the knee; a warm feeling along the lateral side of the lower limbs; pain between GB-40 and GB-41; difficulty moving the fourth toe; paralysis of the legs; cold feet; a discolored patch on the face with loss of luster.

② **Organ-Associated Symptom Patterns**

Aversion to meeting people; timidity and shyness; sighing; chest pain; a sick feeling in the epigastric area; vomiting bitter gastric juices; a bitter taste in the mouth.

6.3   The Heart and Small Intestine   心と小腸

6.3.1 Pathology of the Heart and Small Intestine

It has already been pointed out that there are no patterns of imbalance that arise from Heart deficiency. Therefore, all pathology and symptom patterns related to the Heart result from cold and heat that has spread from other patterns of imbalance. It has also been noted that the Heart is an organ that has an abundance of yang ki. Therefore, it is understood that pathology of the Heart is related to a deficiency or excess of yang ki.

① **Pathology and Symptom Patterns of Heart Heat**

The most common cause of Heart heat is Kidney deficiency. Heat in the Heart increases relative to Kidney deficiency since it is the Kidney, with all its body fluids and yin ki, that normally keeps heat in check throughout the body. Likewise, the yin ki of the Kidney and the yang ki of the Heart exchange yin and yang between the upper and lower halves of the body, so it is only natural that if one [i.e., the Kidney] becomes deficient then the other [i.e., the Heart] will see an increase in heat.

It is also possible for heat symptom patterns to manifest when heat produced by a Liver deficiency heat pattern spreads to the Heart. This was covered in the section on Liver deficiency heat pattern. Heart heat resulting from Liver deficiency is unmistakably indicated by soreness along the Gallbladder channel when there is high blood pressure, palpitations, and a rapid pulse. In this case the Gallbladder channel should be dispersed after tonifying the Liver channel.

In a Liver deficiency cold pattern the body is cold below the level of the middle warmer and there is an abundance of heat in the chest. However, the heat is less than that of a Liver deficiency heat pattern. Also, there will still be symptom patterns such as palpitations, an oppressed feeling in the chest, and arrhythmia. In this case you should tonify both the Liver and Gallbladder channels.

It is also possible to get Heart heat from Spleen deficiency. In this pattern of imbalance there is an abundance of heat in the Stomach due to the Spleen deficiency. That heat becomes heat in the Small Intestine and then affects the Heart. Thus, accurately this should be called Small Intestine heat, and it commonly causes constipation or febrile diarrhea. When the heat spreads to the Heart it causes high blood pressure and a reddish face and tongue. The Small Intestine is part of the bowels, and symptom patterns of the Small Intestine such as abdominal pain and diarrhea are commonly treated as indicating a Spleen deficiency.

② **Pathology and Symptom Patterns of Heart Cold**

There are cases when there is a loss of yang ki of the Heart and the patient complains of such things as chest pain, shortness of breath, and an oppressed feeling in the chest. If the patient has consulted a Western medical practitioner and there is no concern that the condition is a heart attack, then it should be treated as a Spleen deficiency cold pattern. The reason there is a lack of yang ki of the Heart is because of a decline in the production of ki, blood, and fluids by the Spleen and Stomach. Naturally, there is a loss of yang ki of the Small Intestine as well when there is a loss of yang ki of the Heart. This also should be treated as a Spleen deficiency cold pattern.

6.3.2 Symptom Patterns of the Heart and Heart Channel

① **Meridian-Associated Symptom Patterns**

Pain in the sides of the rib cage; pain in the subcostal area; pain in the area where the Heart channel flows from the upper arm to the lower arm; heat in the palms; perspiration and an aversion to wind.

② **Organ-Associated Symptom Patterns**

Shortness of breath, heart pain, and an oppressed feeling in the chest; a dry mouth; hiccups; laughter without a reason; feeling of obstruction in the epigastric area; speech disorders; epilepsy; reddish face; yellowish eyes.

6.3.3 Symptom Patterns of the Small Intestine and Small Intestine Channel

① Meridian-Associated Symptom Patterns

Swollen cheeks; sore throat; hardness of hearing; swollen jaw; inability to rotate the neck due to stiffness; pain in the shoulder as if it were out of joint; pain in the area where the Small Intestine channel flows from the upper arm to the lower arm; warts.

② Organ-Associated Symptom Patterns

Passing of gas when coughing; intestinal sounds; diarrhea that afterwards leaves a dull ache in the lower abdomen and rectum (*rikyūkōjū*, 裏急後重); abdominal pain; belching; a feeling of obstruction in the epigastric area; yellowish eyes; insomnia; reddish face.

6.4 The Pericardium and Triple Warmer 心包と三焦

6.4.1 Pathology of the Pericardium and Triple Warmer

As was previously mentioned, the yang ki of the Heart emerges into the Pericardium. It then functions in the areas of the Triple Warmer by circulating throughout the body. That is why the Pericardium and Triple Warmer are in a paired relationship.

The heat and cold symptom patterns manifested by the Pericardium should be thought of as the same as those of the Heart. However, the treatment consists of tonifying or dispersing the Pericardium channel.

Supposing that the Kidney was deficient and the left distal pulse position was strong and that there were symptoms such as palpitations, then the Heart heat should be reduced by dispersing the Pericardium channel. On the other hand, if the left distal pulse position was deficient and there were palpitations, this would be thought of as Spleen deficiency and treated by tonifying the Pericardium channel. In short, the Pericardium channel is the treatment location for symptom patterns of the Heart.

The Triple Warmer channel reflects any increase of heat in the Heart or the Pericardium. Furthermore, the Triple Warmer channel can also be used to adjust cold and heat in any of the organs and meridians.

For example, when there is an abundance of heat in the Gallbladder channel, heat will also increase in the Triple Warmer channel, both channels of which are lesser yang channels. Likewise, when heat increases in the Stomach, there will also be an increase of heat in the Triple Warmer channel. Conversely, in the case of a body-wide deficiency of yang ki with a cold pattern and a simultaneous stagnation of water, the Triple Warmer channel is still used for treatment.

6.4.2 Symptom Patterns of the Pericardium and Pericardium Channel

① Meridian-Associated Symptom Patterns

Swelling below the axilla; cramping tension in the area where the Pericardium channel flows through the elbow; heat in the palms; a feeling of congestion in the chest as if the thoracic rib cage area were being pushed upwards.

② Organ-Associated Symptom Patterns

Laughter without a reason; heart pain; oppressed feeling in the chest; palpitations; reddish face; yellowish eyes.

6.4.3 Symptom Patterns of the Triple Warmer and Triple Warmer Channel

① Meridian-Associated Symptom Patterns

Pain in the outer canthus of the eyes; hardness of hearing; ringing in the ears; pain behind the ears; pain in the cheeks; a swollen and sore throat; pain along the Triple Warmer channel where it flows through the shoulder, upper arm, elbow, forearm, and fourth finger; curling of the tongue; pain along the Triple Warmer channel so that the hands cannot be raised up (as in fifty-year-old's shoulder); perspiration (due to the deficiency of surface yang ki).

② Organ-Associated Symptom Patterns

Dry mouth; oppressed feeling in the chest; distended abdomen; enuresis; anuria; abdominal edema.

6.5.1   Pathology of the Spleen and Stomach

A Spleen deficiency pattern is a condition in which the essential ki of the Spleen is deficient and in which there is a deficiency of the ki, blood, and fluids of the Spleen due to any of several causes. Within the category of a Spleen deficiency pattern there is a Spleen deficiency heat pattern and a Spleen deficiency cold pattern. The Spleen deficiency heat pattern can be further divided into a Spleen deficiency yang brightness channel excess heat pattern, a Spleen deficiency Stomach excess heat pattern, and a Spleen deficiency Stomach deficiency heat pattern. Additionally, there is also a Spleen deficiency Liver excess heat pattern, and Spleen deficiency Liver excess pattern, but these have already been described.

① Spleen Deficiency Yang Brightness Channel Excess Heat Pattern

This pattern refers to a condition in which deficiency of the yin ki of the Spleen has enabled heat to build up in the yang brightness channel, and dampness (i.e., stagnant water) to accumulate. This pattern of imbalance becomes apparent when there are such disorders as arthritis, rheumatism, and viral warts. There will generally be little urination, and defecation will be easy. Because the heat is only in the channel and does not spread to the Stomach or Intestines, there should be no change in appetite.

This pattern may begin with an aversion to cold or fever. But in any case there will commonly be an increase of heat in the afternoon and a worsening of pain at this time. This is because the ki of the yang brightness channel becomes active after 3:00 P.M., but because it does not become active enough to push heat and water out of the body, ki will then stagnate in the channel, causing fever and pain. If this heat in the yang brightness channel enters the Lung it can cause deformations in the joints that are difficult to cure.

② Spleen Deficiency Stomach Excess Heat Pattern

This is a pattern in which heat, which is generated in the external aspects of the body due to Lung deficiency, becomes stagnant and replete in the fu organs, primarily the Stomach and Intestines (but including the Lung) due to the deficiency of yin ki of the Spleen. When there is substantial heat in the Stomach and Intestines, an aversion to cold disappears and the patient suffers from heat in the body and may have delirious speech. There will also be perspiration from the hands and feet, and in the evening fever will gradually increase like the rising of the tide. In herbal therapy this would be a condition for which the use of a purgative would be appropriate.

This pattern of imbalance is not often seen in the acupuncture clinic. However, some patients do present with constitutional Stomach excess heat. They may present with such symptom patterns as eating inedible substances, perspiration, constipation, a voracious appetite, mania, and a desire to disrobe, all of which are due to a repletion of heat in the Stomach and Intestines. This Stomach excess heat may spread to any other organ or meridian.

③ Spleen Deficiency Stomach Deficiency Heat Pattern

In this pattern there is substantial heat in the Stomach and Intestines, but in this case the heat has arisen due to deficiency of the fluids of the Spleen. Thus, the difference between this pattern and Stomach excess heat is one of deficiency versus excess. In the case of deficient-type heat there will be lethargy either of the whole body or of the extremities, abdominal pain with diarrhea or constipation, and fluctuations in the appetite. The sense of taste will be quite diminished, and the patient may develop a toothache or hemorrhoids. This heat may also spread to any other organ or meridian. While there are certain differences in symptom pattern due to deficiency or excess, there are no essential differences due to the spread of heat when there is Stomach excess heat or Stomach deficiency heat.

Stomach heat may spread to the Liver or Gallbladder resulting in a Spleen deficiency Liver excess heat pattern, which was explained above. However, it is not always necessary to disperse the Liver channel, as it is sometimes sufficient to simply tonify and disperse the Gallbladder channel. People with this pattern often complain of such disorders as tympanitis, cholecystitis (inflammation of the gallbladder), hepatitis, and cholelithiasis (gallstones).

If the heat spreads to the Heart and Small Intestine there will be an increase in the amount of Heart heat. Symptom patterns include laughter without a reason, a feeling of congestion in the epigastric region and oppression in the chest after eating, nosebleeds, hot flushes, and insomnia. Additionally, there is a tendency to go insane, and to develop hypertension, somatitis, gingivitis, and glossitis.

The heat can spread to and fill the Lungs themselves, becoming Lung excess heat. Yet even if the heat does not reach that point, there will still be heat in and drying of the Lung.

The patient may complain of an oppressed feeling in the chest, a dry throat and cough with blood-streaked phlegm, asthma, pleurisy, pneumonia, pulmonary emphysema, lymphadenitis, hives, thyroiditis, or collagen disease.

Urinary abnormalities will appear if the heat extends to the Kidney and Bladder. In this case there will be a tendency to develop such disorders as kidney stones, nephritis, nephrosis, cystitis, pyelitis, and nocturnal enuresis.

④ Spleen Deficiency Cold Pattern

This pattern refers to a condition in which there is Stomach cold due to the simultaneous deficiency of the blood and fluids of the Spleen and yang ki of the Stomach.

The whole body becomes cold when there is a decrease in the production of ki, blood, and fluids due to a lack of yang ki of the Stomach. Sometimes the yang ki in the yang brightness channel will not be greatly affected. But, since it cannot interact with the Stomach, it can cause vomiting, diarrhea, and headaches. If the yang ki of the whole body becomes completely depleted the result is death. In order for the patient to stay alive there will still be some heat retained in the chest even though the whole body becomes cold.

The lips will be white, and there will be copious saliva and no appetite due to the chilled Stomach. Yet since there is no heat, the sense of taste will not be impaired. Additional symptom patterns include stomachache, abdominal pain, diarrhea, low spirits, hypotension, and a feeling of constriction in the epigastric region.

There is a tendency to lose yang ki of the life gate when there is a Spleen deficiency cold pattern. But it can also be said that the lack of yang ki of the Stomach is due to an insufficiency of the yang ki of the life gate, as the existence of these two facets of yang ki are interdependent. That is, a decrease in one will lead to a decrease in the other. Also, it is common for a Kidney deficiency cold pattern to accompany a Spleen deficiency cold pattern because the yang ki of the life gate is dependent on the Kidney. Moreover, there will be difficult urination because the yang ki of the life gate is insufficient, which leads to water accumulation in the Stomach. In short, a Spleen deficiency cold pattern is a pattern in which there is excess water in the Stomach. This gives rise to such symptoms as dizziness, vomiting, and diarrhea.

The cold from a Spleen deficiency cold pattern may affect other organs and meridians.

Dizziness or feeling faint upon standing up will result if there is coldness of the Liver and Gallbladder. There will also be a tendency toward hemorrhaging and insomnia because of blood deficiency that results from Spleen deficiency.

The spread of cold to the Heart is the same as the loss of yang ki of the Heart, as was previously mentioned. Possible symptoms include palpitations, shortness of breath, a feeling as if there were a blockage in the chest, and pain in the chest that radiates to the back. In this case heart pain can be life-threatening.

Coughing and asthma may result if cold spreads to the Lung, but for the most part asthma results from the stagnation of water in the Stomach.

A chilled Kidney can cause diarrhea without abdominal pain. When the Bladder becomes chilled there will be copious urination or loss of the ability to forcefully expel urine. The patient will have little vitality. They will have diarrhea on the day following sexual intercourse.

6.5.2 Symptom Patterns of the Spleen and Spleen Channel

① Meridian-Associated Symptom Patterns

Stiffening of the root of the tongue; a feeling of fatigue throughout the body; lack of strength in the extremities; cold hands and feet; swelling of the medial aspect of the knee upon standing for longer than one can handle; loss of ability to move the big toes; edema of the lower limbs; painful swelling of the cheeks and jaw; heavy-headed feeling; low back pain.

② Organ-Associated Symptom Patterns

Inability to hold down one's food; stomachache; abdominal distension; intestinal sounds; abdominal pain; belching; pain and a congested feeling in the epigastric region; loss of appetite; diarrhea (mucous stool); relief from the above symptoms upon defecation or passing gas; lack of urination; jaundice; insomnia; loss of vitality; feeling of oppression in the chest.

6.5.3 Symptom Patterns of the Stomach and Stomach Channel

① Meridian-Associated Symptom Patterns

Swollen and painful knees; pain along the Stomach channel from the breast to the inguinal area, thigh, lower leg, and second toe; low back pain; Bell's palsy; a rash around the lips; swelling and pain in the neck and throat (tonsillitis); an aversion to cold and then later fever; illnesses with fever but no aversion to cold (excess of internal heat); perspiration and sweaty hands and feet; nosebleeds.

② Organ-Associated Symptom Patterns

State of emotional depression (aversion to cold, groaning, yawning, darkened face, aversion to people, surprise at sudden noises, hiding away with doors and windows closed; manic-depressive state (climbing to high places, going naked, singing, milling about), abdominal distension, intestinal rumblings, abdominal pain, constipation, diarrhea (in which a heat pattern is indicated by diarrhea that brings relief; heat on the anterior surface of the body, abnormal increase in appetite, and yellow urine when the Stomach and Stomach channel become excess (i.e., have an abundance of heat), facial edema, loss of appetite, abdominal edema, yellowish skin; shivering cold on the anterior surface of the body and heavy, bloated abdomen when the Stomach or Stomach channel become deficient (i.e., have an abundance of cold).

6.6   The Lung and Large Intestine   肺と大腸

6.6.1 Pathology of the Lung and Large Intestine

An aversion to cold will arise when there is poor circulation of yang ki, which can occur when there is an invasion by external pathogenic factors (mainly wind or cold) while there is weak release and circulation of yang ki due to a deficiency of Lung ki. Following that, there will generally be an outbreak of fever due to the stagnation of the yang ki that stopped circulating. At this time there may be symptoms such as headache, arthralgia, and an absence of sweating or unnaturally profuse sweating.

The symptom patterns and pathologies given above can, by incorrect treatment or natural processes, develop into either of two broad categories. One is a pattern that has an abundance of heat, and the other is a pattern that has an abundance of cold. The former would be a Lung deficiency heat pattern, and the latter a Lung deficiency cold pattern.

However, a Lung deficiency heat pattern does not mean that there is heat in the Lung itself; it is a pattern in which heat has stagnated and become replete in the greater yang channel (Bladder and Small Intestine channels) and the yang brightness channel (Stomach and Large Intestine channels). Therefore, this pattern is called a Lung deficiency yang channel excess heat pattern. It is treated by dispersing the yang channels, but only after first tonifying the Lung channel to address any remaining aversion to cold.

A Lung deficiency cold pattern refers to a condition in which the illness progresses mainly with cold-related symptom patterns appearing, although there could be fever during the initial stage. Therefore, this pattern could very well be called a Lung deficiency yang channel deficiency heat pattern. But since both the Lung channel and the yang channels are tonified, and since the cold can progress all the way into an invasion of the Lung itself, these points are taken to be included in the term Lung deficiency cold pattern.

Treating Lung deficiency can relieve cold and heat symptom patterns of the Large Intestine or Large Intestine channel, but these are commonly treated as Spleen deficiency.

① Lung Deficiency Yang Channel Excess Heat Pattern

The yang ki in the external aspects of the body is diminished when there is poor circulation and release of Lung ki, and the yang ki that is not released stagnates concurrently in the external areas. As a result an aversion to cold and fever will develop. There will be a lack of perspiration, and coughing, arthralgia, and headache will arise. The pulse will be floating, rapid, and tight.

Heat that has stagnated in the external areas will be transmitted from the greater yang channel to the yang brightness channel. Heat in the yang brightness channel will cause drying of the nose, sore eyes, stiffness and pain in the nape of the neck, and a sore throat. The pulse will be floating, large, rapid, and excessive.

It is also possible for yang brightness channel excess heat to occur as a chronic illness. This time the nose will be blocked (empyema or rhinitis), and there will be stiffness of the shoulders and neck muscles, and neuralgia in the upper body.

② Lung Deficiency Cold Pattern

An aversion to cold will arise when there is poor circulation and release of yang ki due to a deficiency of Lung ki. Immediately thereafter, the yang ki that cannot be released from the body usually stagnates and causes fever. Moreover, there will be a tendency to perspire since there was a deficiency of yang ki to begin with. The pulse will be floating, rapid, and moderate.

At this stage, if there is a large accumulation of stagnated heat there will be a progression into a Lung deficiency yang channel excess heat pattern, as previously described, if there is a large accumulation of stagnated heat. Yet in many cases there is not much stagnation of yang ki, and there are often cold-related symptom patterns due to yang deficiency. For instance, such symptoms can include cold feet, increased perspiration, and frequent urination.

If yang ki is further depleted, perspiration will cease and only an aversion to cold will remain. There will be a loss of spirit and the person will go to sleep. There will also be copious whitish, clear urination. At this stage of a cold pattern the pulse will be sinking and weak.

If there is an ever further depletion of yang ki, the hands and feet will become extremely cold and there will be lientery. On the other hand, there will occasionally be an outbreak of fever, which would indicate the condition known as true cold false heat.

During a cold pattern in which the Lung itself is chilled, the whole body will become cold, and the patient will develop a cough. An aversion to cold and fever will be absent. Even having just a runny nose, light cough, and sore throat could indicate a Lung deficiency cold pattern. In this case the pulse is often weak or minute.

6.6.2 Symptom Patterns of the Lung and Lung Channel

① Meridian-Associated Symptom Patterns

Aversion to cold; aversion to wind; fever; stiffness and pain in the nape of the neck; headache; fever with low back pain or arthralgia; unnaturally profuse sweating or an absence of sweating; runny nose; stuffy nose.

Cold and pain along the Lung channel from the upper arm to the lower arm; heat in the palms; cold and pain in the shoulders and upper back; pain in the supraclavicular fossa; dermatosis.

② Organ-Associated Symptom Patterns

A feeling of expansion of the chest with coughing and difficulty breathing which in severe cases elicits pressing of the chest with both hands; a rush of blood to the head after a coughing fit; blood in the saliva.

Dry mouth; feeling of oppression in the chest; inability to take a deep breath; shortness of breath; nausea after a coughing fit; sore throat; hemorrhoids; lower abdominal pain; pain in the ileocecum; melancholy; frequent urination, but with little volume; whitish urine.

6.6.3 Symptom Patterns of the Large Intestine and Large Intestine Channel

① Meridian-Associated Symptom Patterns

Toothache; swollen neck; yellowish eyes; runny nose; nosebleeds; swollen and sore throat; eye problems; dermatosis.

Pain along the Large Intestine channel from the shoulder to the forearm; difficulty using the index finger; heat and swelling through the Large Intestine channel (in an excess condition); an aversion to cold with the inability to warm up (in a deficiency condition).

② Organ-Associated Symptom Patterns

Intestinal sounds (coldness of the intestines); abdominal pain; dry mouth; stool leakage upon coughing.

6.7   The Kidney and Bladder   腎と膀胱

6.7.1 Pathology of the Kidney and Bladder

The Kidney contains yin ki and is firmed by fluids. At the same time it also contains the yang ki of the life gate so that it does not become chilled with an overabundance of fluids. Therefore, pathology of the Kidney can be thought of in three types: deficiency of yin ki of the Kidney, deficiency of fluids of the Kidney, and deficiency of yang ki of the life gate.

Heat is generated when there is a deficiency of either yin ki or body fluids. Such a condition is called a Kidney deficiency heat pattern. The heat is naturally deficient-type heat. Conversely, coldness is caused by a deficiency of the yang ki of the life gate. Such a condition is called a Kidney deficiency cold pattern.

① Kidney Deficiency Heat Pattern

This pattern of imbalance is one in which a deficiency of Kidney fluids generates deficient-type heat. After Kidney deficiency, the pattern of imbalance will subsequently go through a variety of transformations.

A Liver deficiency heat pattern results when an insufficiency of fluids in the Liver blood is caused by an insufficiency of Kidney fluids. People with constitutional blood stasis readily develop Lung deficiency Liver excess when deficient-type heat is generated by an insufficiency of Kidney fluids. These patterns of imbalance were already explained, but they are mentioned here because they contain some of the pathology and symptom patterns of a Kidney deficiency heat pattern.

When deficient-type heat is produced by an insufficiency of Kidney fluids, there is a tendency to have heat vexation in the soles of the feet and to perspire from the upper body, since heat naturally radiates to the surface of the body and to the Upper Warmer. In such a case the patient may eat a lot but still be slim. However, since the heat is deficient-type heat, if the Kidney deficiency continues for a long time, the surface of the body will tend to become cold even though there is internal heat. This can result in the appearance of symptoms such as pain in the calcaneal tendon, pain in the heel, weak legs, low back pain, nocturnal urination, and loss of vitality.

A Kidney deficiency heat pattern results partly because of a deficiency of yin ki. If this deficiency of yin ki becomes more prominent than the deficiency of Kidney fluids, it causes the running piglet condition, which can be felt as as the sensation of an explosive upsurge of yang ki from the Lower Warmer to the Upper Warmer.

Moreover, the patient may become corpulent if there is a weakening of the contractile or firming power of the Kidney. The deficient-type heat that is produced from yin deficiency heats up the Stomach, causing a robust appetite that accelerates the weight gain.

A patient will perspire if there is a large amount of deficient-type heat leaving the body. However, if there is not enough heat to cause sweating, water is just pushed to the external areas of the body, which is known as a water-ki disease. This is the reason why so many people with Kidney deficiency are overweight.

The heat that is generated in a Kidney deficiency heat pattern can spread to the Lung, Heart, Liver, or other organs or meridians.

Should the heat spread to the Liver, it may cause Liver excess or Liver deficiency. If it goes to the Lung, it may cause coughing or asthma. If it affects the Heart, the patient may develop hypertension. If the Bladder takes on the heat, it may result in copious urination.

② Kidney Deficiency Cold Pattern

This pattern of imbalance is a condition in which the yang ki of the life gate is deficient. This condition can also be described as one in which yang ki cannot be transmitted to the Kidney because a deficiency of yang ki of the Lung causes a lack of yang ki in the Bladder channel. Of course, in Kidney deficiency there is also a deficiency of Kidney fluids, which contributes to the loss of yang ki.

A Kidney deficiency cold pattern may originate as a Spleen deficiency cold pattern or a Lung deficiency cold pattern, or it could also arise directly from an insufficiency of yang ki of the Kidney if that insufficiency of yang ki has become predominant.

People with this pattern of imbalance will have a lack of spirits and vitality even though they present no particular illness. There may be a leakage of semen, copious urination, and constipation accompanied by low back pain that is characterized by a heavy feeling in the lower back. There will be little appetite. The patient will not get a dry mouth, and may in fact spit out saliva.

6.7.2 Symptom Patterns of the Kidney and Kidney Meridian

① Meridian-Associated Symptom Patterns

Lack of luster with a blackish face; corpulence (caused by water retention).

Cold and pain along the Kidney channel from the lower back to the thigh; weak legs; cold feet and lower back; low back pain; heat vexation in the soles of the feet; hot flushes; fatigue with the desire to lie down; lack of perseverance with a tendency to become fatigued.

② Organ-Associated Symptom Patterns

Having a feeling of emptiness in the stomach but quickly becoming full upon beginning to eat; a feeling of emptiness in the epigastric region and lack of a feeling of ease; coughing up blood-streaked sputum; a husky voice; wheezing and coughing; a feeling of faintness upon standing up; spitting out saliva; easily frightened and surprised; dry mouth; sore throat; feeling of oppression in the chest and heart pain; jaundice; diarrhea; facial edema; urinary difficulty or copious urination; lack of vitality; distension of the lower abdomen; ringing in the ears; difficulty hearing.

6.7.3 Symptom Patterns of the Bladder and Bladder Channel

① Meridian-Associated Symptom Patterns

Headache in which the pain shoots up to the head from the neck, and makes the eyes feel like they will pop out and the head fall off; pain in the spine; pain in the lower back as if the back were about to break; stiff hip joints; pain from the popliteal crease down the lower leg; pain along the Bladder channel from the nape of the neck to the back, lower back, buttocks, and lower limbs; difficulty moving the little toe; tendency to shead tears; malarial disease (i.e., attacks of aversion to cold and fever at regular time intervals); pain in the nape of the neck; stuffy nose; nosebleeds.

② Organ-Associated Symptom Patterns

Hemorrhoids; mania; epilepsy; difficulty hearing; blood in the urine; leakage of urine upon coughing; yellowish eyes.

	Table 6–6: Pathology and Symptom Patterns of Ki, Blood, and Fluids
Liver	The Liver contains the essential ki known as the ethereal soul, and has the function of gathering blood. Therefore, there cannot be only ki deficiency of the Liver, since a lack of blood will always occur when there is a deficiency of Liver ki. Since the Liver stores the blood, blood deficiency is the same thing as Liver deficiency, and blood stasis is the same as Liver excess. The blood contains fluids, so blood deficiency results mainly from a deficiency of fluids, or from a loss of blood itself.
Heart	The Heart contains the essential ki known as the spirit. An insufficiency of spirit results in death. The Heart is said to produce the blood. Nutritive ki enters the blood stream, where it becomes blood and is circulated throughout the body by the Heart. Death would result from a deficiency of this blood, so it is not possible to have a blood deficiency of the Heart.
Spleen	The Spleen contains the essential ki known as intention and wisdom. These are the yin ki of the Spleen. A deficiency of these would cause a stagnation and repletion of heat in the Stomach and Intestines and become a Stomach excess heat pattern. A lack of fluids of the Spleen causes cold and heat in the Stomach. Because this heat results from a lack of body fluids, the symptom patterns are different from those of Stomach excess heat that are seen with an acute illness. This type of heat is called deficient-type heat of the Stomach. If the Stomach contracts cold, it results in a Spleen deficiency cold pattern. There is a tendency to hemorrhage when there is blood deficiency of the Spleen.

Lung	The Lung contains the essential ki known as the corporeal soul. Because it also circulates the ki, ki deficiency is the same as Lung deficiency. The Lung circulates ki, and the circulation of ki circulates blood and fluids. If there is poor circulation of Lung ki, it causes a stagnation of blood, which results in blood stasis.
Kidney	The Kidney contains the ki known as the will, and has the functional property of firming. The stability of the Lower Warmer is hindered by a deficiency of ki of the Kidney, which causes the condition known as *running piglet* (the sensation of an explosive upsurge of yang ki from the Lower Warmer to the Upper Warmer.) The Kidney stores the fluids. Heat is generated when there is a deficiency of fluids. There is heat vexation in the feet and pain in the soles of the feet when there is deficient-type heat. Conversely, the whole of the Lower Warmer becomes cold when there is an increase of fluids. In that case there would be diarrhea and Stomach problems.

6.8   Symptom Patterns of Internal and External Illnesses

6.8.1 Symptom Patterns of the Internal Areas

Ri 裏 (internal) refers to the areas of the three yin channels. The three yin channels run adjacent to the fu organs, so that any heat or cold in the three yin channels quickly becomes heat or cold of the fu organs. Therefore, the fu organs are also called internal.

① Internal Heat Pattern

Internal heat is heat of the three yin channels. It is also heat of the fu organs. Lung heat is also included in internal heat since the Lung is considered equivalent to the fu organs. However, because the Stomach and Intestines (yang brightness) are the center of what is designated as internal, in herbal therapy a condition of stagnation and repletion of fu organ heat—that is, internal heat—is called a yang brightness illness. The symptom patterns of the three yin channels as given in the chapter on heat in the *Su Wen* (Chapter 31) are the same as those of yang brightness illnesses in herbal therapy.

Symptoms include constipation; delirious speech; perspiration of the hands and feet; no aversion to wind; fever with sensitivity to heat from the afternoon onward. In herbal therapy a purgative would be used, but in Meridian Therapy one should tonify the Spleen and disperse the yang brightness channel.

② Internal Cold Pattern

An internal cold pattern is a condition in which the yin ki of the three yin channels is flourishing (yin exuberance). There are three types of internal cold patterns: lesser yin illness, greater yin illness, and reverting yin illness. Moreover, in these conditions the yang ki of the fu organs is diminished and those organs are chilled.

Symptoms include abdominal pain; lientery (diarrhea containing incompletely digested material); loss of appetite; cold feet and hands or coldness of the whole body; loss of spirit; drowsiness; copious clear, whitish urine or urinary difficulty; heat and pain in the chest, but cold lower body; sore throat.

In herbal treatment, *fuzǐ* (附子 Aconiti Tuber Laterale) would be the primary herb used to tonify the yang ki. In Meridian Therapy it would be a case of a cold pattern in which one should tonify both yin and yang.

6.8.2 Symptom Patterns of Internal and External Areas

Uchi 内 (internal) refers to the area where the organs are located. *Soto* 外 (external) refers to the areas where the three yang and three yin channels flow—the hair and skin, blood vessels, muscles, sinews, and bones. Normally, internal symptom patterns refer to symptoms of the organs, and external symptom patterns refer to symptoms of the hair and skin, blood vessels, muscles, sinews, and bones. These terms are commonly used when describing chronic illnesses, and the terms external and internal that were explained in this section (6.8) are used when describing acute illness.

6.8.3 Symptom Patterns of External Illness

In a broad sense, the term *hyō* 表 (external) indicates the areas of the greater yang, yang brightness, and lesser yang channels. In the narrow sense it indicates the area of the skin and hair as well as the greater yang and yang brightness channels. The skin and hair are normally included in the greater yang channel. Generally, external illnesses are illnesses of the greater yang and yang brightness channels.

① Symptom Patterns of a Greater Yang Channel Illness (Lung Deficiency)

An aversion to cold; fever; headache; nosebleeds; unnaturally profuse sweating or an absence of sweating; pain in the back of the neck; low back pain. In herbal therapy this condition is called a greater yang illness. A greater yang illness is caused by the deficiency of the Lung, which controls the external surface of the body.

② **Symptom Patterns of a Yang Brightness Illness (Lung Deficiency)**

A lessened aversion to cold; fever with stiffness and pain in the nape of the neck; dry nose; painful eyes; unnaturally profuse sweating or an absence of sweating. In herbal therapy this is included in the category of greater yang illness because the condition will get better if the patient perspires. In Meridian Therapy one would tonify the Lung ki and disperse the yang brightness channel.

6.8.4 Symptom Patterns of Half-External Half-Internal Illnesses

These are illnesses of the lesser yang channel. The greater yang and yang brightness channels are designated as external, and the yin channels are designated as internal. Thus the lesser yang channel, which is in between, corresponds to half-external half-internal.

In cases of lesser yang illness, heat invades all the way to the Liver from the Gallbladder. Symptoms include such things as alternating chills and fever, deafness, loss of appetite, and constipation. In Meridian Therapy one would tonify the Spleen and disperse the lesser yang channel and Liver channel.

6.9 Symptom Patterns of the Extraordinary Vessels 奇経の病証

Table 6–7: Extraordinary Vessel Symptom Patterns	
Governing Vessel	Stiff spine; headache; cold and painful feet; hemorrhoids; upsurges of palpitations from the lower abdomen to the chest; heart pain; edema; enuresis; infertility; insomnia; neuralgia
Conception Vessel	Cramping and pain in the lower abdomen; leukorrhea; menstrual abnormalities; pain and itchiness on the skin of the abdomen
Penetrating Vessel	Counterflow ki (nausea, vomiting, dizziness, headache) with diarrhea
Girdling Vessel	Abdominal pain; cold and pain in the lower back
Yang Heel Vessel	Paralysis of the medial aspect of the lower limbs; flaccidity in the anterior half of the body and cramping tension in the posterior half of the body; eye pain
Yin Heel Vessel	Paralysis of the lateral aspect of the lower limbs; cramping tension in the anterior half of the body and flaccidity in the posterior half of the body
Yang Linking Vessel	Suffering from an aversion to cold and fever
Yin Linking Vessel	Heart pain

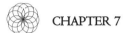 CHAPTER 7

Diagnostic Methods

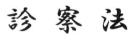

The four diagnostic methods in Meridian Therapy are known as the four examinations: looking, listening and smelling, questioning, and palpation.

- Looking is a method for determining the pattern of imbalance by observing such things as the patient's physique and skin color and luster. Tongue diagnosis is also included in the looking diagnosis.

- Listening and smelling are methods for determining the pattern of imbalance by listening to the condition of the voice and smelling any body odors.

- Questioning is a method for determining the pattern of imbalance by asking the patient about symptoms associated with the pathology.

- Palpation is a diagnostic method of touch and includes palpation of the pulse, abdomen, back, and meridians. Pulse diagnosis will be discussed in Chapter 8.

  Palpation of the abdomen (fukushin) is a diagnostic method whereby the practitioner touches the whole of the abdomen and chest while feeling for any cold or heat, dampness or dryness, depressions, protuberances, pain on pressure, indurations, or resistance.

  Palpation of the back (haishin) focuses on palpating the governing vessel and back transport points while touching the whole back and feeling for the same signs as on the abdomen.

Palpation of the meridians focuses on palpating the meridians on the extremities for depressions, protuberances, pain on pressure, and indurations.

In this chapter we will discuss the specifics of the above-mentioned diagnostic methods. However, in order to understand this material, it is necessary to first have a strong grasp of the fundamental principles, flow of the meridians, visceral manifestations, etiology, pathology, and symptom patterns.

It is critical to understand pathology, as it is not possible to determine the pattern of imbalance by only gathering information. For instance, when using questioning, it is not sufficient to simply ask what the symptoms are; you must always keep pathology in mind when questioning. The same holds true for palpating the pulse and abdomen.

7.1   Looking   望診

Looking refers to what would today be termed a visual examination. But as it is used in acupuncture, looking implies observing the patient from a slight distance. The classics say, "Those who look and know [the patient's condition] are called spirit (神 *kami* or *shin*)." (*Nan Jing*, Chapter 61) This means that those who can perform an examination by only looking have divine or superhuman skills. It is actually very difficult to make a complete diagnosis by just looking because the information that can be obtained from looking is intertwined with information related to constitutional factors and any chronic illnesses. Yet, even though it is difficult, there is extremely important elemental information to be gathered from looking—which is known as examining the spirit.

7.1.1 Examining the Spirit *Kami (Shin)* 神

Those who have spirit will recover, and those without spirit have a poor prognosis. So, what exactly is spirit? Simply, spirit can be called the life force. It also refers to the presence of luster in the skin. Even when there is some imbalance in the body, if there is vigor in the body and luster in the skin, then spirit is present. The presence of spirit in a patient can be judged by the following factors.

① **Physique and Color**

The strength and weakness of the skeletal structure, muscles, blood vessels, flesh, and skin are observed during the looking examination. For instance, spirit is judged to not be present if the flesh is wasted away and weak, and if there is a dark complexion about the face. Conversely, spirit is present if the flesh is in excellent condition and the complexion of the face is bright.

② **Sparkle in the Eyes**

Spirit is present if the eyes are penetrating and have life in them. Spirit is not present if there is a dullness and a vague look in the eyes.

③ **Emotional State**

Spirit is present when there is a healthy countenance and the speech is clear.

④ **Condition of the Breathing**

Spirit is present if the breathing is deep and even and is not present if the breathing is irregular.

⑤ **Luster in the Skin**

Spirit is present if there is luster to the skin and not present if there is no luster to the skin. However, if someone is wearing makeup the condition of the facial skin cannot be determined, and thus the so-called cubit skin around LU-6 can be observed in lieu of the facial skin. It is also possible to judge the vivacity of the body by the condition of the skin on the neck.

The area of the face in which the presence of spirit is read is from the area between the eyebrows to the tip of the nose.

7.1.2 Condition of the Eyes

When examining each part of the body it is important to always consider whether or not that part shows the presence of spirit. Following are lists of factors to know about the color and shape of each part of the body, starting with the eyes. The eyes are associated with the Liver, Gallbladder, and the yang brightness channel.

Table 7–1: Indications and Patterns Associated with the Eyes		
Color and Shape	**Indication**	**Pattern**
Large eyes	Constitutionally there is an abundance of blood	Liver excess pattern
Eyes that are almond shaped or that have long slits at the outer corners		Constitutional Liver deficiency heat pattern
Small eyes		Constitutional Liver deficiency cold pattern
Overly penetrating	High-strung nerves	Liver deficiency heat pattern
Lack of strength in the eyes		Liver deficiency cold pattern
Bluish conjunctiva	The "irascibility bug" (*Kan no mushi* 疳の虫)*	Liver deficiency pattern in young children and failure of sexual maturation in adults
Yellowish conjunctiva	Possibly jaundice	Spleen deficiency Liver excess heat pattern
Bloodshot eyes	Abundance of blood in the Upper Warmer Commonly seen with hypertension or stiff shoulders	Any heat pattern Excess heat in the Stomach
Desire to close the eyes	Deficiency of yang ki	Cold patterns
Darkness around the eyes	Fatigue Overindulgence in sex	Liver excess pattern Kidney deficiency heat pattern
Edema of the upper eyelids		Kidney deficiency pattern
Edema of the lower eyelids		Spleen deficiency pattern
Twitching of the eyelids		Liver deficiency cold pattern
Trichiasis and hordeolum (inflammation of sebaceous gland of the eyelid)		Spleen deficiency Liver excess pattern
Moist eyes during a febrile disease		Lung deficiency yang channel excess heat pattern
discoloration under the eye or on the cheek		Liver excess pattern or a Liver deficiency pattern
pink color (under the eye)	Transformation of true cold False heat	Liver deficiency cold pattern
painful eyes	Heat in the Large Intestine channel	

* A syndrome of children that is traditionally recognized in Japan, the general characteristics of which include crying at night, loss of appetite, and frequent irritability

The most important aspect of the art of healing is to not make a misinterpretation of [the patient's] complexion or pulses. It is a great principle of the art of healing [i.e., is imperative] to have no doubt or confusion as to the application of these [diagnostic techniques]. If one acts counter [to this principle] then one will not comprehend the manifestation [symptoms] or the root [i.e., causes of disease], and will cause the decay of the spirit and the ruin of the country [i.e., body]…

Qibo said, "Unity is the highest matter in the art of healing."

The Yellow Emperor asked, "What is meant by unity?"

Qibo answered, "Unity means 'connection,' which is ascertained [by the presence or lack of spirit]."

The Yellow Emperor asked, "How does one do that?"

Qibo said, "Close the doors and shut the windows [i.e., enter a state of concentration] and [establish] a bond with the patient. Observe [their] condition [state of mind-heart-body], and follow [your] intuitive sense. Those [who are] judged to have spirit will thrive, and those [who are] judged to have lost spirit will die." (*Su Wen*, Chapter 13)

7.1.3 Condition of the Tongue

The tongue is associated with the Heart, Small Intestine, Spleen, and Stomach. The amount of ki and blood can be judged by the color of the tongue. For instance, a pale tongue indicates a lack of blood and a red tongue indicates an abundance of blood or an abundance of deficient-type heat.

Table 7–2: Indications and Patterns Associated with the Tongue		
Color and Shape of the Tongue	**Indication**	**Pattern**
Inability to fully extend the tongue during examination and a shriveled coated tongue without luster	Absence of spirit	
Dark red tongue		Liver excess pattern
Overall paleness	Anemia	Liver deficiency cold pattern
Teeth marks around the perimeter	Phlegm retention	Spleen deficiency cold pattern
Disappearing lingual papilla, or redness upon splitting of lingual papilla		Liver deficiency heat pattern or a Kidney deficiency heat pattern
Aversion to cold or fever with a normal tongue that does not show a coating, redness, or anemia		Lung deficiency yang channel excess heat pattern

Coating on the tongue that is moist on top	Heat in the Stomach and Intestines	Deficiency-type heat
Coating on the tongue that is dry on top	Heat in the Stomach and Intestines	Spleen deficiency Stomach excess heat pattern or a Spleen deficiency Liver excess heat pattern
Tongue coating progresses from whitish to yellowish	Increasing abundance of heat	
Tongue with blackish coating	Poor prognosis	

7.1.4 Condition of the Lips

The lips and the surrounding area reveal the condition of the Spleen and Stomach, as well as the condition of the blood.

Table 7–3: Indications and Patterns Associated with the Lips		
Color and Condition of the Lips	**Indication**	**Pattern**
Reddish lips		Spleen deficiency and either deficient-type heat or excess heat
Blackish lips		Kidney deficiency heat pattern or a Liver excess pattern
A yellowish color around the mouth		Spleen deficiency/Stomach deficiency heat pattern
Pimples or small boils around the lips		Spleen deficiency pattern
Chapped lips following a febrile disease		Spleen deficiency pattern
Chronic chapped lips		Liver deficiency cold pattern
Cracked lips	Hemorrhoids	Spleen deficiency
Pimples or small boils in the philtrum	Urethritis	
Well-defined philtrum	In women, may indicate ease of conception	
Angular cheilitis (corners of the lips inflamed)	Stomach heat	Spleen deficiency heat pattern or a Kidney deficiency heat pattern
Bluish lips	Sudden onset of coldness	
Gum problems		Kidney deficiency heat pattern or a Spleen deficiency heat pattern
Stained teeth	Stomach heat	Spleen deficiency pattern

7.1.5 Condition of the Nose

The nose is associated with the Lung, Large Intestine, and yang brightness channel.

Table 7–4: Indications and Patterns Associated with the Nose		
Color and condition	**Indication**	**Pattern**
Large nostrils	Constitutionally large Large Intestine	
Thick nasal mucus and empyema (sinus infection)		Heat in the yang brightness channel
Watery nasal mucus		Lung deficiency cold pattern or a Spleen deficiency cold pattern
Rhinitis		Spleen deficiency with heat in the Large Intestine channel
Redness on the tip of the nose		Spleen deficiency Stomach heat or a Liver deficiency heat pattern
A blackish color at the root of the nose	Chronic constipation with blood stasis	
Redness between the eyebrows	Heat in the Heart	Kidney deficiency heat pattern
Whitish nose		Lung deficiency cold pattern
Blackish forehead	Blood stasis	
No luster between the forehead and the nose	Poor prognosis	
Too much luster in the forehead		Kidney deficiency heat pattern

7.1.6 Condition of the Ears

The ears are associated with the Kidney and the lesser yang channel.

Table 7–5: Indications and Patterns Associated with the Ears		
Color and Condition	**Indication**	**Pattern**
Small ears	Constitutionally weak Kidney	Kidney deficiency cold pattern
Large ears	Constitutionally strong Kidney	Kidney deficiency heat pattern
Reddish or blackish ears		Kidney deficiency heat pattern
Wrinkly ears	Poor prognosis in chronic disease	
Ringing in the ears and difficulty hearing		Kidney deficiency pattern or a Liver deficiency pattern
Tympanitis	Heat in the lesser yang channel	Spleen deficiency

7.1.7 Condition of the Skin and Hair

The skin and hair are under the control of the Lung.

Table 7–6: Indications and Patterns Associated with the Skin and Hair		
Condition of the Skin and Hair	**Indication**	**Pattern**
Soft and smooth hair on the hands and feet	Tendency to be healthy	
Men with thick hair and body		Tendency to constitutional Lung deficiency; Lung deficiency yang channel excess heat pattern
Women with abundant peach fuzz		Tendency to constitutional Lung deficiency
Abundant peach fuzz or body hair in the interscapular area		Tendency to easily develop Lung deficiency
Abundant peach fuzz or body hair around BL-25		Tendency to easily develop Kidney deficiency pattern
Body hair that is hard and bristly	Heat in the internal organs; poor prognosis	
White hair		Kidney deficiency cold pattern
Balding		Kidney deficiency heat pattern
Alopecia areata		Liver deficiency cold pattern
Whitish skin over the whole body		Constitutional Lung deficiency
Tough skin		Constitutional predisposition to develop a Liver deficiency heat pattern
Rough skin		Spleen deficiency heat pattern
Dry skin and wrinkles on young people	Poor prognosis	
Itchy eczema	(Often) atopic dermatitis	Lung deficiency Liver excess pattern
Rash* accompanied by a fever, often seen in small children		Lung deficiency pattern or Spleen deficiency pattern

*Localized moxibustion is good for pustules. Additionally, moxibustion is appropriate for many skin problems.

7.1.8 Condition of the Blood Vessels

The Heart controls the blood vessels.

Table 7–7: Indications and Patterns Associated with the Blood Vessels		
Condition	**Indication**	**Pattern**
Varicose viens		Kidney deficiency heat pattern or Liver deficiency heat pattern
Vascular spiders	Commonly seen with circulation problems, respiratory problems, neuralgia, rheumatism, and digestive problems, or appearing even when there is no particular abnormality	
Vascular spiders on the chest or abdomen	Commonly seen with hepatic cirrhosis	

7.1.9 Condition of the Flesh

The flesh is under the control of the Spleen and Stomach.

Table 7–8: Indications and Patterns Associated with the Flesh		
Condition of the Flesh	**Indication**	**Pattern**
Flaccid skin		Tendency to Spleen deficiency cold pattern
Robust and corpulent flesh		Spleen deficiency Stomach excess heat pattern
Extremely emaciated flesh	Poor prognosis	

7.1.10 Other Conditions

Table 7–9: Indications and Patterns Associated with Other Conditions		
Other Conditions	**Indication**	**Pattern**
Muscle cramps		Liver deficiency heat pattern or cold pattern
Weak nails		Tendency to Liver deficiency
Curved lower back		Tendency to Kidney deficiency or Liver deficiency
Demented countenance	Poor prognosis	
Edema due to water retention		Kidney deficiency
Edema in the lower limbs		Kidney deficiency or Spleen deficiency
Abdominal edema	Poor prognosis	
Edema of the dorsum of the hands	Poor prognosis	
Facial edema		Spleen deficiency

[Speaking of complexions, those who] appear [malachite] greenish like a rush mat will die.

Those who appear reddish like dried blood will die.

Those who appear yellowish [more specifically a darkish marigold color] like a trifoliate orange will die.

Those who appear whitish like old dry bones will die.

Those who appear blackish like soot will die.

Those who appear bluish-green like the feathers of a kingfisher will live.

Those who appear reddish like a cock's comb will live.

Those who appear yellowish like the belly of a crab will live.

Those who appear whitish like lard will live.

Those who appear black like the feather of a raven will live.

(*Su Wen*, Chapter 10)

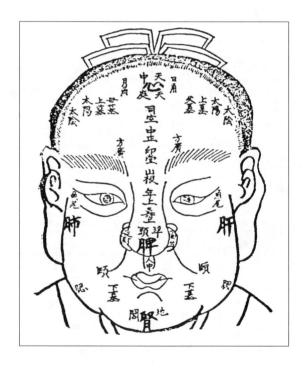

Figure 7–1: Areas of the face used in looking diagnosis

Listening and smelling are diagnostic methods for gathering information used to help determine the pattern of imbalance by smelling any body odors and listening to the sounds of the voice and breathing.

7.2.1 Body Odors

Table 7–3: Patterns Associated with Body Odors	
Body Odor	**Pattern**
Rancid, fatty, fleshy odor	Liver deficiency or Liver excess
Burnt	Often heat
Fragrant; sweet-and-sour	Spleen deficiency
Fleshy	Heat in the Lung
Rotten	Kidney deficiency heat pattern

7.2.2 Five Phonations

① **Tusk Sound (Liver)** represents wood; the shrill, strong sounds heard in the Japanese phonemes *ka*, *ki*, *ku*, *ke*, *ko*, *ga*, *gi*, *gu*, *ge*, and *go*. These sounds are made as if thrusting the front teeth out. People who have this kind of vocalization tend to have Liver deficiency.

② **Tongue Sound (Heart)** represents fire; the powerful sounds made by pressing the tongue against the teeth such as in *ta*, *chi*, *tsu*, *te*, *to*, *na*, *ni*, *nu*, *ne*, *no*, *ra*, *ri*, *ru*, *re*, *ro*, *da*, *ji*, *zu*, *de*, and *do* from the Japanese phonemes. These are sounds that seem to fly out of the mouth with force. People with this form of vocalization tend to have an abundance of fire in the Heart. Conversely, those who lack strength in their voice tend to have deficient yang ki of the Heart and a poor prognosis.

③ **Throat Sound (Spleen)** represents earth; the sounds that emanate directly from the throat made by opening the mouth wide, as in *a*, *i*, *u*, *e*, *o*, *ya*, *yu*, *yo*, *wa*, and *wo* from the Japanese phonemes. A Spleen deficiency heat pattern is indicated in people who speak in a loud voice. A lack of strength in the voice itself and indistinct pronunciation indicates a Spleen deficiency cold pattern.

④ **Teeth Sound (Lung)** represents metal; the pure, crisp sounds such as heard in the Japanese phonemes *sa*, *shi*, *su*, *se*, *so*, *za*, *ji*, *zu*, *ze*, and *zo*. People with clear vocalization and yet deep toned voices tend to have Lung deficiency.

⑤ **Lip Sound (Kidney)** represents water; the soft, non-forceful sounds such as *ha*, *hi*, *fu*, *he*, *ho*, *ma*, *mi*, *mu*, *me*, and *mo* from the Japanese phonemes. A feeling as if something were missing from the voice or as if the voice were trapped inside indicates Kidney deficiency.

7.2.3 Five Sounds

These five sounds represent the tonal scale, and can be applied in the following way: A person's normal voice corresponds to the sound *kyū*. Taking that as the standard, if their voice sounds like it has gone up by two tones, that would indicate trouble with the Heart, or if it went up by four tones, that would indicate trouble with the Liver. Conversely, a drop by two tones would indicate trouble with the Lung, and a drop by four tones would indicate trouble with the Kidney.

| Table 7–11: Tones and Associated Organs ||
Tone	Organ
Kaku (角)	Liver
Bi (微)	Heart
Kyū (宮)	Spleen
Shō (商)	Lung
U (羽)	Kidney

7.2.4 Other Considerations

| Table 7–12: Patterns Associated with Other Conditions ||
Conditions to Consider	Pattern or Indication
Those who always sound like they are angry, or those who talk as if they were ordering others to do their bidding	Constitutional Liver deficiency heat pattern
Those who talk with a smile on their face even under unhappy circumstances	Kidney deficiency heat pattern with heat in the heart
Delirious speech in conjunction with a febrile disease condition	Spleen deficiency Stomach excess heat pattern
People who tend to complain a lot	Constitutional Lung deficiency
Wet coughing or wheezing	Spleen deficiency and Lung heat
Dry, irritating cough	Deficiency and Lung heat
Groaning while inflicted with a febrile disease	Kidney deficiency
People who like to sing or those who tend to hum	Spleen deficiency heat pattern

Questioning is an examination method whereby various questions that may be of help in determining the pattern of imbalance are asked of the patient. Questioning is a very important and fundamental part of an examination, but many beginners are uncertain what to ask. Many are also poor questioners and ask irrelevant questions or ask questions in a rote manner, such that the patient feels uncomfortable or offended.

Some patients, for instance, who come for a fairly simple low back treatment, may think it intrusive to be asked for information beyond the basics of name, address, and age, such as profession, previous illnesses, home and family environment, and family medical history. To them, such seemingly overly detailed questioning can make them dislike the practitioner. Questioning, in a sense, involves eliciting some secrets from the patient, so appropriate discretion should be used while asking only those questions that are related to the symptom pattern.

Poor questioners usually get poor answers from their patients. Some patients may really dramatize their situation and others may go on and on about their condition. This can reach the extent that some practitioners even think the patient is telling nothing but lies. But all these problems arise from unskilled questioning.

In order to be a competent questioner it is essential to have a wealth of knowledge about numerous diseases—both from the contemporary medical perspective and the traditional medical point of view. It is of course even better to have experience examining and treating those diseases.

7.3.1 Basic Questions

① Name, Address, Age, and Occupation

This is the bare essential information to be asked. Sometimes it may be necessary to ask the patient's gender if it is not apparent.

Some patients may not wish to reveal their occupation. Depending on the circumstances, the question may be phrased in a general manner such as, "Do you do office work?" Or, you may ask in a chatty manner while giving the treatment.

② Family Structure and Family Medical History

Some patients may dislike being asked in a formulized manner for this information if they have only come for treatment of something like low back pain or stiff shoulders. On the other hand, some patients may develop a sense of mistrust if they are not asked for this information when they know it is relevant to their illness and should have been asked for it up front.

It is essential to ask about family structure if you are giving advice to parents with a child having a psychological block about going to school or are treating patients who have had a nervous breakdown.

While conducting the pulse diagnosis it may be good to ask questions concerning family medical history to confirm any suspicions gathered from the pulse, such as, "Would either of your parents happen to have high blood pressure?" Other common conditions to which family medical history is relevant include diabetes, asthma, and atopic dermatitis.

③ Previous Illnesses

It is also best, if possible, to ask about any previous illnesses based on insights gained while conducting the pulse diagnosis or abdominal diagnosis. Or, if you do not perceive anything through these examinations you may ask, "Have you ever had any serious illnesses?"

Liver deficiency or Spleen deficiency Liver excess are common when the patient has previously had diseases such as hepatitis, cholecystis, or cholelithiasis (gallstones). Spleen deficiency Liver excess or Kidney deficiency are common when there has been a case of gastric or duodenal ulcer. Spleen deficiency is common when there has been an intestinal disease. Patients who have had lung diseases tend to develop Lung deficiency or Lung heat.

Therefore, asking about previous illnesses can give useful information for helping to determine the pattern of imbalance. However, it should be kept in mind that this information is first and foremost only for reference, and that mistakes can be made due to diagnoses based on preconceived ideas. Acute conditions in particular almost always are unrelated to previous illnesses.

7.3.2 Chief Complaint

The chief complaint refers to the symptoms that cause the most suffering. Questions pertaining to the chief complaint include such things as its location, when the patient contracted the illness, its progression since then, what the patient thinks might be the cause, and times or seasons when the symptoms become aggravated.

① Confirming the Localized Area of Illness

All illnesses stem from a deficiency of essential ki of the zang organs. Localized symptoms appear when heat and cold arise due to a deficiency of ki, blood, and fluids (pathological deficiency) caused by the combination of any of a number of possible factors in combination with the underlying deficiency. The majority of localized symptoms that patients convey as their chief complaint are the areas affected by cold and heat. That is to say, it is common for the area of the chief complaint to lie along the meridian(s) that should be used for the local treatment.

For instance, suppose that a patient presents with a complaint of stiff shoulders due to age (i.e., fifty-year-old's shoulder). This ailment is commonly caused by Liver deficiency. Blockage of the meridians in the area of the shoulder joint gives rise to it being the specific area of the chief complaint. So, first of all you should diagnose whether or not the problem is due to Liver deficiency, and at the same time you must assess which meridian(s) have blockage that may be causing the difficulty in raising the arm. In order to do that you should palpate each of the channels and have the patient raise the arm. But, before having the patient raise the arm, ask exactly where the pain is felt. This should be done with precision, politeness, and gentleness. This information will help in determining the meridian(s) and points to be used for the local treatment.

Obviously one must learn the flow of the meridians in order to be able to confirm the specific locations of complaint, but this should also be thought about together with yin and yang theory and the five phases theory when determining the pattern of imbalance.

For instance, pain and indurations focused near LI-15 on the shoulder might be due to the appearance of a disharmony of the Large Intestine channel caused by Lung deficiency, since the Large Intestine channel and Lung channel are in a paired yin-yang relationship. Or, the Large Intestine channel disharmony could be caused by Spleen deficiency because of the

Spleen channel's association with the yang brightness channel, of which the Large Intestine channel is a part. Or, the cause could lie in the controlling cycle relationship so that Liver deficiency causes deterioration in the flow of the Lung and Large Intestine channels.

② **Ask About Conditions that Aggravate the Symptoms**

Acute problems are aggravated in relation to the time of day and physical posture, and chronic problems are aggravated in relation to the seasons. A simple listing of conditions is as follows:

Table 7–13: Seasonal and Temporal Aggravations and Associated Patterns or Indications	
Aggravation	**Pattern or Indication**
Aggravation in the afternoon, during the rainy season, or from overeating	Spleen deficiency
Aggravation in the spring and difficulty moving in the morning	Liver deficiency
Aggravation in the nighttime	Liver excess or any of the heat patterns
Aggravation in the summer	Kidney deficiency heat pattern or a Spleen deficiency cold pattern
Aggravation in the autumn	Lung deficiency or Lung heat
Aggravation in the winter	Liver deficiency cold pattern or a Spleen deficiency cold pattern
Aggravation caused by warming up or applying heat	Heat pattern
Improvement from cooling off or applying cold	Heat pattern
Aggravation caused by cooling	Any of the cold patterns

Moreover, it is possible to surmise which meridians are afflicted according to the worsening of pain felt with certain movements.

③ **Classification of the Chief Complaint by Yin/Yang, Deficiency/Excess, and Cold/Heat**

Yin & Yang: Classification of the symptoms of the chief complaint by yin and yang means differentiating whether the disorder is chronic and unchanging or acute and varying in its symptom pattern.

For instance, treatment should focus on tonification of the yin channels with retained needles, moxa-on-the-handle needles, and direct moxibustion for chronic conditions in which there is little change in the symptom pattern. On the other hand, rapid insertion and removal with shallow needling is necessary when there are acute symptoms such as fever or asthma.

Deficiency & Excess: Classification by deficiency and excess means differentiating whether the area to be given the local treatment is deficient or excess.

Suppose, for instance, that you have tonified a deficient Kidney for low back pain. Next you must tonify or disperse the localized area of pain (e.g., the Bladder channel) depending on whether that area is deficient or excess.

However, it should be noted that palpation and the pulse qualities are used in addition to the symptom pattern for making the final determination of whether the local area is deficient or excess.

Cold & Heat: Classification by cold and heat means to differentiate the patient's chief complaint by whether it is a cold pattern or a heat pattern.

For a patient with low back pain and Liver deficiency, for example, it would be important to differentiate whether the pain is caused by a Liver deficiency cold pattern or a Liver deficiency heat pattern. At the same time, you should think about which meridian (i.e., the area of local treatment) is being affected by the cold or heat. Cold should be treated by tonification, and heat should be differentiated by whether it needs to be reduced by tonification or dispersion. It is imperative to reduce heat by tonification if there is no excess.

7.3.3 Etiology

When talking with patients concerning when their illness began, one usually asks if they know the cause of their illness. If this can be ascertained, it often leads to knowing which yin channel deficiency caused the illness. In other words, you can surmise which meridian is to be used for the root treatment. This demonstrates the importance of etiology. For more details, please refer to the chapter on etiology.

7.3.4 Questions Related to Particular Areas and Conditions

It should be no surprise that, depending on the chief complaint, there are questions that should be asked and those that are not necessary to ask. Below is a list of general things to ask about and information related to particular areas of the body and certain conditions.

Head	Complaints include headache, heavy-headed feeling, dizziness, and faintness upon standing.
	Question whether the pain is chronic or acute.
	If the pain is chronic, ask the specific location. Migraine headaches (pain on the lateral sides of the head) are related to the Gallbladder channel. Pain in the occipital region is related to the Bladder channel. Pain in the prefrontal region is related to the yang brightness channel. Pain in the region of the parietal bone is caused by either Liver deficiency or Liver excess. Pain in the nighttime and pain that feels like the head is being squeezed is caused by Liver excess.
	In cases of acute headache, ask whether there is an aversion to cold or fever. Regardless of whether there is an aversion to cold or fever, a splitting headache with nausea may indicate a serious condition such as a subarachnoid hemorrhage.
	A headache with a puffy, swollen feeling upon touching the head is caused by Kidney deficiency. A heavy-headed feeling is often caused by Spleen deficiency. Dizziness upon standing is commonly caused by Liver deficiency.

Eyes	Illnesses of the eyes are usually treated as Liver deficiency, and the Large Intestine channel is commonly used for the local treatment.

Ears	Many patients have complaints such as a ringing in the ears, difficulty hearing, sudden deafness, and inner ear infections.
	Ringing in the ears is treated as Kidney deficiency with attention given to the Triple Warmer. Chronic hearing difficulty is treated as Kidney deficiency. Sudden deafness is treated as a Spleen deficiency Liver excess pattern with attention given to TW-17. Inner ear infections also indicate a Spleen deficiency Liver excess pattern, and either the Triple Warmer channel or the Small Intestine channel is used for treatment.

Mouth and Tongue	Patients may come with chief complaints such as stomatitis, angular cheilitis, herpes labialis, or ulceration of the mouth. Most of these are caused by heat in the Stomach. The Stomach heat could in turn result either from Spleen deficiency or Kidney deficiency. Stomatitis can be caused by Behcet's Syndrome, in which there will also be ulceration of the genitals and erythema nodosum (red and painful nodules on the legs). A Liver deficiency cold pattern is commonly seen with Behcet's Syndrome.

Nose	Patients may have chief complaints such as rhinitis or empyema (sinus infections). A runny nose, sneezing, itchy eyes, and seasonal occurrence indicate allergic rhinitis. It is treated as Spleen deficiency using the Large Intestine channel. A heavy or oppressed feeling around BL-2 and in the occipital region, and a stuffy nose with occasional thick mucus discharge indicates an empyema. It is treated as Lung deficiency with heat in the yang brightness channel or Spleen deficiency with heat in the yang brightness channel. Rhinitis symptoms with an aversion to cold or fever should be considered as Lung deficiency and treated using the yang brightness channel.

Throat	Patients may have a sore throat as the chief complaint. Confirm whether there is an aversion to cold and fever, or only an aversion to cold, or neither an aversion to cold nor fever. Next, confirm whether the pain is on the Conception Vessel (anterior midsagital line) or the yang brightness channel. Pain along the Conception Vessel with mainly an aversion to cold and little fever is treated as Kidney deficiency. A swollen and painful yang brightness channel with an aversion to cold, a subjective feeling of fever, and a high fever that is measured with a thermometer indicates tonsillitis. This condition is treated as Lung deficiency or Spleen deficiency by dispersing the yang brightness channel.

Throat (cont.)	Kidney deficiency or the disharmony known as *running piglet* (in which there is an explosive upsurge of yang ki from the Lower Warmer to the Upper Warmer) may be indicated if there is a clogged feeling in the throat that is unrelated to an aversion to cold or fever. Confirm whether the patient has the sensation of something welling up from below the navel. Melancholy is indicated if this sensation is absent, but there is still a choked-up feeling in the throat. This is treated as Spleen deficiency Liver excess or as Lung deficiency Liver excess.

Face	The main facial complaints are trigeminal neuralgia and Bell's palsy. In either case they are quite obvious, and if given as the chief complaint they do not require any special questioning. However, finding out how long the patient has had the disorder and the possible cause can help determine the prognosis. Bell's palsy is treated as Liver deficiency, and trigeminal neuralgia is treated as Lung deficiency Liver excess.

Shoulder Joint	Liver deficiency is common when there is a limited ability to elevate the arm at the shoulder joint. You should ask common questions such as whether or not there is spontaneous pain, the exact location of pain when moving, and to what extent the patient can move the arm. A case of Spleen deficiency is sometimes seen when the patient can raise the arm but feels pain in the joint.

Stiff Shoulders	Stiff shoulders can accompany any patterns of imbalance, and thus are not a decisive factor for determining the pattern of imbalance based on questioning. Nonetheless, it can be useful to inquire about the type of work the patient was doing at the time of onset of stiff shoulders. Stiffness in the shoulders that accompanies work that uses the extremities can indicate Spleen deficiency, and stiffness in the shoulders that accompanies doing something with unremitting diligence can indicate Liver deficiency.

Chest	Chief complaints include such things as coughing, asthma, shortness of breath, palpitations, oppressed feeling in the chest, and heart pain.

Disorders of the Lung are often caused by Lung deficiency or by heat in the Lung (Lung heat) that spread from a Liver deficiency heat pattern or Spleen deficiency heat pattern. If heat has spread to the Lung, the throat will be dry and the patient may bring up sticky sputum. The mouth could be dry and there may be constipation. Or, there could be coughing with blood rushing to the head. Symptoms that are aggravated by cold indicate Lung deficiency. Likewise, Spleen deficiency is indicated if coughing or asthma is aggravated by high humidity.

A Kidney deficiency heat pattern is indicated when climbing stairs causes palpitations and shortness of breath. The sensation of something welling up from below the navel to the chest causing palpitations also indicates a Kidney deficiency heat pattern. To confirm this it is usually necessary to ask the patient, as they seldom mention this. You must refer the patient to a medical specialist if they have a feeling of oppression in the chest and palpitations for no apparent reason with accompanying pain and difficulty breathing. It is even more critical if the pain has sudden onset and is intense. |

Upper Abdomen	Disorders of the upper abdomen include such things as cholecystitis (inflammation of the gallbladder), cholelithiasis (gallstones), gastric and duodenal ulcers, and inflammation of the pancreas. Many patients come for acupuncture treatment after having been diagnosed with these conditions by medical specialists. Because these disorders are treated as many different patterns of imbalance, you must ask questions to determine whether there is pain or not, when the pain is felt, whether the mouth is dry, whether there is appetite or nausea, the condition of the bowel movements, whether there is full body fatigue or not, and whether there is fever.

Lower Abdomen	Lower abdominal pain is often seen in small children, and it is almost always due to a Spleen deficiency heat pattern.

Lower Abdomen (cont.)	If the pain is in the ileocecal area, you must be careful to ask about the progression of the pain, as it could be appendicitis. A Spleen deficiency Liver excess pattern is often seen when there is appendicitis.
	Pain in the lower left part of the abdomen is possibly constipation or a buildup of gas. The problem will go away after having a bowel movement. Ileus (intestinal obstruction) may be suspected if there is abdominal pain but no excretion of stool or gas.
	A Liver deficiency cold pattern is common with serious illnesses of the intestines.
	Abdominal pain coming from coldness of the feet is common in women. It is usually due to Kidney deficiency or Liver deficiency.
	Pain in the area of the uterus that is unrelated to menstruation may be inflammation of the uterine tubes or other parts of the uterus.

Back	Stiffness and pain in the interscapular area and around BL-20 can appear in any pattern of imbalance. It is useful to ask about the condition of the bowel movements and urination to help in determining the pattern of imbalance.

Lower Back	Pain from below BL-23 down to the buttocks is seen in lower back problems and sciatica. Determine the pattern of imbalance by confirming any cold areas and the cause of the pain. It is also important to confirm the exact location of the pain for purposes of giving precise local treatment. When the patient has acute low pack pain you should also confirm which particular movements elicit pain.

The Four Limbs	Patients may not mention a feeling of fatigue in the extremities unless asked, but such a condition unmistakably indicates Spleen deficiency. However, weak legs indicate Kidney deficiency. Cold hands and feet indicate the cold pattern of Liver deficiency or Spleen deficiency, and rushes of blood to the head with onset of coldness of the feet indicates Liver deficiency, Kidney deficiency, or a Lung deficiency Liver excess pattern.

The Four Limbs (cont.)	Rheumatism throughout the joints of the whole body commonly indicates a Spleen deficiency heat pattern or a Spleen deficiency cold pattern. Joint pain of the knee could be due to Liver deficiency, Kidney deficiency, or Spleen deficiency. You should also ask about any other symptoms before determining the pattern of imbalance.

Fever	This fever refers to the subjective feeling of fever and not to fever that is measured by taking the patient's temperature with a thermometer. If it is accompanied by an aversion to cold it indicates a Lung deficiency heat pattern, but if there are symptom patterns related to the internal organs it indicates Spleen deficiency. A Spleen deficiency Stomach excess heat pattern is indicated if a thermometer shows a high fever and the patient has delirious speech and constipation in addition to having the subjective feeling of fever. A Liver deficiency heat pattern is indicated if there is no fever shown on a thermometer but the patient has the subjective feeling of sudden alternations between getting very hot and then becoming very cold. A Spleen deficiency Liver excess heat pattern is indicated when there is a fever shown on a thermometer as well as the subjective feeling of alternating fever and chills.

Aversion to Cold	The cold pattern of Lung deficiency or other such deficiencies is indicated when there is only the subjective feeling of an aversion to cold even though a fever temperature registers on a thermometer gauge.

Defecation	People who suffer from even a single day of constipation tend to have a Spleen deficiency heat pattern. The heat pattern of any pattern of imbalance tends to cause constipation. Lung deficiency Liver excess and Spleen deficiency Liver excess tend to cause constipation in which the stool will be firm and dark.

Defecation (cont.)	People with copious urination due to a Kidney deficiency cold pattern will develop constipation.
	A Spleen deficiency heat pattern is indicated when diarrhea gives relief.
	A Spleen deficiency cold pattern is indicated when diarrhea is physically tiring.
	Diarrhea accompanied by abdominal pain indicates Spleen deficiency, and diarrhea that is not painful indicates Kidney deficiency.
	Abdominal pain that does not cease upon defecating indicates a Spleen deficiency heat pattern with excess-type heat in the Intestines or a Spleen deficiency cold pattern.
	Diarrhea that afterwards leaves a dull ache in the lower abdomen and rectum indicates a Spleen deficiency Stomach excess heat pattern.
	Defecation soon after eating indicates a Spleen deficiency Stomach deficiency heat pattern.

Urination	A cold pattern of any of the patterns of imbalance is indicated when there is frequent and copious urination.
	Frequent urination, even though the amount is small, indicates a Kidney deficiency heat pattern, and often appears as urination during the nighttime. Infrequent and small amounts of urination (i.e., urinary difficulty) indicate a Spleen deficiency heat pattern and heat in the Bladder or Kidney. This condition is common with nephritis.
	Pain on urination and the feeling of having residual urine may indicate such things as cystitis, urethritis, prostatomegaly, prostatitis, or kidney stones.
	Dark-colored urine indicates internal heat, and whitish urine indicates coldness due to deficient yang ki.

Appetite	Overeating indicates Kidney deficiency with heat in the Stomach or Spleen deficiency with heat in the Stomach.
	An upset stomach immediately following overeating indicates a Spleen deficiency heat pattern.

Appetite (cont.)	A small appetite indicates a Spleen deficiency cold pattern. Inability to distinguish the flavors of foods indicates that there is heat in one of the organs. Having an ability to clearly distinguish the flavors of foods indicates a cold pattern. A complete lack of appetite or nausea and vomiting commonly indicate a Spleen deficiency Liver excess heat pattern. People who do not feel like eating but who can eat if they sit down to a meal, or those who must force themselves to eat tend to have Liver deficiency. Getting full almost immediately upon starting to eat even though one had the feeling of an empty stomach indicates a Kidney deficiency cold pattern. The five tastes were introduced in the chapter on etiology. It is important to ask about any likes or dislikes of the five tastes.
Menses	Menstrual cramps indicate a Liver deficiency cold pattern or a Spleen deficiency Liver excess pattern. The menstrual cramps of multiparous women indicate a Spleen deficiency Liver excess pattern. A woman may experience menstrual cramps after a menstrual period that came during a fever, or if a fever induced a menstrual period. Such a condition also indicates a Spleen deficiency Liver excess pattern. Generally, late menses indicate a Liver deficiency cold pattern or Liver excess, and early menses indicate a Liver deficiency heat pattern. Profuse bleeding and discharge during menstruation indicates a Liver deficiency cold pattern, and light bleeding indicates a Liver excess pattern.
Sleep	Difficulty falling asleep indicates a Spleen deficiency heat pattern. Waking up in the middle of the night is caused by an abundance of heat in the chest—either heat in the Lung or heat in the Heart. Inability to sleep is caused by blood deficiency and indicates a Liver deficiency cold pattern. Excessive dreaming with the feeling that one has not slept properly indicates a Liver deficiency heat pattern. Waking up early indicates a Kidney deficiency heat pattern. Oversleeping indicates a Spleen deficiency cold pattern.

Dry Mouth	It is difficult to confirm a dry mouth, so it should be examined in relation to the tongue. A dry mouth and tongue indicate a Spleen deficiency Liver excess heat pattern or a Spleen deficiency Stomach excess heat pattern. A dry mouth with a moist tongue usually indicates the heat pattern of a disharmony such as Liver deficiency. Teeth marks around the perimeter of the tongue in a mouth that is not dry indicate phlegm retention. This condition is common in people with a Spleen deficiency heat pattern. Not drinking even though one has a dry mouth indicates a Liver excess pattern. The complete lack of a dry mouth even though in actuality one does not drink anything indicates one of the cold patterns. Abundant saliva in the mouth indicates a Spleen deficiency cold pattern.

7.4 Palpation 切診

Palpation is the method for examining the patient through touching. It includes pulse diagnosis and palpation of the abdomen, back, and meridians. As was previously mentioned, pulse diagnosis will be covered in a separate chapter. This section will cover the other palpation methods.

7.4.1 Abdominal Diagnosis

In abdominal diagnosis the chest and abdomen are palpated to see if there is any dampness or dryness, cold or heat, resistance, depressions, protuberances, pain on pressure, indurations, or palpitations, any of which are used to help determine the pattern of imbalance. The patterns of imbalance found in the abdomen are referred to as abdominal patterns.

Because signs of constitutional and chronic conditions are revealed in the abdominal patterns, an accomplished practitioner can determine not only the present condition, but can also guess past ailments and anticipate possible future illnesses. On the other hand, in the case of an acute febrile disease, such as in what are referred to as external diseases, the pattern of imbalance is determined while ignoring the abdominal patterns.

① **Posture of the Patient During the Abdominal Examination**

Have the patient lie in a comfortable supine position with the arms and legs naturally extended. Western style medical doctors have their patients bend the knees during palpation of the internal organs. The Meridian Therapy practitioner, on the other hand, is looking for imbalances of ki, blood, and fluids, so the patient is asked to extend the legs in a natural posture during examination.

② **Method and Procedure of Abdominal Examinations**

The practitioner should stand on the left side of the patient and palpate using the left hand because the left hand is used as the supporting hand while needling, and thus is employed more often as the diagnostic hand. To palpate with the right hand, the practitioner should stand on the right side of the patient. However, it will be more difficult to needle from this position.

The hand used to palpate should be warm and soft.

Step One: Gently slide the whole palm over the skin to see if there is any dampness or dryness, cold or heat, depressions, protuberances, or resistance. The practitioner's fingers should not be spread apart and there should not be any gaps between the practitioner's palm and the patient's skin.

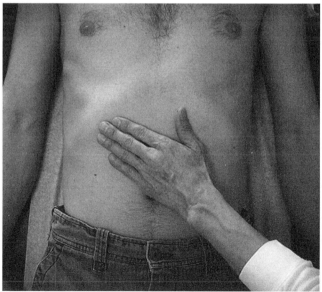
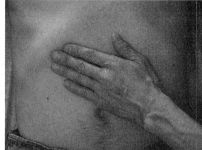
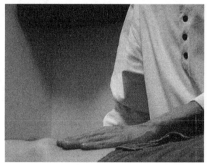

Photos 7–1 A, B, C: Step One Abdominal Palpation

Step Two: Press with the whole palm on areas where any of the above mentioned disharmonies were felt in order to check the degree of disharmony.

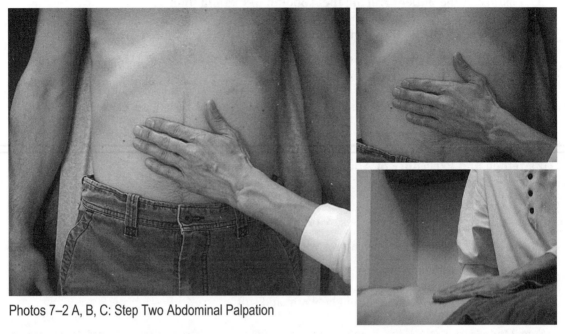

Photos 7–2 A, B, C: Step Two Abdominal Palpation

Step Three: Raise the palm slightly and press the fingers into the body to examine the degree of resistance and condition of depressions, as well as to look for pain on pressure and indurations. If there is any pain on pressure, distinguish whether it is deficient or excess.

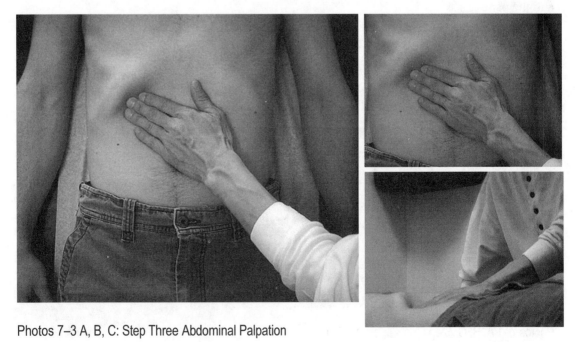

Photos 7–3 A, B, C: Step Three Abdominal Palpation

Step Four: For areas that show resistance or indurations, raise the palm further and press deeper into the body in order to ascertain the depth and whether or not there is any pain on pressure.

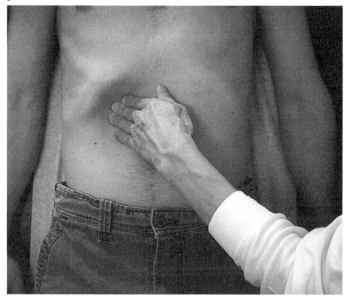
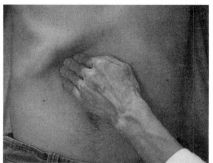
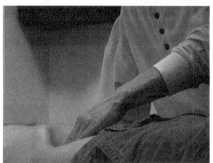
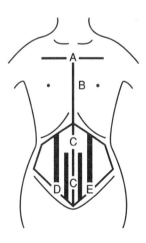

Photos 7–4 A, B, C: Step Four Abdominal Palpation

③ **Areas and Procedure of Abdominal Examination**

A. Palpate from the area near CV-22 to LU-1 on the left and right sides, and down to the area around SP-21.

B. Return to the midline and palpate from CV-17 to the xiphoid process.

C. Palpate with one movement from CV-14 down to below the navel while paying attention to the condition of the area around CV-14, CV-12, the navel, CV-4, and CV-3. Also check the condition of the upper aspect of the pubic bone.

D. Palpate from the top of the pubic bone (CV-2) through the superior aspect of the right inguinal area, then from the ileocecal area up along the Stomach and Spleen channels to below the costal arch (LR-14, GB-24), and then check above and below the costal arch. Next, examine the right side of the abdomen (LR-13, GB-25).

Figure 7–2: Areas and Procedure for Abdominal Examination

E. Palpate the left side in the same manner through the superior aspect of the inguinal area, from the sigmoid colon up along the Stomach and Spleen channels to below the costal arch, and then check above and below the costal arch. Next, examine the left side of the abdomen.

The order of the examination can be a little different from the one given above, but in order to glide the palm smoothly, you should practice a set order. First the skin is stroked, then the palm is raised and fingers pressed into the body; such that the same areas are examined two or three times. Pay attention to those areas that particularly stand out.

The alarm points must also be examined during the abdominal examination, and as a matter of course the areas around the alarm points must also be examined, not just the points themselves.

7.4.2 Abdominal Patterns of Each Pattern of Imbalance

① Abdominal Pattern of a Liver Deficiency Heat Pattern

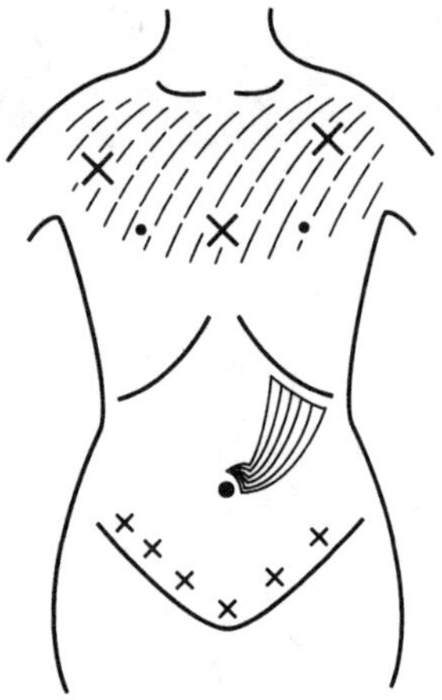

Figure 7–3: Abdominal Pattern of a Liver Deficiency Heat Pattern

There will be resistance below the costal arch on the left side. This is referred to as subcostal tension, and in the *Nan Jing* as Liver accumulation (*shaku* 積). There will be no pain on pressure. When it is difficult to determine if there is Liver accumulation, comparing the left and right sides can be helpful.

Pulsations may be felt from the left side of the navel up to CV-9 above the navel, in which case the patient will be irritable and will experience hot flushes in the upper body and have a cold lower body.

There will be resistance and pain on pressure extending from the superior aspect of the pubic bone through the superior portion of the inguinal area. This indicates changes in the Liver channel and appears when there is a Liver deficiency heat pattern, a Liver deficiency cold pattern, a Spleen deficiency Liver excess pattern, or a Lung deficiency Liver excess pattern. Tension will extend from here up through the lateral extremes of the abdomen.

Deficient-type heat is generated in a Liver deficiency heat pattern. This heat will rise up to the chest, causing LU-1 and CV-17 to exhibit pain on pressure and feel hot to the touch.

② **Abdominal Pattern of a Liver Deficiency Cold Pattern**

There will be coldness in the chest. Even if the surface feels warm to the touch, when the palm is pressed firmly to the chest it will feel cold.

The whole of the upper abdomen will be tense and feel stiff on the surface, but will not show any resistance underneath.

There will be a little resistance and pain on pressure around ST-25 on both sides of the navel, but not enough to be a defining feature in this pattern of imbalance.

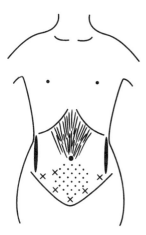

Figure 7–4: Abdominal Pattern of a Liver Deficiency Cold Pattern

There will be resistance and pain on pressure in the ileocecal area due to the presence of longstanding cold. This cold may extend up as far as the right subcostal area, causing pain on pressure there as well.

There may be tension in both lateral extremes of the abdomen, in which case pain on pressure will be found from there extending through the superior portion of the inguinal area to the superior aspect of the pubic bone.

The whole of the lower abdomen will be soft, weak, and cold.

③ **Abdominal Pattern of a Spleen Deficiency Stomach Excess Heat Pattern**

The entire chest will feel very hot to the touch.

The whole abdomen will be distended to such a degree that it will be difficult to depress the abdomen because of strong resistance. The strongest resistance will be felt in the epigastric region around CV-14.

The patient will feel fullness in the chest and abdomen.

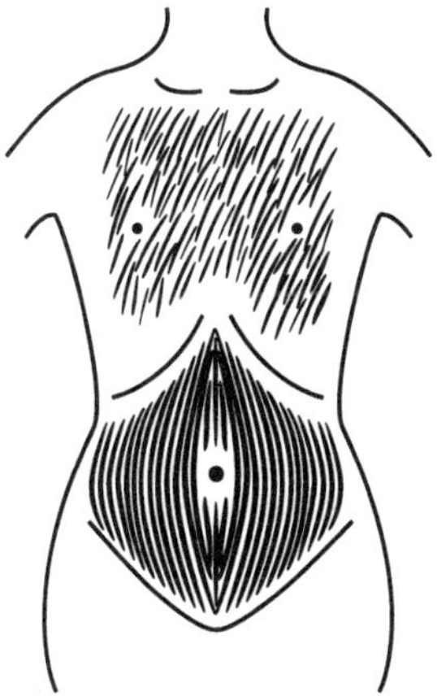

Figure 7–5: Abdominal Pattern of a Spleen Deficiency Stomach Excess Pattern

The lower abdomen along the CV line will feel slightly less resistant in most cases due to a deficiency of Kidney fluids caused by heat in the Stomach and Intestines.

④ Abdominal Pattern of a Spleen Deficiency Stomach Deficiency Heat Pattern

There will be resistance and pain on pressure in the epigastrium, centering on CV-12. A serious illness is indicated if the area of resistance extends out to CV-14.

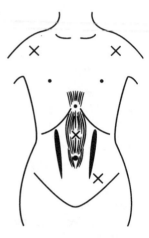

The Stomach channels on both the left and right sides will be tense from ST-19 to below ST-25.

Moreover, the area around the navel may reveal pain on pressure upon light pressure, in which case the patient has a predisposition to abdominal pain.

Pulsations may be felt at CV-9 in some patients. If they extend up as far as CV-14 the condition will be difficult to cure.

The area around the xiphoid process may feel hot to the touch, in which case the patient will have rumbling intestines and belch a lot.

Figure 7-6: Abdominal Pattern of a Spleen Deficiency Stomach Deficiency Heat Pattern

If heat from a Spleen deficiency Stomach deficiency heat pattern spreads to the Lung, the LU-1 points will reveal pain on pressure.

There will be pain on pressure from ST-25 on the left to the area of the sigmoid colon.

⑤ Abdominal Pattern of a Spleen Deficiency Cold Pattern

In a severe cold pattern the whole abdomen will be depressed and will show absolutely no resistance. In extreme cases it is possible to feel the internal organs.

The skin may feel like a thin covering stretched over the internal organs. Such an abdominal pattern carries with it a poor prognosis. This condition may be seen occasionally in elderly patients.

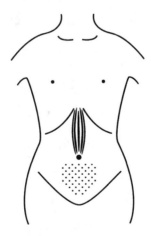

Figure 7-7: Abdominal Pattern of a Spleen Deficiency Cold Pattern

When the cold pattern is relatively light, a little resistance will be felt in the area centering on CV-12. If there happens to be phlegm retention at this time, then resistance and pain on pressure will also appear at CV-14. However, the lower abdomen will be soft, weak, and cold.

⑥ **Abdominal Pattern of a Spleen Deficiency Liver Excess Heat Pattern**

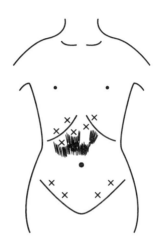

There will be edema (water retention) and pain on pressure above and below the costal arch on both the left and right sides, but especially on the right. Below the costal arch there will be resistance that may extend from LR-14 to the area around CV-14. Such a condition is caused by Liver excess heat. If there is only resistance and no pain on pressure, then the Liver excess was caused by blood stasis and not by heat.

There will be resistance and pain on pressure in the epigastric region centering on CV-12, which is caused by the Spleen deficiency.

Figure 7-8: Abdominal Pattern of a Spleen Deficiency Liver Excess Heat Pattern

In the superior portion of the inguinal region there will be pain on pressure as well as spontaneous pain that may radiate to the lower back. This condition is caused by heat in the Liver channel.

⑦ **Abdominal Pattern of a Spleen Deficiency Liver Excess Pattern**

Two abdominal patterns are seen in this pattern of imbalance. In the first one there is an area of tension like a rod extending from ST-19 in the subcostal area down to ST-25 at a width of ST-19 to LR-14. There will be no pain on pressure, and the tension will be mainly on the right side. This is also considered subcostal tension, and in the *Nan Jing* is referred to as Lung accumulation. This condition is caused by blood stasis.

There may be resistance and pain on pressure in the area centered on CV-12.

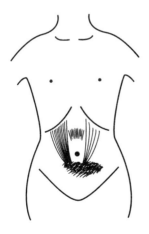

Figure 7-9: Abdominal Pattern of a Spleen Deficiency Liver Excess Pattern

In the other pattern there is blood stagnation in the lower abdomen. There will be resistance, indurations, and pain on pressure extending from below ST-25 on the left, going under the navel, and over to below ST-25 on the right. New blood stasis will show signs mainly on the left while longstanding blood stasis will show signs extending from just below the navel to the area below ST-25 on the right.

⑧ Abdominal Pattern of a Lung Deficiency Liver Excess Pattern

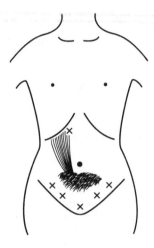

There will be subcostal tension on the right side, which corresponds to Lung accumulation.

ST-19 on the right side will manifest resistance and pain on pressure, a condition that is caused by overeating. This condition is especially common in patients who enjoy raw fish or a diet rich in meat.

The superior portion of the inguinal region and the area above the pubic bone will have resistance and pain on pressure, which is due to changes in the Liver channel.

There will be lower abdominal blood stasis just below and to the sides of the navel.

There will be resistance and pain on pressure in the ileocecal area.

Figure 7-10: Abdominal Pattern of a Lung Deficiency Liver Excess Pattern

⑨ Abdominal Pattern of a Kidney Deficiency Heat Pattern

The CV line will be deficient below the navel due to the Kidney deficiency. At the same time the Stomach channel will feel tight on both the left and right sides, which is due to the spread of deficient-type heat from the Kidney to the Stomach channel.

The CV line below the navel may feel like it has a pencil-sized core, which is literally called in Japanese the *pen-case below the navel*. This is commonly seen in young people with Kidney deficiency. Moreover, patients who have this condition will have a history of cystitis or urethritis.

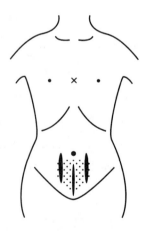

Figure 7-11: Abdominal Pattern of a Kidney Deficiency Heat Pattern

When the Kidney is deficient, heat will increase in the chest. If CV-17 reveals pain on pressure and the whole chest feels hot to the touch, special care needs to be taken since this is a precursor to heart disease.

Because ki naturally rises to the Upper Warmer when there is Kidney deficiency, there may be resistance in the epigastric region.

⑩ **Abdominal Pattern of a Kidney Deficiency Cold Pattern**

The whole of the lower abdomen will be protruding yet will lack strength. The patient will be aware of intestinal movements.

When palpating the abdomen of some patients who have very little flesh it may feel like their skin is directly attached to the internal organs, in which case the skin will of course be quite wrinkled.

The whole abdomen will feel rather cold to the touch, which is caused by the lack of sufficient heat to create resistance.

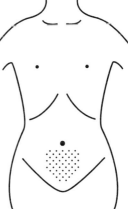

Figure 7-12: Abdominal Pattern of a Kidney Deficiency Cold Pattern

7.4.3 Back Examination

Depressions, protuberances, indurations, pain on pressure, and cold and hot areas on the back, mainly on the back transport points, are used both as examination points and treatment points. However, if a practitioner simply uses these points for treatment without determining the pattern of imbalance, then he will be performing "acupoint therapy" and not Meridian Therapy. If there is pain on pressure, then the practitioner should try to connect these signs with the pattern of imbalance, try to understand why there is pain on pressure, and only then use those points for treatment. The remainder of this section will list important clinical indications that can be gathered from back examinations.

① Lung deficiency is indicated when the skin around BL-13 is rough and cold and the patient has lost flesh in that area.

② There are cases when pain on pressure and indurations appear in the scapular area at points such as SI-14, BL-13, BL-42, BL-14, and BL-43. Stiffness can extend from here up to the neck, making BL-10 and GB-20 stiff. These signs tend to appear when there is an increase of heat in the Heart or Lung, which indicates a Kidney deficiency heat pattern, a Liver deficiency heat pattern, or a Lung deficiency Liver excess pattern.

③ Many patients with pain on pressure along the governing vessel from GV-12 to GV-9 are afflicted with a neuropsychiatric disorder such as neurosis or emotional depression. The most common symptom among these individuals is insomnia. The pattern of imbalance could be Liver deficiency, Lung deficiency Liver excess, or Spleen deficiency Liver excess.

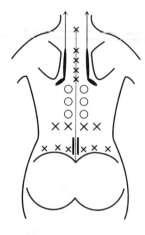

Figure 7-13: Back Examination and Treatment Points

④ It is common for BL-17 to be puffed up and to reveal pain on pressure when there is cholecystopathy (gallbladder disease), hepatitis, or manifest gastritis. In such a condition the pattern of imbalance is usually Spleen deficiency Liver excess heat.

⑤ Cases in which the area around BL-20, BL-21, and BL-22 protrudes, but turns into a depression when pressed, and even shows deficient-type pain—that is, it feels good when pressed—are seen in individuals with a chronic Spleen deficiency heat pattern or a chronic Spleen deficiency cold pattern.

⑥ People who have pain on pressure or indurations at BL-23 and BL-52 usually have Liver deficiency or Kidney deficiency.

⑦ People in whom there are indurations medial to the line between BL-23 and BL-25—in other words the paravertebral points—usually have chronic low back pain. This condition should be treated as blood stasis with a Lung deficiency Liver excess pattern.

⑧ Indurations and pain on pressure along the superior border of the ilium reaching around to the superior aspect of the inguinal area tend to appear when there is Liver deficiency or Liver excess.

⑨ Gynecological disorders and hemorrhoids are indicated when there are indurations and pain on pressure between BL-25 and the area around BL-30. This condition could be due to various patterns of imbalance, but is commonly seen with Liver deficiency or Spleen deficiency.

⑩ Patients who have pain on pressure on BL-35 have a Liver deficiency cold pattern.

⑪ Patients who have water stagnation in the sacral area and in whom it is difficult to discern the *yāo yǎn* point (腰眼穴 *yōgan ketsu*) have a Kidney deficiency heat pattern.

⑫ If a portion of the governing vessel is hot to the touch and manifests pain on pressure, then the organs associated with the back transport points in that portion have heat in them.

7.4.4 Meridian Palpation

Meridian palpation is an examination method whereby the channels are palpated to find any cold or heat, dampness or dryness, depressions, protuberances, indurations, or pain on pressure, any of which can be used to help determine the pattern of imbalance. Further detail was given about this in the "explanation" subsections of Chapter 3, The Flow of the Meridians.

The method of meridian palpation should be performed the same as that for abdominal palpation. The palpation should not be too rough, nor should the practitioner press too strongly in an attempt to find pain on pressure. Gently stroke the skin, and when necessary lightly press deeper into the body. Pain on pressure tends to appear on the yang meridians and depressions tend to appear on the yin meridians.

CHAPTER 8	Pulse Diagnosis
	脉 诊

Since ancient times many pulse diagnosis methods have been formulated. Some of these ancient methods that are presently known include the "three-positions nine-indicators pulse diagnosis" found in the *Su Wen*, the "carotid pulse diagnosis" from the *Ling Shu*, and the "radial artery pulse diagnosis" from the *Nan Jing*. Various other pulse diagnosis methods are introduced in the *Mai Jing* (*Classic of Pulses*).

While each method of pulse diagnosis has its own characteristics, we believe the "six-position pulse diagnosis" (radial artery pulse diagnosis) is the only diagnostic method whereby one can perceive all pathological conditions of the organs and meridians, and can thus demonstrate the effectiveness of this ancient medicine at its best. The proof of this conviction lies in the fact that the six-position pulse diagnosis has been continuously practiced until the present day without flagging in its popularity.

There are some controversial discussions in the literature regarding the meaning of the six-position pulse diagnosis. However, since that topic is not a critical concern for clinical practitioners it will not be discussed here. Yet, a few points about the six-position pulse diagnosis will be mentioned so as to dispel any misunderstandings there may be.

Because some people think the six-position pulse diagnosis is the same as the "pulse-strength comparison diagnosis," they mistakenly think that the "pulse-quality diagnosis" is something altogether different. This is a misunderstanding. The pulse strength comparison diagnosis and the pulse quality diagnosis are necessarily related to each other. This is discussed in detail later in the text, but a general explanation will be given here.

The six-position pulse diagnosis is a method used to examine the six positions as a whole and each of the six positions individually in order to determine whether there is any deficiency, excess, cold, or heat in the ki, blood, and fluids of the organs and meridians. This is the original purpose of the six-position pulse diagnosis, and it is explained as such in all the pulse diagnosis manuals written after the *Classic of Pulses*.

However, it is very difficult to ask beginners to understand how to do this. Therefore, to begin with, we start by teaching only how to differentiate deficient and excess (weak and strong) qualities, according to the method of pulse-strength comparison diagnosis or the pulse comparison diagnosis methods.

The pulse-strength comparison diagnosis is useful only for determining deficiency and excess in the meridians. As this method is the origin of the pulse-position/pulse-quality diagnosis, which will be discussed later, it is meaningful to us as such. But it cannot be used to understand pathology that includes the organs. If one wishes to have a detailed comprehension of the clinical conditions of a disease, one must have a thorough understanding of the kinds of pulse qualities that accompany a deficient pulse or excess pulse. Moreover, the most important thing to remember is that while the pulse-strength comparison diagnosis can be used to select which meridian(s) to treat, it will not help in determining which technique is the most appropriate to use. To that end it was natural to develop the six-basic-pulses diagnosis.

The six-basic-pulses diagnosis is a method for classifying various pulse qualities into six categories. Through the utilization of this method it is possible to grasp the general pathology as well as to determine the appropriate tonification or dispersion insertion technique.

However, even though a floating pulse, for example, within the six basic pulses, can be determined, that does not help in addressing the fact that there are many *degrees* of a floating quality that can be seen from pulse to pulse. The same thing can be said about the other five basic pulses. Therefore, in order to comprehend pathology in even greater detail, and to accordingly apply precise techniques, it is necessary to further divide the six basic pulses into more detailed pulse categories. The pulse-quality diagnosis was developed to achieve that goal.

When pulse qualities are examined on the left and right wrists, the same overall quality often may be found in all six positions, although sometimes a single position shows a different quality from the rest. At those times, the entire pulse quality must be taken into account as a whole, although it goes without saying that attention should be paid to any unusual characteristics in individual pulses among the six positions. In other words, the pattern of imbalance should be determined by considering the pulse qualities in each of the six positions. Note that the pulse-strength comparison diagnosis is used only to ascertain deficiency or excess within the pulse. In this way the location of disease (i.e., the meridian(s) to be treated), the pathology, and needling techniques all become that much more precisely determined.

The beginner can learn six-position pulse diagnosis in a step-by-step manner, as outlined above, and rest assured that each method is not an extraordinarily different way of diagnosis, but rather a part of a unified whole.

8.1 Pulse Diagnosis Positions and Pulse Diagnosis Techniques
脉診部位と脉診方法

8.1.1 The Diagnosis Position and Its Meaning

The pulse is taken mainly on the pulsating part of the radial artery of both wrists. In the classics, this area—between the crease of the wrist and a point 1.9 cùn proximal to the crease—is called the "inch mouth" (寸口 *sunkō*) or "ki opening" (気口 *kikō*). In standard practice, this area is divided into three positions: "inch mouth" (寸口 *sunkō*), "bar top" (関上 *kanjō*), and "cubit center" (尺中 *shakuchū*), which we will call the distal, middle, and proximal positions, respectively, in this text.

The distal position is located directly below the carpal crease. The middle position is located medial to the radial eminence (called the "high bone" in the classics). The proximal position is just proximal to the middle position.

Therefore, there are six positions—three on each wrist—with each position having its corresponding organ and meridian.

Table 8–1: Wrist Postion and Corresponding Organ		
Left Hand	**Position**	**Right Hand**
Small Intestine Heart	**Distal** **Upper Warmer**	Large Intestine Lung
Gallbladder Liver	**Middle** **Middle Warmer**	Stomach Spleen
Bladder Kidney	**Proximal** **Lower Warmer**	Triple Warmer Pericardium

1. The distal positions on both wrists are used to diagnose areas of the body between the diaphragm and head (the Upper Warmer).

2. The middle positions on both wrists are used to diagnose areas of the body between the diaphragm and navel (the Middle Warmer).

3. The proximal positions on both wrists are used to diagnose areas of the body below the navel (the Lower Warmer).

8.1.2 Basics of Pulse Diagnosis

① As a rule the pulse should be taken while the patient is in the supine position. The patient's hands should be positioned slightly below the navel in such a way that they naturally lie on the lower abdomen. The patient's elbows should touch the sides of his/her abdomen. There is no need to hold the patient's hands up or put stress on them. It is good if the palms are facing toward the patient's head or tilted slightly upwards. (Photo 8–1) As a rule the practitioner should stand by the left side of a patient when taking the pulse. Moreover, the pulse should not be taken immediately, but rather taken after the patient has been lying on the treatment table for about five minutes to relax.

② Place your left index finger on the patient's right distal position, your left middle finger on the patient's right middle position, and your left ring finger on the patient's right proximal position. The corresponding ordering of fingers and positions follows for the opposite wrist as well. The proper way to place your fingers is as follows: First put your middle finger on the patient's middle position, then place your index finger between the patient's middle position and the carpal crease. Because it is not good positioning if your index finger is touching the patient's trapezium, if this is the case then you may slightly move your finger proximally. Next place your ring finger beside your middle finger.

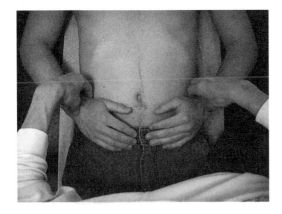

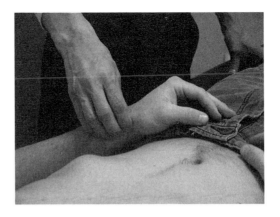

Photo 8–1: Correct positioning of the patient's hands and body for pulse taking

Photo 8–2: Position your fingers at a 90° angle to the artery.

③ The three fingers used for each pulse should be positioned uniformly to match the distance between the index and middle fingers; i.e., the ring finger should be placed next to the index finger to duplicate the distance between the index and the middle fingers. In this way you can find the appropriate distance between the fingers even for a person of large build.

④ The fingers should be placed at an angle 90° to the artery. Be careful not to put the fingers on a diagonal. (Photo 8–2)

⑤ Place the most sensitive part of your finger on the artery where the pulse will be taken. In general most individuals are more sensitive on the pads of the fingers than on the tips of the fingers. You should follow your own sensitivity. However, if you sense your own pulse in the tips of your fingers then you should use the pads of your fingers, so as not to be confused between the patient's pulse and your own pulse.

⑥ The time for taking the pulse should not be too long. As practitioners tend to squeeze the patient's wrist when taking a pulse for a long time, some patients do not like having their pulse taken for very long.

⑦ When taking the pulse you should intermittently apply both harder and lighter pressures. At first you should practice putting pressure on all six fingers evenly and simultaneously. After you get used to this method, you can apply a very light pressure to the distal position, a mid-pressure to the middle position, and a slightly harder pressure to the proximal position. The pulse always seems to be deficient at the distal position and stronger at the proximal position if you do not distribute the pressure correctly.

⑧ If you apply excessive pressure with your fingers you will not be able to read the pulse. It is better to relax your fingers and just let them feel whatever they feel. The fingers always tend to get tense when you press hard on the pulse. Therefore, instead of putting strength into the six fingers, it is better to put strength into your thumb, which is placed on TW-4.

⑨ Pulse diagnosis should be done at the depths of *floating*, *middle*, and *sinking*. But this should not be confused with the floating and sinking pulse qualities. Therefore, in order to avoid this confusion, we shall call the level at which you "float" your fingers on the pulse the superficial level, and the level at which you "sink" your fingers into the pulse the deep level. We will skip an explanation of how to put your fingers into the middle level, as this tends to be too confusing.

⑩ The superficial level is palpated to examine conditions of the yang meridians and fu organs, diseases of which can be differentiated by the pulse quality and symptom pattern.

When palpating the pulses at the superficial level, the fingers only very gently touch the artery. Even if the pulse cannot be detected at this level, you should not press deeper in an attempt to feel something, as this lack of a pulse sensation indicates deficiency.

However, if the pulse is clearly felt at the superficial level, you should consider this information in regard to the pathological condition while also taking into account the pulse quality at the deep level.

⑪ The pulse is palpated at the deep level to examine yin meridians and zang organs, again, diseases of which can be differentiated by the pulse quality and symptom pattern.

As previously noted, slightly more pressure is applied to the proximal position than the distal position when examining the pulse. But care should be taken to not press so hard that blood flow in the artery is cut off.

If the pulse at one position cannot be felt at all at the deep level, it can be regarded as showing a deficiency of essential ki in the zang organ that corresponds to that pulse position. At the same time, in order to determine the pattern of imbalance and method of treatment, the pulse qualities within this specific pulse and the overall pulse should be considered for whether they show signs of ki, blood, or fluid deficiency, or the generation of any heat or cold.

If the pulse at one position can be strongly felt at the deep level, it can be regarded as indicating stagnation of blood or heat in the zang organ or yin meridian of that pulse position. Here, the pattern of imbalance and treatment method should be decided by taking into account the degree of excess or heat present, as revealed in the pulse qualities of that specific pulse position and in the overall pulse.

When shifting from the superficial level to the deep level some practitioners' wrists and fingers tend to straighten up so that they feel the pulse with their fingertips instead of the pads of their fingers. Great care should be taken to avoid this since it causes the fingers to end up palpating at an incorrect location [on the artery] at the deep level.

The pulse should be examined at both the superficial and deep levels as explained above. The pulse *quality* should be ascertained at the position that displays the clearest pulse.

8.1.3 Introductory Pulse Comparison Method

Absolute beginners should follow the steps outlined below for learning pulse diagnosis.

① Memorize which positions of the six-position pulse diagnosis correspond to which organs and meridians.

② Master how to apply your fingertips to the pulse. This may require some training and practice.

③ First place your fingers on the pulse and then repeatedly try to feel the pulse at both the superficial and deep levels. Pay attention to any pulse position(s) that are clearly felt at the superficial level, as these are often the positions that are found to be deficient at the deep level.

Table 8–2: Pulse Comparison of Deficiency Patterns					
Liver Deficiency Pattern			**Spleen Deficiency Pattern**		
Left		Right	Left		Right
	Distal		O	Distal	
O	Middle			Middle	O
O	Proximal			Proximal	O

Lung Deficiency Pattern			Kidney Deficiency Pattern		
Left		Right	Left		Right
	Distal	O		Distal	O
	Middle	O		Middle	
	Proximal		O	Proximal	

Next, look for the weakest position among the six at the deep level. For example, Liver deficiency is indicated if the weakest position is found at the middle position of the left wrist. In this case attention should also be paid to the proximal position of the left wrist, as Kidney deficiency often appears along with Liver deficiency.

In Spleen deficiency the left distal position and the right middle position are commonly both weak. Additionally, pay attention to the right proximal position when examining deficiency and excess in the meridians only.

The right distal and middle positions are often both weak when there is Lung deficiency.

In Kidney deficiency the left proximal position and the right distal position tend to both be weak.

④ A cold pattern with dual yin and yang deficiency is often indicated when there is a pulse position at which nothing is felt at the superficial level even though that position was deficient at the deep level.

It is possible that all the pulse positions may feel weak, and hence do not match any of the typical patterns as shown in the above diagram. In that case, the pattern of imbalance would be determined according to the pulse qualities. However, since this is too much of a stretch for beginners, you should make a judgment by placing more emphasis on the symptom pattern. Note that it is not possible to have a doubling up a Liver deficiency pattern with a Lung deficiency pattern or a Spleen deficiency pattern with a Liver deficiency pattern.

⑤ Pay attention to any positions where the pulse can be felt strongly at the deep level. This strongly felt pulse is caused by the stagnation of heat or blood in the area corresponding to that pulse position. However, such a pulse will not always appear in the suspected area even though there may be stagnation of heat or blood, since heat can move to any other organ or meridian.

⑥ The pulse diagnosis method explained above is termed the pulse-strength comparison diagnosis. It is possible to make a misdiagnosis using only this method. However, it is useful to begin learning by placing an emphasis on finding the deficiency, since all disorders start from a deficiency of essential ki of the zang organs. It should be noted that if you are preoccupied with only finding the strong and weak positions of the pulse, it is possible that you will clumsily grasp the artery. It is best to first and foremost follow the proper methods of observing the superficial and deep levels; otherwise you may make impaired judgments concerning the pulse qualities, which will be explained later.

8.1.4 Intermediate Six-Basic-Pulses Diagnosis

There are 24 pulse qualities mentioned in the *Classic of Pulses*. Including other pulse qualities that were added during later periods, all pulse qualities can be loosely classified into six categories: floating, sinking, slow, rapid, deficient, and excess. These six categories are termed the "six basic pulses." That is, they are the basis of all the other pulse qualities. Some examples are given in the following table.

Table 8–3: Basic Pulse Categories	
Pulses in the Floating (浮 *Fu*) Category	Floating, hollow, large
Pulses in the Sinking (沈 *Chin*) Category	Sinking, hidden, thin
Pulses in the Slow (遲 *Chi*) Category	Slow, moderate
Pulses in the Rapid (数 *Saku*) Category	Rapid, moving
Pulses in the Deficient (虚 *Kyo*) Category	Deficient, hollow, minute, thin, soft, weak
Pulses in the Excess (実 *Jitsu*) Category	Excess, flooding; and slippery, wiry, and tight pulses that are powerful

It must be stressed that the terms floating and sinking, slow and rapid, and deficient and excess have slightly different meanings when they are used to refer to the basic pulses and when describing the pulse qualities.

For instance, a deficient pulse in the sense of a basic pulse includes all the pulse qualities that fall in the deficient pulse category. A weak pulse in the pulse-strength comparison diagnosis should be thought of as the same as a deficient pulse in terms of the six basic pulses. However, a deficient pulse in the sense of pulse qualities is a narrower concept related to a specific pathology.

Accordingly, one must master the pulse qualities to achieve a detailed understanding of pathology. It is nevertheless important to classify pulses according to the six basic pulses, as this will help determine which techniques are appropriate for treating the pattern of imbalance that was diagnosed when finding the weakest pulse using the pulse-strength comparison technique.

Following is a list of the general pathologies that can be gathered from the basic pulses and the associated tonification and dispersion techniques. Note, however, that since all diagnoses and their corresponding treatment methods are based first of all on deficiency and excess, the other four basic pulses should be understood in combination with deficiency and excess. Therefore, even though deficiency and excess are listed individually as two of the six basic pulses, they are given below in conjunction with the other basic pulses.

① The Floating Basic Pulse	
Pathology	**Tonification & Dispersion**
The floating basic pulse appears when an abundance of ki gathers in the yang meridians. The pathology can vary, but a floating and excess pulse is caused by external pathogenic influences and a floating and deficient pulse is caused by yin deficiency (i.e., blood or fluid deficiency).	Primarily tonify with shallow insertion. If the pulse is floating and excess, the yang channels could be dispersed after tonifying the yin channels. If the pulse is floating and deficient, either only tonify the yin channels, or sometimes tonify the yang channels as well.

② Sinking Basic Pulse	
Pathology	**Tonification & Dispersion**
The sinking basic pulse appears when there is an abundance of ki in the yin channels or organs. The pathology can vary, but a sinking and excess pulse indicates blood and heat stagnation. A sinking and deficient pulse indicates an excess of water or a lack of yang ki with an abundance of cold.	Primarily use slightly deep insertion. However, if the pulse is sinking and deficient, both the yin and yang channels must be tonified with shallow insertion. The yin channels can be dispersed if the pulse is sinking and excess.

③ Slow Basic Pulse	
Pathology	**Tonification & Dispersion**
The slow basic pulse appears when there is chronic coldness that has extended to the blood. A slow and excess pulse indicates blood stagnation. A slow and deficient pulse indicates coldness and water stagnation.	Primarily use slow insertion and retained needles. However, if the pulse is slow and excess, retain the needle a little deeper. When the pulse is slow and deficient it is necessary to tonify for a long time or tonify with moxibustion.

④ Rapid Basic Pulse	
Pathology	**Tonification & Dispersion**
The rapid basic pulse appears when there is heat. When the pulse is rapid and excess the heat is stagnated somewhere in the body. Blood and fluids are deficient if the pulse is rapid and deficient.	Primarily use the rapid insertion and removal needling technique in order to reduce the heat. However, focus on tonification if the pulse is rapid and deficient.

8.1.5 Advanced Pulse-Quality Diagnosis

By using the six basic pulses it is possible to make rough classifications of the pulses. But each of the six basic pulses has a variety of different pulses that fall within its range of description. Therefore, the pulse-quality diagnosis is used to make further classifications within each of the six basic pulse categories. Detailed explanations about each pulse quality will be given later, so here we will just mention the significance of differentiating pulse qualities.

① Knowing the pulse qualities presented by a patient enables you to understand in greater detail the location of disease, etiology, pathology, and the pattern of imbalance, and makes it easier to comprehend the clinical conditions of the disease.

② When you understand the location of disease, etiology, pathology, and the pattern of imbalance, you will be able to appropriately employ a variety of techniques, reduce treatment mishaps, and speed healing time.

③ Misdiagnoses of patterns of imbalance that are undeterminable by the pulse-strength diagnosis because of multiple deficiencies can be avoided by considering the pathology in terms of the pulse qualities.

8.1.6 Most Advanced Pulse-Position/Pulse-Quality Diagnosis

In his book, the *Essence of Acupuncture Treatment*, Okabe Sodō concluded his discussion of what we now term the six-basic-pulse diagnosis technique with the following statement:

> Even if the six-position pulse diagnosis is not to be found in the *Su Wen*, *Ling Shu*, or *Nan Jing* in its present form, I think it is a good thing that it was developed and perfected. I do not know whether or not there is a more advanced form [of pulse diagnosis], but I feel that [the six-position pulse diagnosis] has served our generation well as it is now. Yet, if it is possible to develop an even greater [pulse diagnosis method], then I think it should be done.

We propose that the pulse diagnosis technique that goes beyond the six-position pulse diagnosis of the six-basic-pulses technique is what is called pulse-quality diagnosis, or the pulse-position/pulse-quality diagnosis. Okabe Sodō wrote about the pulse-position/pulse-quality diagnosis very early on.

The pulse-position/pulse-quality diagnosis is meaningful for the following reasons:

① It is uncommon to see only one kind of pulse quality appearing by itself in the overall pulse. Rather, it is usual for a combination of two or three kinds of pulse qualities to appear. By categorizing these pulse qualities by position as well, it is possible to gain a more detailed understanding of the pathology and to form a prognosis.

② Later in the text we will go into a description of the pulse conditions for each pattern of imbalance. That information is based on the pulse-position/pulse-quality diagnosis. Your understanding of etiology, pathology, and symptom patterns, which we have already introduced, will deepen as you practice the pulse position/pulse quality diagnosis.

③ You will come to know which among ki, blood, and fluids is deficient through having a greater understanding of the significance of the weak pulse positions. It will also become easier to distinguish between cold and heat.

④ By understanding the pulse quality of the strong positions you will be able to know what (i.e., ki, blood, or fluids) is excess and where (i.e., which meridian or organ) that excess is located. By knowing this information, you will be less likely to miss any serious illnesses.

⑤ Determining the pattern of imbalance and accurately selecting the appropriate techniques will become easier with the detailed understanding of pathology gained from utilizing the pulse-position/pulse-quality diagnosis.

Each of the pulse diagnosis methods mentioned above—pulse-strength comparison, six basic pulses, pulse-quality, and pulse-position/pulse-quality—are conducted at the superficial and deep levels. The different methods represent a gradual progression in observed detail, but they are in no way contradictory. As was stated at the beginning of this chapter, it is a misunderstanding to think that the six-position pulse diagnosis and the pulse-quality diagnosis are different.

8.2 The Normal Pulse (The Healthy Person's Pulse)
平脉 （健康人の脉）

The Chinese classic *Gatherings from Eminent Acupuncturists* (*Zhěn Jiā Shū Yào*) states, "As a rule, [to do] pulse diagnosis one must first know the [seasonal pulses and] time pulses, Stomach pulse and normal pulse of the organs, and thereafter may proceed to diseased pulses." Other pulse diagnosis books say much the same thing—basically that it is important to know a healthy pulse before one can understand a diseased pulse. However, one hardly ever meets someone with the ideal normal pulse, as each person's pulses reflect their own peculiar constitutional imbalances. Nevertheless, since it is still important to have a standard, this section will present the classic picture of a healthy person's pulse.

8.2.1 Stomach Ki Pulse *I-Ki no Myaku* 胃気の脉

The presence of a Stomach ki pulse is considered a normal pulse. A Stomach ki pulse refers to a pulse that is supple and soft. A floating pulse, for instance, should have a softness that is peculiar to a floating pulse.

Moreover, a soft pulse that does not incline toward either floating or sinking, slow or rapid, or deficient or excess is considered to have Stomach ki.

Stomach ki is judged to be bountiful if there is a large depth to the pulse between the superficial level and the deep level. A sinking pulse, for example, is a pulse that can be easily felt at the deep level. Thus, a sinking pulse that has an abundance of Stomach ki would be slightly felt at the superficial level and felt very clearly at the deep level. A pulse that cannot be felt at all at the superficial level, and that can only be felt at the deep level, would be a sinking pulse with very little Stomach ki.

These are the three methods for evaluating the Stomach ki pulse. If by any of these methods Stomach ki is found to be lacking, that person is judged as having weak life energy and little natural healing ability. The prognosis of a patient with a serious illness is judged by the amount of Stomach ki. Moreover, a treatment is considered successful when after the treatment the pulse shows an improvement in Stomach ki.

8.2.2 Seasonal Pulses *Kisetsu no Myaku* 季節の脉

① A spring pulse is soggy-weak and long, and is also called wiry-like. Wiry-like means a soft wiry pulse that has Stomach ki. A healthy person should have this kind of pulse during the springtime. Spring is the time when yang ki arises from the power of the blood. Because the yang ki is not yet full, it is called soggy-weak. However, at this time yang ki is hidden inside; hence it is called long. Such a pulse is also called wiry. Because it is not taut like the string of a newly strung bow, it is termed wiry-like.

② A summer pulse is said to arise with a sudden surge and then slowly taper off. Such a pulse is called a flooding pulse, but of course it is not a diseased flooding pulse. It can be thought of as a pulse that floats and is easily felt because it is a soft flooding pulse that has Stomach ki. The appearance of this kind of pulse during the summertime is a sign of health.

Summer is the time when yang ki is abundant. In the human body as well, it is best to have an abundance of yang ki and to release it along with sweat. That is why the pulse should be floating and why it is called a flooding pulse.

③ It is best to have a slow-moderate pulse during midsummer (the *doyō* 土用 of summer). A moderate pulse means that the Spleen and Stomach are working well and the production of ki and blood is active. A slow pulse means that summer yang ki has not retreated to the inside, and there is also not much heat in the Heart. When this slow-moderate pulse accompanies any of the seasonal pulses, those pulses are soft pulses that have Stomach ki.

④ An autumn pulse is lightly deficient and floating, and is likened to a hair. It is floating, but when pressure is applied there is no strength in the middle. However, because it has Stomach ki, it is not too soft. This is a healthy pulse for the autumn.

Autumn is the time everything gathers together. In the body as well, yin ki becomes prosperous and yang ki hides inside. However, some yang ki remains in the external areas of the body as leftover traces of summer. That is why a floating pulse appears, but feels like a hair because the inside is empty.

⑤ A winter pulse is sinking, soggy, and slippery and is likened to a stone. The term stone here conveys the meaning of sinking but does not refer to a diseased pulse. It is a soft sinking pulse that has Stomach ki. This is a healthy pulse to have during the winter.

Winter is the time when everything hides. In the body as well, yin ki becomes abundant and yang ki hides inside. The sinking pulse indicates that yin ki is abundant. But, the pulse becomes slippery because yang ki increases inside. Of course it is not a diseased slippery pulse, and that is why it is a soggy pulse that is slippery.

A healthy person would have each of the pulses described above during the appropriate season. Moreover, it is said that the clinician should aim at creating these kinds of pulses in the patient according to the season. Realistically speaking, however, there are very few patients who have such ideal pulses. Nevertheless, there are some who do have pulses that are close to these, such as those who, for example, show a floating pulse in the summer and a sinking pulse in the winter.

In clinical usage this concept is adopted as follows: People who show a sinking pulse in the summer, a flooding pulse in the winter, a wiry pulse in the autumn, and a floating pulse in the spring will likely have a slow recovery or a bad prognosis.

8.2.3 Normal Pulses of the Five Zang Organs *Gozō no Hei Myaku* 五臓の平脉

According to Chapter 4 of the *Nan Jing*, the Lung shows a floating, choppy, and short pulse, the Heart shows a floating, large, and scattered pulse, the Spleen shows a moderate and large pulse, the Liver shows a wiry and long pulse or a sinking, firm, and long pulse, and the Kidney shows a sinking, soggy, and excess pulse or a sinking, soggy, and slippery pulse. In general, it is said that these pulses appear when the five zang organs are healthy and that these standards should be kept in mind when using the six-position pulse diagnosis. So, for example, the right distal position should show a floating, choppy, and short pulse, while the left distal position should show a floating, large, and scattered pulse.

However, to continue with our example of the right distal position, we must next face the question of how to distinguish a healthy, floating, choppy, and short pulse from a diseased pulse. If the pulse is floating, choppy, and short *and* has Stomach ki, then it is a healthy pulse and really should not be called floating, choppy, and short, but should rather be called by some other name. Therefore some practitioners primarily use these terms to describe pulses that appear when there is a zang organ disease.

Compared to the proximal positions, it is best for the Heart and Lung pulses to be slightly floating, and compared to the distal positions, it is best for the Liver and Kidney pulses to be slightly sinking. That is why we press a little harder on proximal positions than the distal positions when performing pulse diagnosis.

8.2.4 Pulses of the Corpulent and the Slender

A heavyset person's pulse tends to be sinking and difficult to read and a thin person's pulse tends to be floating and easy to read. This must be taken into account when examining pulses.

A heavyset person's overall pulse tends to be sinking. In brief, this condition points to a water toxin (i.e., chronic water stagnation) or blood stasis and is an indication of the individual's physical constitution. When we try to ameliorate the conditions of patients with chronic diseases or constitutional irregularities—such as obesity—the pattern of imbalance should be determined by considering a sinking pulse as a diseased pulse. In the case of an acute illness, even if the pulse appears to be sinking, it could be a floating pulse for that person. This must be taken into consideration when examining the pulse.

Men who exercise or perform physical labor tend to be among those who are slender and have a floating pulse. This also is a manifestation of their physical constitution. By nature this type of person tends to have blood deficiency. Therefore, when treating patients with such chronic diseases or constitutional irregularities, we should use this floating pulse as a reference in order to decide the pattern of imbalance. However, in an acute case that shows signs of cold, the pulse could still be floating. In this case you should pay attention to the deficiency and excess in the pulse and be careful not to misdiagnose the pattern as a yang excess pattern.

8.2.5 Normal Pulses of the Individual

It is practical to consider that almost no one has an ideally healthy pulse. However, it is important to quickly become familiar with the regular healthy pulse of each patient.

Imagine, for an instance, someone who is in excellent condition even though they regularly present with a Liver deficient pulse. Such a person may feel sick if they develop Lung deficiency or Spleen deficiency, but not so much if they develop Kidney deficiency. Therefore, the goal of treatment in this case would be to bring about a return to a Liver deficiency condition.

In his seminar about the *Nan Jing*, Inoue Keiri said that it is possible to make a so-called ideal pulse, but that doing so does not make people feel better; on the contrary, people usually feel worse.

8.3   Pulse Qualities, Pathology, and Insertion Techniques
脉の形状と病理・刺法

For the following descriptions of pulse qualities we have followed the *Classic of Pulses*, and for those pulse qualities that made their appearance during later periods—firm, long, short, large, small, and racing—we have used the *Gatherings from Eminent Acupuncturists* and the *Zēng Bǔ Mài Lùn Kǒu Jué* as references.

The following subsections give an explanation of each pulse quality as adopted from the *Classic of Pulses*. Following that are comments on pathology based on other references. Lastly, insertion techniques based on Okabe Sodō's descriptions from the *Oriental Medical Journal* are introduced.

8.3.1 Floating Pulse *Fu Myaku* 浮脉

Quality	A floating pulse is clearly felt at the superficial level and disappears at the deep level.

Pathology	A floating pulse that is powerful is one that is caused by an external pathogenic influence and that results from the accumulation of ki in the external areas (i.e., the yang meridians). Ki accumulation in the external areas is caused by the fever produced by external pathogenic influences such as cold damage or wind stroke. A floating pulse that is not powerful is one that results from yin deficiency. The lack of blood or fluids due to fatigue produces deficient-type heat, which is what causes the floating pulse. This pulse is common in a Liver deficiency heat pattern. A floating pulse appears when the source ki of the Triple Warmer is almost gone. At this time there will be a marked deficiency. A floating pulse at the distal positions indicates either yang excess or yang deficiency, and a floating pulse at the middle or proximal positions indicates a yin (i.e., blood or fluids) deficiency of the corresponding area. During the autumn it is a sign of health to have a floating pulse that is neither deficient nor excess nor slow nor rapid.
Needling	Use dispersion with the rapid insertion and removal technique for a floating and rapid pulse that is powerful. Use shallow tonification for a pulse that is floating and rapid but that is not powerful. Use tonification with needles that are retained for a pulse that is floating but is not powerful.

8.3.2 Sinking Pulse *Chin Myaku* 沈脉

Quality	A sinking pulse is not felt at the superficial level but is clearly felt at the deep level.
Pathology	A sinking pulse that is powerful indicates blood stasis (i.e., Liver excess). This pulse tends to appear at the left middle position. Heat in the corresponding organ is indicated if a sinking pulse that is powerful appears at one of the other positions.

	A sinking pulse that is not powerful indicates a water toxin (pathogenic dampness) condition, such as phlegm retention, or coldness (cold pattern). This pulse tends to appear when the patient has any of the cold patterns.
	During the winter it is a sign of health to have a sinking pulse that is neither deficient nor excess nor slow nor rapid.
Needling	Tonify yang and disperse yin if there is a sinking pulse that is powerful. Retain the needles or use warming needles on the lower abdomen if there is a sinking pulse that is not powerful.

8.3.3 Slow Pulse *Chi Myaku* 遲脉

Quality	A slow pulse is one that beats three times or fewer during one breath.
	Both slow and rapid pulses are examined in relation to the patient's breath, but can be measured against the clinician's breath if he or she has a normal (i.e., calm) breathing rate.
Pathology	A slow pulse that is powerful is usually seen when there is chronic coldness or pain resulting from dampness.
	A slow pulse that is not powerful indicates blood or fluid deficiency with coldness. This pulse is common with a Kidney deficiency cold pattern.
Needling	Tonify for a long time. If the pulse is powerful, find the strong pulse position and slightly disperse the corresponding meridian.

8.3.4 Rapid Pulse *Saku Myaku* 数脉

Quality	A rapid pulse is one that beats six or seven times during one breath.
Pathology	A rapid pulse that is powerful usually results when there is an acute febrile disease, when there is internal heat such as from Liver excess heat, or when there is heat in the yang channels or fu organs.
	A rapid pulse that is not powerful usually results when there is an abundance of deficient-type heat due to fluid deficiency, when there is a lack of yang ki due to an incorrect treatment, or when the patient has boils.

Needling	Disperse the excess areas when the pulse is rapid and powerful. Use only tonification when the pulse is rapid but is not powerful.

8.3.5 Deficient Pulse *Kyo Myaku* 虚脉

Quality	A deficient pulse is slow, large, and soft. It disappears from under the fingers at the deep level.
Pathology	Please pay close attention to the description of a deficient pulse taken from the *Classic of Pulses*. This does not simply mean that the pulse is weak, and it is not the same as a deficient pulse in terms of the six basic pulses. It refers to an extremely specific pulse quality. The classics say that this kind of deficient pulse appears when there is blood or fluid deficiency due to fatigue, or when the meridians have been injured by summerheat. They also say that the symptom pattern includes being easily frightened and having a tendency to feel uneasy. Considering this fact, it would seem that a deficient pulse is caused mainly by fluid deficiency, in particular that of the Kidney.
Needling	Tonify the fluids. In other words, use one of the water points on the yin channels and one of the earth points on the yang channels.

8.3.6 Excess Pulse *Jitsu Myaku* 实脉

Quality	An excess pulse is large and continuous from the superficial level to the deep, and feels slightly strong. At the deep level it feels like the pulse is gathering into a knot under the fingers. An excess pulse does not have to be so strong that it seems to deflect the finger; it can be taken to mean a pulse that does not disappear at the deep level and that becomes very knotted and hard.
Pathology	An excess pulse results from a stagnation of heat usually created by an external influence in the yang meridians or fu organs. Blood stasis can also cause an excess pulse, as can heat that spreads from any of the heat patterns.
Needling	Use quick insertion and removal for yang channel heat, and use deep insertion for yin channel heat.

8.3.7 Slippery Pulse *Katsu Myaku* 滑脉

Quality	A slippery pulse is smooth and seems to roll along nicely. It resembles a rapid pulse.
	The name slippery was used to invoke the image of smooth coming and going, in the sense of gliding. It does not incline toward floating or sinking, slow or fast, nor deficient or excess. However, it is more likely than not to appear with a rapid pulse or an excess pulse.
Pathology	A slippery pulse appears when the influence of heat reaches all the way to the blood, the heat being produced when yang ki becomes bottled up due to mucus and food trapped in the stomach. Or, it is also common in individuals who naturally have an abundance of blood.
	Nowadays it is often seen among individuals with hypertension. If the patient does not have high blood pressure, one should considere that heat is trapped somewhere in the body.
Needling	After tonifying yin, apply a slightly long dispersion in the area that has the heat.

8.3.8 Choppy Pulse *Shoku Myaku* 濇脉

Quality	A choppy pulse is thin and slow. The pulsation is not smooth and seems to stumble along. It can also feel scattered or sometimes interrupted.
	The choppy pulse contrasts with the slippery pulse. Here as well, the word choppy was used to invoke the image of difficulty in coming and going.
Pathology	A choppy pulse appears when there is a deficiency and stagnation of ki or when there is blood stasis due to ki deficiency.
	Ki deficiency is common when there is a choppy pulse in the right distal position, and Liver excess is common when there is a choppy pulse in the left middle position.
Needling	Tonify ki and disperse if there is any blood stagnation.

8.3.9 Wiry Pulse *Gen Myaku* 弦脉

Quality	A wiry pulse is not felt at the superficial level and feels like a bowstring at the deep level. It is said to be one of the seven external pulses, which means that it is related to heat.
Pathology	A wiry pulse appears because of heat that is trapped somewhere in the body. It tends to arise when there is a lack of blood in the muscles (Liver deficiency) or when the patient has sore muscles or neuralgia. In the case of internal illnesses it tends to appear when there is Spleen deficiency with Liver excess heat. A wiry pulse that is not powerful indicates blood deficiency with the resultant deficient-type heat in the corresponding meridian. A wiry pulse that is powerful indicates a stagnation of heat in the corresponding organ. In the spring a wiry pulse that does not incline toward deficiency or excess and is neither slow nor fast should be considered a healthy pulse.
Needling	Tonify yin and disperse areas when necessary where heat is trapped in the blood.

8.3.10 Tight Pulse *Kin Myaku* 緊脉

Quality	A tight pulse is very tense and feels like a tautly pulled straw rope. The analogy of a straw rope is used because the sensation on the finger is somewhat rough.
Pathology	A tight pulse appears when there is a sudden and severe invasion of coldness (Jpn: *kanrei*, Chn: *hán lěng*) or when there is pain or boils. Be cautious if the patient shows a tight pulse with an internal illness and pain. A tight pulse in one of the six pulse positions should be considered an indication that there is a lack of Stomach ki in the organ that corresponds to that position.
Needling	Tonify both yin and yang, and remove the tight pulse by increasing yang ki or by increasing Stomach ki through tonification of the Spleen and Stomach. If this does not remove the tight pulse, disperse the excess if there is any.

8.3.11 Hollow Pulse *Kō Myaku* 芤脉

Quality	A hollow pulse is floating, large, and soft. It is empty between the superficial and deep levels, although the pulse can be felt encompassing this central emptiness. It is said to resemble the feeling of a scallion stalk.
Pathology	The hollow pulse is one of the floating and deficient basic pulses. It has no central core and is weak overall. Hemorrhaging that produces bloody stools or blood in the urine causes this pulse quality. A hollow pulse in one of the six pulse positions due to some other loss of blood should be considered as indicating a lack of blood in the corresponding organ or meridian.
Needling	Tonify in great measure, focusing on yin ki.

8.3.12 Flooding Pulse *Kō Myaku* 洪脉

Quality	A flooding pulse feels extremely large and thick at the superficial level. It is one of the floating and excess basic pulses. In the summer it is healthy to have a flooding pulse that is not too strong. After the *Classic of Pulses* was written the flooding pulse became known as a large pulse.
Pathology	A flooding pulse appears when there is an abundance of heat in the yang channels or when the patient has a very vigorous illness. Naturally it indicates a heat pattern and an excess pattern. It can be caused by external pathogenic influences or yin deficiency, which produces a milder condition.
Needling	Disperse areas that have heat. Use bloodletting when appropriate.

8.3.13 Hidden Pulse *Fuku Myaku* 伏脉

Quality	A hidden pulse is felt only at such a deep level that it is as if one were feeling the bone. It is one of the sinking basic pulses.
Pathology	A hidden pulse appears when there is extreme ki and blood deficiency due to over- thinking, when there is a chronic cold pattern (with dampness), or when there is a stiff lump in a yin channel or zang organ due to blood stasis.
Needling	Tonify with deep insertion. Retaining the needles is the most appropriate.

8.3.14 Leathery Pulse *Kaku Myaku* 革脉

Quality	A leathery pulse, like the sinking pulse and the hidden pulse, can only be felt at the deep level. It is excess, large, and so long that it protrudes out from the normal pulse positions. It is also slightly wiry.
	The leathery pulse is one of the sinking and excess basic pulses. However, it is not a real excess pulse; it just feels hard because of deficient and dried out fluids. Applying further pressure reveals that it is deficient at the bottom.
Pathology	A leathery pulse appears when there is an abundance of internal heat due to a lack of fluids or when there is stagnation of ki and blood due to emotional depression. The left proximal position can show a leathery pulse quality when there is a Kidney deficiency heat pattern.
Needling	Tonify the yin channels.

8.3.15 Minute Pulse *Bi Myaku* 微脉

Quality	A minute pulse is extremely fine and soft. It fades in and out of perceptibility. Like the thread of a spider's web, it disappears when pressure is applied.
Pathology	The minute pulse is one of the deficient basic pulses.
	It appears when there is extreme ki and blood deficiency or when ki and blood are not being produced in the Middle Warmer. Both cases should be treated as a cold pattern.
Needling	Tonify both yin and yang for quite a long time with thin needles using only a few acupuncture points.

8.3.16 Thin Pulse *Sai Myaku* 細脉

Quality	A thin pulse is a slender pulse that is slightly larger than a minute pulse. Unlike a minute pulse, it does not fade in and out of perceptibility.
Pathology	A thin pulse appears when both ki and blood are deficient and when there is a lack of Stomach ki. It is one of the deficient basic pulses. It appears with each of the cold patterns.
Needling	Gently and slowly tonify both yin and yang.

8.3.17 Soft Pulse *Nan Myaku* 軟脉

Quality	A soft pulse is floating and slender. It is one of the floating and deficient basic pulses. Some books use the term "soggy pulse" (*nan myaku* 濡脉) instead of soft pulse, but these terms are equivalent.
Pathology	A soft pulse appears when both yin and yang are deficient due to a deficiency of the yang ki of the Lower Warmer. It is seen with greater frequency when there is a Kidney deficiency cold pattern.
Needling	Gently tonify both yin and yang of the Kidney channel for a long time.

8.3.18 Weak Pulse *Jaku Myaku* 弱脉

Quality	A weak pulse is extremely soft, and is sinking and thin. It feels like it will disappear at the deep level. It is one of the sinking and deficient basic pulses.
Pathology	A weak pulse appears when both ki and blood are deficient, but especially when there is a lack of yang ki due to blood deficiency. In other words, it tends to appear when there is a Liver deficiency cold pattern.
Needling	Tonify both yin and yang. A touching needle is most appropriate.

8.3.19 Scattered Pulse *San Myaku* 散脉

Quality	A scattered pulse is irregular and amorphous. The pulsation can be felt at the superficial level, but the shape of the artery cannot be determined. Naturally it cannot be felt at the deep level.
Pathology	A scattered pulse indicates the condition in which ki that has gathered in the external areas of the body due to extreme blood deficiency. The prognosis is bad if it seems like the scattered pulse is going to continue. It also indicates that there is Kidney deficiency and deficiency of the source ki of the Triple Warmer.
Needling	Firmly tonify the Kidney and tonify the source ki of the Triple Warmer.

8.3.20 Moderate Pulse *Kan Myaku* 緩脉

Quality	A moderate pulse is slow and relaxed, but it is faster than the slow pulse.
Pathology	A diseased moderate pulse appears when the circulation of ki and blood is sluggish due to their dual deficiency or when there is a deficiency of yang ki. If a person is healthy and has a moderate pulse, that pulse is said to be full of Stomach ki.
Needling	Tonify the Pericardium channel and the Spleen channel to activate the Stomach ki.

8.3.21 Hasty Pulse *Soku Myaku* 促脉

Quality	The beat of a hasty pulse is rapid, and yet it stops sometimes, so it is irregular.
Pathology	A hasty pulse is rapid because ki is circulating quickly in an effort to restore deficient blood to normal. It is sometimes irregular because there is not enough blood and it seems to spin around in aimless circles. This pulse quality tends to appear when there is Heart heat or Lung heat due to a heat pattern from Kidney deficiency or Liver deficiency.
Needling	Tonify the fire point on the Kidney channel, the metal point on the Liver channel, and the fire points on both the Lung and Heart channels.

8.3.22 Knotted Pulse *Ketsu Myaku* 結脉

Quality	As the name implies, the beat of a knotted pulse is slow and sometimes irregular.
Pathology	A knotted pulse appears when accumulation (積 *shaku*) or emotional depression causes yin ki to flourish and causes ki and blood to circulate poorly. It tends to be seen when there is Spleen deficiency Liver excess or Lung deficiency Liver excess.
Needling	Disperse the excess area after tonifying both yin and yang.

8.3.23 Intermittent Pulse *Tai Myaku* 代脉

Quality	The beat of an intermittent pulse will stops so that the rhythm of the pulse is disrupted then suddenly it will start beating again.
Pathology	An intermittent pulse appears when the source ki of the Triple Warmer is about to diminish and there is a deficiency of ki, blood, and fluids of the zang organs.
Needling	Because this is one of the death pulses (*shi myaku* 死脉). In principle treatment should not be performed.

8.3.24 Moving Pulse *Dō Myaku* 動脉

Quality	A moving pulse is like loose marbles. It only appears in the middle position.
Pathology	A moving pulse appears when there is blood deficiency due to exhaustion, bloody stools, or menstrual bleeding.
Needling	Treat as a Kidney deficiency heat pattern.

8.3.25 Firm Pulse *Rō Myaku* 牢脉

Quality	A firm pulse is solid at the deep level and is powerful; the beating can always be felt at the deep level, as if it were stuck to the bottom of the pulse.
Pathology	"When the internal [areas] are excess and the external [areas] are deficient, and [there is] hasty ki [rapid breathing with short breaths] in the chest, physical fatigue, and extreme weakness of the sinews, at that time the pulse will almost always be close to having no stomach ki, so all practitioners regard this pulse as very dangerous. Moreover, there will be pain in the bones and ki will be deficient in the external areas." *(Gatherings from Eminent Acupuncturists)*
Needling	It is common to tonify both yin and yang while giving treatment for cold patterns due to Liver deficiency or Kidney deficiency.
Note	In the centuries after the *Classic of Pulses* was written, some people referred to a leathery pulse as a firm pulse. Because there seems to be considerable confusion about this, below we will give the description of a leathery pulse as explained in the *Gatherings from Eminent Acupuncturists.*

	A leathery pulse is "sinking, hidden, excess, and large, and [it] feels like [the leather covering of a] drum."

Furthermore the *Qiānjīn Yìfāng (Supplement to A Thousand Gold Pieces Prescriptions)* says, "A firm pulse is a leathery pulse that has changed qualities." |

8.3.26 Long Pulse *Chō Myaku* 長脉

Quality	Everyone has his or her own length for the three pulse positions on each wrist. Usually these can all be felt separately, but in the case of a long pulse, it feels as if each position were intruding into the neighboring position(s). The *Gatherings from Eminent Acupuncturists* says, "The position goes beyond the [area] beneath [each] finger."
Pathology	A long pulse appears when there is an abundance of ki and blood, internal stagnation of heat, or a feeling of fever all over the body due to heat in the Triple Warmer.
Needling	It is common to disperse the Triple Warmer channel as a treatment for Spleen deficiency Stomach excess heat.

8.3.27 Short Pulse *Tan Myaku* 短脉

Quality	A short pulse is the opposite of a long pulse; it has insufficient length in each of the pulse positions. For instance, in the middle position it would be in the center of the position and would feel separated from the distal and proximal positions.
Pathology	A short pulse appears when there is a deficiency of ki. It also appears when there is great heat in the yin channels due to a stagnation of blood, which is caused by the deficiency of ki. But, the symptom pattern appears mainly as ki deficiency. It can also appear when the patient has difficulty digesting food. It tends to appear when there is Spleen deficiency or Lung deficiency.
Needling	Gently tonify.

8.3.28 Large Pulse *Dai Myaku* 大脉

Quality	A large pulse is floating and flooding at the superficial level and large with no strength at the deep level. This is a kind of flooding pulse, but it has the unique characteristic of no strength at the deep level.
Pathology	A large pulse appears when an abundance of ki has gathered in the yang areas of the body due to yin deficiency (i.e., blood and fluid deficiency).
Needling	Give the yin channels a good tonification, since the large pulse indicates a yin deficiency pattern. One does not usually disperse the yang channels.

8.3.29 Small Pulse *Shō Myaku* 小脉

Quality	A small pulse feels small at both the superficial and deep levels.
Pathology	A small pulse appears when both ki and blood are deficient.
Needling	Tonify both yin and yang.

8.3.30 Racing Pulse *Shitsu Myaku* 疾脉

Quality	A racing pulse is faster than a rapid pulse.
Pathology	A racing pulse appears when there is an abundance of heat. When a racing pulse appears with heat that is mainly in the yang channels the patient will recover. But, if a racing pulse appears with heat in the organs, recovery is difficult.
Needling	Tonify the yin channels and disperse the yang channels. In the case of heat in the organs, reduce it by tonifying the yin channel.

8.4   Pulse Condition for Each Pattern of Imbalance   証別の脉象

Each of the pulse qualities appears in the overall pulse, but during a chronic illness a certain pulse quality or combination of pulse qualities appear in specific pulse positions. These characteristic pulses and combinations of pulses allow the practitioner to form an image of the pulse condition. This section introduces the pulse conditions that correspond to each of the patterns of imbalance.

Tables summarizing the pulse conditions are also given, but as these are merely formulaic in nature it is best to read and understand the text first.

8.4.1 Liver Deficiency Heat Pattern Pulse *Kan-Kyo Nesshō no Myakushō* 肝虚熱証の脉象

Overall Pulse	The overall pulse is most often large (floating yet deficient at the deep level) or wiry. When there is a great deal of deficient-type heat, the pulse is floating, wiry, and rapid or it is floating, slippery, and rapid. As the heat decreases the pulse becomes sinking and slows down. If the pulse also has a tight quality then there is not much Stomach ki and recovery will be difficult.
Left Distal Position	When the Heart takes on heat this pulse becomes wiry with power at the deep level. In this situation the overall pulse can become hasty.
Left Middle Position	Even if the other positions are sinking, this pulse is easily felt at the superficial level and deficient at the deep level. In cases of extreme insufficiency of Liver fluids this pulse becomes leathery.
Left Proximal Position	Like the left middle position, this pulse is easily felt at the superficial level and deficient at the deep level even though the other positions are sinking. It becomes leathery in the case of an extreme insufficiency of Kidney fluids.
Right Distal Position	When the Lung takes on heat, at the deep level this pulse is either wiry or slippery with power or it is choppy and excess. However, if this pulse is slightly floating then the heat is in the Large Intestine or Large Intestine channel rather than in the Lung.
Right Middle Position	A rather serious illness is indicated when the Spleen pulse is powerful at the deep level. Normally the Spleen pulse is wiry or choppy and is neither deficient nor excess. However, when heat has increased in the Stomach or Stomach channel, the Stomach pulse can become strong although it will not be floating.
Right Proximal Position	It is normal for the Pericardium pulse at the deep level to be weak. Yet, the Triple Warmer pulse at the superficial level may be detectable since the overall pulse will be floating when there is an abundance of heat. This condition is an indication that the yang ki of the life gate is dangerously depleted.

Table 8–4: Liver Deficiency Heat Pattern Pulse Condition		
Left Wrist		**Right Wrist**
Wiry with power	**Distal**	Wiry with power
Large – Deficient	**Middle**	Wiry or Choppy
Large – Deficient	**Proximal**	Large – Deficient

8.4.2 Liver Deficiency Cold Pattern Pulse *Kan-Kyo Kanshō no Myakushō* 肝虚寒証の脉象

Overall Pulse	The overall pulse is weak (sinking, thin, and deficient) and slow or rapid. It is slow when the patient is rather cold and is rapid when the source ki of the Triple Warmer is deficient. When the pulse is rapid there could be a stagnation of heat somewhere in the body, but it must not be removed by dispersion since the overall pulse is weak. Moreover, there could be a hidden pulse.
	Alternatively the pulse could be hollow, soft, or scattered. These pulse qualities are easily felt at the superficial level but they are not indicative of heat.
Left Distal Position	Although the overall pulse is weak, this pulse can seem strong when compared to the other pulse positions. This is due to onset of coldness from the Middle Warmer down and a simultaneous increase in heat in the Upper Warmer.
Left Middle Position	This pulse is invariably weak. It is not detectable at the superficial level and is deficient at the deep level.
Left Proximal Position	This pulse is weak or soft (floating and thin as well as deficient at the deep level).
Right Distal Position	Again, this pulse can feel strong compared to the other positions even though the overall pulse is weak. This is due to a little bit of heat remaining in the chest.
Right Middle Position	The Spleen pulse is choppy (thin), but does not disappear even when pressure is applied beyond the deep level.
Right Proximal Position	The Pericardium pulse is weak (sinking, thin, and deficient).

Table 8–5: Liver Deficiency Cold Pattern Pulse Condition		
Left Wrist		**Right Wrist**
More powerful than others	**Distal**	More powerful than others
Weak	**Middle**	Choppy - Thin
Weak or Soft	**Proximal**	Weak

8.4.3 Spleen Deficiency Yang Brightness Channel Excess Heat Pattern Pulse *Hi-Kyo Yōmeikei-Jitsu Nesshō no Myakushō* 脾虚陽明経実熱証の脉象

Overall Pulse	This pulse is either floating, large, and excessive or sinking, thin, and excessive. Either way the overall pulse is powerful. However, there are also cases when the pulse is not so excessive. The pulse will also be rapid when there is an abundance of heat. When the pulse is sinking and excessive, meridian diseases and fu organ diseases can be differentiated by the symptom patterns.
Left Distal Position	This pulse can be felt at the superficial level and is deficient at the deep level.
Left Middle Position	Like the overall pulse this pulse is either floating or sinking, but it is neither deficient nor excess at the deep level. If it does happen to feel strong it is unlikely that there is any accompanying symptom pattern and it can therefore be disregarded.
Left Proximal Position	This pattern of imbalance characteristically occurs with urinary difficulty. Given that a function of the Bladder is expelling heat through the urine, if it is unable to perform this function, heat will build up in the Bladder and cause this pulse to feel strong. If the pulse is sinking and excessive, then heat generated by dampness is invading inwardly.
Right Distal Position	This pulse is easily felt at the superficial level and normally does not change when more pressure is applied to reach the deep level. However, if heat has invaded the Lung, then the pulse is stronger at the deep level. Deformations of the joints can result if this condition continues without being treated.

Right Middle Position	This pulse is easily felt at the superficial level and is deficient at the deep level.
Right Proximal Position	This pulse is floating or sinking. At the deep level it is neither deficient nor excessive, or tends toward being slightly deficient.

<table>
<tr><td colspan="3">Table 8–6
Spleen Deficiency Yang Brightness Channel Excess Heat Pattern Pulse Condition</td></tr>
<tr><td>Left Wrist</td><td></td><td>Right Wrist</td></tr>
<tr><td>Deficient</td><td>Distal</td><td>Excess</td></tr>
<tr><td>Normal</td><td>Middle</td><td>Deficient</td></tr>
<tr><td>Occasionally Excess</td><td>Proximal</td><td>Deficient</td></tr>
</table>

8.4.4 Spleen Deficiency Stomach Excess Heat Pattern Pulse *Hi-Kyo I-Jitsu Nesshō no Myakushō* 脾虚胃実熱証の脉象

Overall Pulse	The pulse feels strong even under the slightest pressure. At the deep level it is even stronger, and as well is tight and excessive or slippery and excessive. If the patient has a fever the pulse will be long (large and connected across all three positions on the wrist) and rapid. The pulse is often rapid even when there is no fever detected by a thermometer.
Left Distal Position	In theory this pulse will be deficient. But, it is often difficult to distinguish the deficiency because the overall pulse is strong.
Left Middle Position	Liver excess heat can develop from Stomach excess heat. In that case this pulse will be sinking and excessive.
Left Proximal Position	This pulse is often deficient at the deep level. At such times distinguishing whether the pattern of imbalance is Kidney deficiency or Spleen deficiency can be perplexing. In order to make the distinction, compare the pulses at KI-3 and ST-42. If the pulse at KI-3 is floating and larger than the pulse at ST-42, the pattern is Kidney

	deficiency. If the pulse at ST-42 is large and that at KI-3 is sinking, the pattern is Spleen deficiency.
	If the pulse has an excess quality when felt slightly deeper than the superficial level, the Bladder has taken on heat.
Right Distal Position	This pulse is felt at the superficial level and is even stronger at the deep level, which is due to the Lung taking on heat.
Right Middle Position	This pulse is strong at the superficial level and deficient at the deep level, although it may be difficult to discern since the overall pulse is strong.
Right Proximal Position	This pulse is strong when lightly palpated, but upon closer examination is found to be deficient at the deeper level.

Table 8–7: Spleen Deficiency Stomach Excess Heat Pattern Pulse Condition		
Left Wrist		**Right Wrist**
Flooding	**Distal**	Flooding – Excess
Sinking – Excess	**Middle**	Superficial level: Excess Deep level: Deficient
Hollow – Deficient	**Proximal**	Large

8.4.5 Spleen Deficiency Stomach Deficiency Heat Pattern Pulse *Hi-Kyo I-Kyo Nesshō no Myakushō* 脾虚胃虚熱証の脉象

Overall Pulse	This pulse does not display extremes of the floating or sinking qualities. Only when there is heat is it likely to approach being floating. When there is not much heat the pulse can be distinctly felt at the deep level.
	With light palpation the pulse never feels excessive, but it can feel surprisingly strong when there is an abundance of heat. However, at the deep level it may be wiry and deficient or slippery and deficient.
	As heat decreases the pulse will become moderate or hollow.

Left Distal Position	This pulse is often deficient, or more specifically minute or thin, at both the superficial and deep levels. If the pulse in this position is distinctly felt at the superficial level then there is heat in the Small Intestine.
Left Middle Position	This pulse is wiry, but is never deficient. This is because it is more likely that the Liver and Gallbladder will take on heat when the Spleen is deficient.
Left Proximal Position	If the Kidney pulse is tight or choppy and excessive, then there is heat in the Lower Warmer. If the overall pulse is floating the heat is in the Bladder. If it is sinking the heat is in the Kidney. If this pulse has a striking pulse quality (like a stone being flicked against the skin) and the patient has a renal disease the prognosis is not good. However, generally this pulse is close to a normal pulse.
Right Distal Position	If this pulse is wiry with power at the deep level then there is Lung heat, and if it is slippery with power then there is even more heat. The patient will most likely have a disorder in the lungs or in the upper third of the body.
Right Middle Position	This pulse is distinctly felt at the superficial level. At the deep level it is deficient and seems hollow.
Right Proximal Position	It is better if this pulse is deficient at the deep level, but if it feels strong then the Spleen deficiency is due to overwork and fatigue.

Table 8–8: Spleen Deficiency Stomach Deficiency Heat Pattern Pulse Condition		
Left Wrist		**Right Wrist**
Minute or Thin	**Distal**	Wiry or Slippery
Wiry	**Middle**	Moderate or Hollow
Normal	**Proximal**	Deficient

8.4.6 Spleen Deficiency Cold Pattern Pulse *Hi-Kyo Kanshō no Myakushō* 脾虚寒証の脉象

Overall Pulse	The pulse is weak (sinking and deficient), or choppy (thin and slow), or thin. The pulse is normally slow, but as a reaction to becoming cold the patient may develop a fever, in which case the pulse will become rapid. The overall pulse could also be floating, weak, and deficient in all positions. This condition is described as hollow, scattered, or soft pulse qualities.
Left Distal Position	This pulse is barely perceptible at both the superficial and deep levels, and has qualities of being minute or thin.
Left Middle Position	Because the yang ki of the Gallbladder channel is deficient and because there is blood deficiency, this pulse is sinking, wiry, and weak.
Left Proximal Position	This pulse is often weak (sinking and deficient), because it is easy to develop a Kidney deficiency cold pattern from a Spleen deficiency cold pattern.
Right Distal Position	This pulse is sinking, choppy, and weak.
Right Middle Position	Although the overall pulse may be weak, the Stomach pulse can often be felt at the superficial level. If the Stomach pulse is entirely absent the illness is grave.
Right Proximal Position	This pulse is deficient at the deep level.

Table 8–9: Spleen Deficiency Cold Pattern Pulse Condition		
Left Wrist		**Right Wrist**
Minute or Thin	**Distal**	Sinking – Choppy
Sinking – Wiry	**Middle**	Weak – Deficient
Weak	**Proximal**	Weak – Deficient

8.4.7 Spleen Deficiency Liver Excess Heat Pattern Pulse *Hi-Kyo Kan-Jitsu Neshhō no Myakushō* 脾虚肝実熱証の脉象

Overall Pulse	The pulse is wiry and rapid, or choppy, excessive, and rapid at the deep level. Even when there is not much heat the pulse is still wiry with surprising strength at the deep level.
Left Distal Position	This pulse is deficient at both the superficial and deep levels.
Left Middle Position	At the deep level this pulse is wiry and excessive or choppy and excessive. The Gallbladder pulse can also be strong when there is substantial heat in the Liver.
Left Proximal Position	The pulse in this position will be strong if Liver heat spreads all the way to the Kidney. If that happens and the patient has a renal disease the situation requires special care.
Right Distal Position	Respiratory symptoms can manifest if the Liver heat spreads to the Lung. However, the Lung pulse will not be so strong. If the Lung pulse is strong at the same time that there is Liver heat, the patient will often have pneumonia or pleurisy.
Right Middle Position	This pulse is wiry with strength, but is deficient at the deep level.
Right Proximal Position	As might be expected, this pulse is wiry, but deficient at the deep level. If it is wiry and excessive then there is heat in the Lower Warmer, indicating a condition such as appendicitis or pregnancy. A wiry and excessive pulse in this position during any other pattern of imbalance has the same implications.

Table 8–10: Spleen Deficiency Liver Excess Heat Pattern Pulse Condition		
Left Wrist		**Right Wrist**
Wiry - Deficient	**Distal**	Wiry
Wiry - Excess	**Middle**	Wiry - Deficient
Wiry	**Proximal**	Wiry - Deficient

8.4.8 Spleen Deficiency Liver Excess Pattern Pulse *Hi-Kyo Kan-Jitsu Shō no Myakushō* 脾虚肝実証の脉象

Overall Pulse	At the deep level the pulse is wiry and powerful. It may be slow if there is blood stasis. The pulse could also be sinking, thin, and minute, or sinking, thin, and choppy. This may look like a cold pattern, but there will be no signs of onset of coldness (Jpn: *rei;* Chn: *lěng*) of the Stomach and Intestines. Such a pulse is characteristic of this pattern of imbalance.
Left Distal Position	This pulse is minute and deficient at both the superficial and deep levels.
Left Middle Position	At the deep level this pulse is wiry and excessive or choppy and excessive.
Left Proximal Position	This pulse has the same qualities as the overall pulse, but is not often deficient or excessive.
Right Distal Position	This pulse also has the same qualities as the overall pulse, but is not often deficient or excessive.
Right Middle Position	This pulse is wiry or choppy and is deficient at the deep level.
Right Proximal Position	As might be expected, this pulse is wiry or choppy and is deficient at the deep level.

Table 8–11: Spleen Deficiency Liver Excess Pattern Pulse Condition		
Left Wrist		**Right Wrist**
Minute	**Distal**	Normal
Sinking – Excess	**Middle**	Wiry – Deficient
Normal	**Proximal**	Wiry – Deficient

8.4.9 Lung Deficiency Yang Meridian Excess Heat Pattern Pulse *Hai-Kyo Yōkei-Jitsu Nesshō no Myakushō* 肺虚陽経実熱証の脉象

Overall Pulse	The pulse is floating, rapid, and excessive (tight). So, it can be difficult to determine which position is the most deficient. One or two days after developing a fever the pulse may be floating, rapid, and flooding (large or long), which is due to an increase in stagnated heat. On occasions when there is no heat the overall pulse is floating and powerful, but at the deep level the Lung and Spleen will clearly be deficient.
Left Distal Position	This pulse is floating and tight. If it is floating more than the other positions then there is an abundance of heat in the Small Intestine channel.
Left Middle Position	This pulse is floating and tight. If it is stronger than the other positions then heat is moving from the lesser yang channel to the Liver and Gallbladder.
Left Proximal Position	Again, this pulse is floating and tight. If it is floating more than the other positions then there is an abundance of heat in the Bladder channel.
Right Distal Position	This pulse is floating and excessive at the superficial level. At the deep level it can be so strong as to seem to bounce off the finger. But, the core of this pulse is deficient. When there is no heat this pulse is distinctly felt at the superficial level and is clearly deficient at the deep level, but the overall pulse is powerful.
Right Middle Position	This pulse is distinctly felt at the superficial level and is deficient at the deep level. However, it is also possible that the deficiency will not be very clear.
Right Proximal Position	This pulse is floating and tight.

Table 8–12: Lung Deficiency Yang Meridian Excess Heat Pattern Pulse Condition		
Left Wrist		**Right Wrist**
Floating – Tight	**Distal**	Superficial level: Floating – Excess
Floating – Tight	**Middle**	Superficial level: Floating – Excess
Floating – Tight	**Proximal**	Floating – Tight

8.4.10 Lung Deficiency Cold Pattern Pulse *Hai-Kyo Kanshō no Myakushō* 肺虚寒証の脉象

Overall Pulse	The pulse is floating, rapid, and deficient. As heat decreases the overall pulse becomes thin and tends to become sinking. If there is a further decrease in heat the pulse will become completely sinking. Moreover, as cold becomes predominant the pulse will become thin and weak. If ki deficiency is the primary pathology the pulse will be choppy.
Left Distal Position	This pulse is rarely deficient or excessive, but can become deficient when cold becomes predominant.
Left Middle Position	This pulse is either floating or sinking, but it is neither deficient nor excessive. However, it can be choppy and close to being excessive when ki deficiency is the primary pathology. This indicates that blood stagnation is about to develop.
Left Proximal Position	This pulse also tends to be neither deficient nor excessive, but it can become deficient when there is a lack of the yang ki of the life gate due to a predominance of cold. In other words, the pattern of imbalance is transforming into a Kidney deficiency cold pattern.
Right Distal Position	This pulse is floating when the patient has a fever, but it is clearly deficient at the deep level. If ki deficiency is the primary pathology then a choppy quality will be more conspicuous than a deficient quality.
Right Middle Position	Again, this pulse is deficient at the deep level, but on occasion a choppy quality will be more prominent, making it difficult to detect the deficiency.
Right Proximal Position	This pulse tends to be neither deficient nor excessive, but it can become deficient when cold is predominant.

Table 8–13: Lung Deficiency Cold Pattern Pulse Condition		
Left Wrist		**Right Wrist**
Floating - Deficient	**Distal**	Floating - Deficient
Floating	**Middle**	Floating - Deficient
Floating	**Proximal**	Floating

8.4.11 Lung Deficiency Liver Excess Pattern Pulse *Hai-Kyo Kan-Jitsu Shō no Myakushō* 肺虚肝実証の脈象

Overall Pulse	The pulse has strength and at the deep level is either slippery and excessive or wiry and excessive.
Left Distal Position	Patients with constitutional Lung deficiency subsequently tend to develop Kidney deficiency. Therefore, during the transition period a wiry and excessive pulse or a slippery and excessive pulse can be felt in this position.
Left Middle Position	This pulse is slippery and excessive or wiry and excessive.
Left Proximal Position	The overall pulse tends to be excessive, but this pulse alone is deficient at both the superficial and deep levels.
Right Distal Position	Because the pattern of imbalance is Lung deficiency, this pulse is usually deficient, yet there are a number of variations. It could be floating and easy to distinguish, with a deficient pulse at the deep level, or it could constitutionally have an overflowing pulse quality (a quality in which the pulse overflows in the direction of LU-10). Conversely, the Lung pulse could also be strong, in which case the patient could have diabetes.
Right Middle Position	This pulse can be felt at the superficial level and is powerful at the deep level. This is due to spreading of deficient-type heat from the Kidney to the Spleen and Stomach. Again, the patient could have diabetes. The prognosis is grave if the pulse gets increasingly stronger toward the deep level and the patient has recently lost weight very suddenly. On the other hand, the prognosis is more favorable in conditions where the pulse is deficient at the deep level and the Stomach pulse is strong.
Right Proximal Position	Like the left proximal position this pulse is deficient at the deep level.

Table 8–14: Lung Deficiency Liver Excess Pattern Pulse Condition			
Left Wrist		**Right Wrist**	
Slippery - Excess	**Distal**	Overflowing	
Slippery - Excess	**Middle**	Excess	
Deficient	**Proximal**	Deficient	

8.4.12 Kidney Deficiency Heat Pattern Pulse *Jin-Kyo Nesshō no Myakushō* 腎虚熱証の脉象

Overall Pulse	The pulse is commonly floating and slippery or leathery, or it is sinking, slippery, and deficient. It is unlikely that this overall pulse will be as strong as the overall pulse in a Liver deficiency heat pattern. Nor will the pulse be thin. Occasionally it will be slow, but most of the time it will be slightly rapid.
Left Distal Position	When this pulse has strength at the deep level it indicates that the patient could have hypertension or related circulatory disorders.
Left Middle Position	This pulse tends to be neither deficient nor excessive. If it does happen to be deficient it indicates Liver deficiency, and if it is excessive it indicates Liver excess. However, when the left proximal position is deficient and the distal position is strong, the pulse forms an inverted triangle. Hence the Liver pulse, which is in the middle, will often be close to excessive.
Left Proximal Position	This pulse can be deficient at both the superficial and deep levels and may feel thin at the center. Or, it could be distinctly felt at the superficial level and slippery and deficient at the deep level. It could also be undetectable at the superficial level and leathery at the deep level.
Right Distal Position	This pulse could be deficient at both the superficial and deep levels and minute at the center. It could also be distinctly felt at the superficial level and deficient at the deep level. Conversely, it could have strength at the deep level if there is an abundance of heat.
Right Middle Position	This pulse could be wiry with strength at both the superficial and deep levels, in which case the patient may tend to overeat or have diabetes.
Right Proximal Position	This pulse is invariably deficient and may be slippery or wiry.

Left Wrist		Right Wrist
Table 8–15: Kidney Deficiency Heat Pattern Pulse Condition		
Slippery – Excess	**Distal**	Minute
Slippery – Excess	**Middle**	Wiry
Slippery – Deficient	**Proximal**	Slippery – Deficient

8.4.13 Kidney Deficiency Cold Pattern Pulse *Jin-Kyo Kanshō no Myakushō* 腎虚寒証の脉象

Overall Pulse	The pulse is often thin, weak, and soft or floating; when pressed, it is weak and hollow. Furthermore, the pulse is almost always slow.
Left Distal Position	Even though the overall pulse is soft or hollow this pulse alone may often be surprisingly powerful.
Left Middle Position	This pulse is weak, but it tends to be neither deficient nor excessive.
Left Proximal Position	Even if the overall pulse is thin and sinking this pulse alone is often easily felt at the superficial level. Of course at the deep level it is deficient.
Right Distal Position	This pulse is minute and is deficient at both the superficial and deep levels.
Right Middle Position	Normally this pulse tends to be neither deficient nor excessive, but in this pattern of imbalance the yang ki of the life gate is deficient, and thus this pulse is, more than anything, close to being a deficient pulse.
Right Proximal Position	This pulse is deficient at the deep level.

Table 8–16: Kidney Deficiency Cold Pattern Pulse Condition		
Left Wrist		**Right Wrist**
Soft	**Distal**	Minute – Deficient
Normal	**Middle**	Deficient
Soft – Deficient	**Proximal**	Deficient

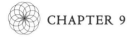 CHAPTER 9

Treatment

治 療 法

We have at last reached the chapter on treatment. So far we have covered a lot of material, but it will be of little use unless you learn to apply it in the clinic.

The first step in the clinic is to determine the pattern of imbalance. To do that you must understand the basic principles, visceral manifestations, etiology, and pathology, and you must master each of the examination methods. Likewise it is crucial that along with determining the pattern of imbalance you must be able to ascertain the correct treatment area(s) and appropriate tonification or dispersion techniques as well as be able to assess the prognosis.

Next, after determining the pattern of imbalance you must be able to skillfully perform the treatment techniques if the goal of healing is to be attained. It is not good enough to only be able to use standard needles, and to not know how to use such techniques as intradermal needles or moxibustion. As a professional practitioner you must master all the techniques of your art.

This chapter covers such topics interspersed with notes from a clinical case study.

9.1 Determining the Pattern of Imbalance (Determining the Treatment Strategy)　証の決定（治療方針の決定

9.1.1　Clinical Case Study

①　Looking

The patient was a slightly plump woman of 50 years of age and was somewhat on the short side. She had a number of blotches under her eyes. Such blotches are common in patients with a Liver deficiency pattern or a Liver excess pattern.

The patient had large eyes, which is an indication of a Liver excess constitution. Her lips were slightly dark (blackish). These signs pointed toward possible blood stasis. Her facial complexion was not poor, but her countenance clearly revealed that she was troubled by illness. Also, she seemed somewhat hesitant upon entering the treatment room, coming perhaps from a sense of uncertainty about acupuncture treatment.

Essential Points for Observation

Observe the patient from the time they enter the examination or treatment room.

Are they slim or overweight? Do they look healthy? How is their facial complexion? Do they seem cheerful or aloof? Do they appear nervous or relaxed or skeptical? This does not mean that you should stare at people with a scrutinizing eye, but rather just casually make keen observations. Later you will observe the pulse and the abdomen, at which time the question becomes: do all the signs fit together? You must also consider the patient's build and consider whether deep needling can be used or only shallow needling. As well, personality characteristics must be taken into account. Is the patient the kind of person who requires full explanations or one who needs to be treated extra gently?

9.1.2　Questioning

①　Chief Complaint

The patient normally worked at a part-time job, but had taken three days off over the New Year's holiday. The following day she had difficulty moving her right shoulder, and forcing it caused pain. She somehow continued to work in that condition, but from about three months prior to this visit it had become nearly impossible to raise her right arm. At first there was spontaneous pain, but now it hurt only when she moved her arm. However, it hurt if she moved the shoulder only slightly, and on days when she pushed herself too much it hurt at night as well. She asked if acupuncture could help her.

② **Questioning**

Upon asking whether she had already received any kind of treatment, she replied that she had been receiving injections and electrotherapy at the hospital. That treatment only eased the pain somewhat.

She had experienced acupuncture previously and had no notable illnesses in the past. She remarked that her bowel movements, urination, and appetite were all normal. But this would need to be confirmed again later, as she made a face that expressed something like, "What does that have to do with shoulder pain?"

Essential Points for Questioning

Ascertain the patient's chief complaint. At first you should ask about the most bothersome symptoms are and where they are located, what the possible causes are, and what has been the progress of the condition.

If there is pain, ask the degree of pain. For instance, is there no pain at all if the patient does not move? Is it somewhat painful at night? Is there pain with only slight movement? Moving in which direction causes pain?

Additionally you should ask general questions such as the condition of the bowels, urination, appetite, sleep, and any previous illnesses. If the patient is employed, what kind of work do they do? Have they ever had acupuncture before?

9.1.3 Treatment Preparations

It was explained to the patient that even though it was her shoulder that was hurting, the treatment would encompass her whole body. That is, remedying the condition would be difficult without treating both the whole body and the area of complaint.

The patient was informed that she had fifty-year-old's shoulder, a condition afflicting people around 50 years old (her present age) at which time there is often hormone imbalance. Overuse of the shoulder was explained as another part of the cause. Of course she was also advised that the disorder would definitely get better by treating the shoulder *and* by improving the overall circulation of blood. Since she had some reservations about acupuncture, it was important, in addition to simply explaining the disorder, to reassure her that she would definitely recover.

Explanation of Treatment Preparations and Illnesses

After asking all the initial questions concerning the chief complaint, have the patient lie down on the treatment table. A warm, quiet room is preferable as a treatment space. It is best if the patient wears loose-fitting clothing that allows for easy access to all areas of the body that may be treated, such as the abdomen or legs. They may also strip to their underwear and use a sheet or gown as a cover.

Often it is necessary to provide explanations to the patient about their illness. This can be done at the end of the treatment. This holds true for both contemporary biomedicine and traditional medicine. It is fine, if not preferable, to use common, everyday language. It is important to give explanations that satisfy the patient.

In technical terms an acupuncture treatment encompasses both a root treatment and a local treatment. That these are important aspects of traditional acupuncture should be explained to the patient without using overly technical terms.

9.1.4 Examining the Afflicted Area

Once our patient had reclined comfortably on the table we made a closer examination of the afflicted area, calling upon our sharpest observational skills. It was clear that the patient had cramping of the muscles between her right shoulder joint and scapula, and that the right shoulder was thinner than the left. This was indicative of a difficult case of fifty-year-old's shoulder.

When asked to raise her arm, she was only able to move her arm slightly to the front, back, and side. It was as if her arm were stuck to the side of her body. The shoulder was very painful, and she could not move it any further.

9.1.5 Palpation

① Pulse Diagnosis

The middle and proximal positions on the left wrist were both deficient at the deep level. The overall pulse was a bit wiry, but it was close to being leathery, as it was sinking and tight. This indicated that there was not much depth to the pulse. The width was neither large nor thin, indicating a primary pathology of fluid insufficiency. Categorized by cold and heat, it was more of a heat pattern. The mouth of patient with a heat pattern would be somewhat dry. When asked about this she replied that it was not exactly dry, but that she did have a craving for fruit. A craving for fruit can be considered as having a heat pattern. In further queries concerning appetite, she said that she had a tendency to overeat.

Careful scrutiny of the pulse revealed that the right distal position was slightly sinking and wiry and was slightly powerful. In relation to fifty-year-old's shoulder, this could mean that the Lung channel excess was a result of the spreading of heat. Excess in the Lung channel will spread to the Large Intestine or to the Large Intestine channel. Therefore, when asked about the condition of her bowels, the patient said that she was constipated, which confirmed the diagnosis.

② Abdominal Diagnosis

A routine abdominal diagnosis showed that the area around CV-17 was hot to the touch. This is associated with a strong Lung pulse. People tend to wake up during the night when there is heat in the chest. When asked about the condition of her sleep, the patient said that when she rolled over in bed her shoulder would hurt and wake her up.

Next, resistance in the left subcostal area was found to be stronger than in the right when the two were compared. Palpitations could be felt on the left side of the navel. Liver deficiency is clearly indicated by this abdominal examination. In asking the patient if there were certain times when she tended to become irritated, or if she was the kind of person who never quits once starting something, she confirmed that to be true. There was resistance and pain on pressure on the left and right edges of the inferior side of the navel. This is an indication of blood stasis, but in this case it was ignored since a condition of Liver excess did not seem possible. There was pain on pressure in the superior aspect of the inguinal area on both the left and right sides, likely also related to the Liver channel.

③ **Meridian Palpation**

There was pain on pressure at LU-1, LU-2, and ST-12, all on the right side, indicating that the Lung and yang brightness channels were clogged. Accordingly, pressing on the right Lung channel and focusing on LU-3, LU-4, and LU-6 showed that all these areas had pain on pressure. There was also pain on pressure at LI-10, LI-4, LI-14, and LI-15, and less at LI-11.

On the lower limbs there was intense pain on pressure at LR-8 and LR-5 on both sides. Men who have pain on pressure at LR-5 often have had prostatitis, and women who have pain on pressure at LR-5 often have had cystitis. In this case, our patient confirmed a tendency to get cystitis.

The examination revealed a conflict between the answers to the initial questioning and the general symptom patterns. In this case our study patient said everything (except her shoulder) was fine, yet it turned out that she had constipation, tended to wake up during the night, and also has a predisposition toward cystitis even though she claimed to have not had any major previous illnesses. This kind of response is common and is most likely the result of the patient thinking that her bowel movements had nothing to do with a painful shoulder.

Essential Points for Examination: Part II

First examine the pulse. Check to see if the overall pulse is strong or weak, or fast or slow, to determine the patient's present level of tension or nervousness and constitutional tendencies. Of course you should be able to understand the pulse condition well enough to determine the pattern of imbalance. Remember that the pulse condition will change later.

Next examine the abdomen. If possible it is also good to reexamine the pulse after using a light *sanshin* technique (see page 324) or retaining the needles on the abdomen. Often the patient's pulse will change after this, and if it does change you should use the new pulse condition for the diagnosis.

Normally, questioning concerning the overall condition continues while examining the pulse and abdomen. The pulse diagnosis of our case study patient revealed that she had a Liver deficiency heat pattern and that the local treatment should focus mainly on the Lung and Large Intestine channels. To make doubly sure of the diagnosis, the abdomen is examined and the meridians are also palpated. Then there still remains the questions of whether acupuncture or moxibustion is more appropriate, what gauge needles to use, and at what depth of insertion.

Often a patient may not reveal their full condition until a second round of questioning after the practitioner performs the pulse and abdominal examinations.

9.1.6 Treatment Strategy

The pattern of imbalance was diagnosed as a Liver deficiency heat pattern with excess Lung and Large Intestine channels. This condition required tonification of the Liver and Kidney channels and local treatment was given on the Large Intestine and Lung channels. The local pain on pressure was determined to be excess pain. In other words, the root treatment was to focus on tonification and the local treatment would add dispersion.

The patient's build was normal and the diagnosis was a heat pattern. Since she had also had previous experience with acupuncture, it was decided that slightly deep insertion would be fine.

① Root Treatment

KI-10 and LR-8 were tonified with 40mm #0 needles. The needles were removed when the practitioner sensed that ki had arrived. The pulse was checked to see that it had become slightly floating and soft.

Treatment points for the root treatment were selected in accordance with the principles given in Chapter 69 of the *Nan Jing*.

② Local Treatment

A moxa-on-the-handle needle was used on LI-15 with the patient in the supine position. The needle was a 40mm #4 needle. At the same time 40mm #0 needles were extremely shallowly retained at LU-1, LU-2, LU-3, LU-4, LU-5, LU-6, and ST-12. They were left in for 30 minutes. The treatment was completed with a dispersal *sanshin* technique where there was stiffness on the back along the medial edge of the scapula. After the treatment the patient said that her shoulder felt warm and good.

The rationale for the local treatment (moxa-on-the-handle needle and sustained retention of needles) was the necessity to treat the blood so as to restore the ability to move a joint that is nearly frozen. It would be possible to do this treatment with *okyū* (お灸) moxibustion, but many patients do not like *okyū* these days, so as a rule needling treatments have increased. If required it may be good to massage LU-3 and LU-4.

Essential Points for Treatment

Once you determine the constitution of the patient and the hot/cold yin/yang aspects of the patient's condition, you can decide on the type of needling to perform.

Root treatment points can be selected according to the principles from one of the *Nan Jing* chapter protocols (see pages 291 and 296).

For the local treatment choose procedures that address the patient's strongest discomforts, based on the symptom patterns and diagnostic considerations outlined in pervious chapters.

9.1.7 Prognosis

The patient was told that her condition required treatment three or more times per week for a minimum of three months. However, she was assured that after a few treatments she would see improvement, since conditions that exhibit pain on pressure tend to be more easily alleviated. Moreover she was advised to move her arm and shoulder within the limits of comfort, and that drinking alcohol or soaking in hot baths should be avoided since they cause an onset of coldness after initially warming up the body, but that there were no restrictions on types of foods she could eat.

> ### Explaining the Prognosis
>
> It takes experience to become good at explaining the prognosis. If you do not know what the prognosis should be, then you must be honest and tell the patient that the determination of the prognosis will become much clearer after two or three treatments.
>
> Be aware that many patients cannot follow through with strict or detailed advice concerning lifestyle changes such as diet and exercise.

9.2   Treatment Basics   治療方法の基礎

In the example case that we just used, the most important detail in regards to the treatment is determining which meridians and which points are to be used. These points must be divided into root treatment points and local treatment points. This will require some explanation, but first an explanation of basic treatment methods is given for beginners.

9.2.1   Basic Treatment Methods

① First use extremely shallow retained needles on the abdomen or head. Points to use are: GV-20, GB-5, and TW-17 on the head, and CV-12, ST-25 (left and right), and CV-4 or CV-6 on the abdomen. The needles should be retained for about 15 minutes.

Because retaining the needles at these points reduces tension and hot flushes and improve the circulation of Stomach ki, such treatment should make the pulse stand out more clearly. After needling, reexamine the abdomen and pulse. You can also use the time while these needles are retained to do the questioning examination.

② The root treatment is performed after determining the pattern of imbalance. But if the cold and heat patterns cannot be differentiated, then points may be selected using only the principles set forth in Chapter 69 of the *Nan Jing*, (see page 291). Execute tonification to the extent you know how. If there is excess and you think that the treatment will require dispersion but you do not have the confidence to undertake dispersion techniques, then you should only do the tonification.

③ Next, retain needles on the back. Needles are retained on the back at areas that are found to be deficient (depressions). If you are confident of your diagnosis, you may also disperse excess areas (indurations) with a single needle technique.

④ Finish the treatment with the *sanshin* technique on the upper back and shoulders with the patient in the supine position or seated. Deep needling should never be performed on the upper back and shoulders.

While you have the patient in the supine or prostrate position, use that opportunity to also retain the needles in any areas that are painful in addition to doing the root treatment. For instance, if the patient has knee pain, retain the needles there when the patient is in the supine position. If the patient has sciatica, retain the needles while the patient is in the prostrate position. If neither position is possible, have the patient lie on the side. Fifty-year-old's shoulder, for example, is treated with the patient lying on the side.

After learning the one-pattern treatment given above you may next start selecting the root and local treatments based on the pulse condition, and also try using cone moxibustion, direct moxibustion, moxa-on-the-handle needles, or intradermal needles when appropriate.

Basically, extremely shallow insertion is just fine, but if you have a good grasp of the pathology and have confidence, you should try touch needling or deeper insertion. You can also try varying the number of points used. However, the most basic facet to needling is doing it in such a way that it does not hurt.

9.2.2 Root Treatment and Point Selection

In our example case the patient had a Liver deficiency heat pattern and fifty-year-old's shoulder. In this case there was deficiency of the essential ki of the Liver and simultaneous blood deficiency. Moreover, heat had been generated, and that affected the Lung and Large Intestine channels, which caused the fifty-year-old's shoulder.

In order to treat this condition the first thing required was to tonify the deficient Liver, as Liver deficiency was the primary pattern of imbalance and the underlying cause of the illness. The next question, then, is which points to use for this kind of pattern. Basically the five phase points are used, and they are employed under the following principles. This use of points for treating the primary pattern of imbalance is what is known as the root treatment.

① For Deficiency, Tonify the Mother

The "mother" refers to the generating cycle of the five phases and the relationship between each pair of phases—the phase that gives rise to the following phase being the "mother" and the one that is given rise to being the "child." (See page 20 for a diagram of the generating cycle of the five phases.) In the case of the Liver, its mother is the Kidney. Thus, for a Liver deficiency pattern, tonify the Kidney channel.

Next, within each meridian there are points that are divided according to the five phases. Thus the principle, "for deficiency, tonify the mother," is relevant here as well. Applying this to our Liver deficiency pattern, the point selection becomes KI-10, which is the water point (or mother of wood/Liver) within the Kidney channel, and LR-8, which is the water point within the Liver channel.

② For Excess, Disperse the Child

Here as well, "the child" refers to the generating cycle of the five phases. So, for instance, the Kidney is the child of the Lung. Again, just as was the case for deficiency, this principle is applicable to acupuncture points and to meridians. Thus, for Lung excess, LU-5 would be selected since it is the water point or child within the Lung channel. In the same way, for Large Intestine excess, LI-2 would be selected since it is the water point within the Large Intestine channel.

9.2.3 Local Treatment and Point Selection

It would be great if a case of fifty-year-old's shoulder got better after improving the flow of the Kidney and Liver channels with the root treatment. But, for the quickest and most fundamental treatment the practitioner must also consider whether or not to treat the meridians that have been affected by heat and the meridians that flow into the affected area of the body. If there are indurations or pain on pressure, then the flow of the meridians through that area has deteriorated, and treatment becomes necessary. The local treatment aims to improve the local flow of the meridians or to adjust meridians that have been affected by cold or heat.

In the local treatment one need not adhere to the five phase points, but should mainly select points where there are indurations or pain on pressure, while also using points that were mentioned in the classics for specific patterns or the experience of teachers and senior students as a reference. However, points must not be selected arbitrarily. If you think the flow of the Lung and Large Intestine channels has deteriorated with a Liver deficiency heat pattern, then points should be selected focusing on those channels.

9.2.4 Root Treatment Supplementary Points

In any disorder the alarm points (*boketsu* 募穴) and back transport points (*haibu yuketsu* 背部俞穴) frequently display deficiency or excess. These are basically local treatment points, but the pulse can be brought into order simply by retaining the needles at these points. Therefore, the Society of Traditional Japanese Medicine decided to use these points not simply as local treatment points, but rather, thinking that they aid the root treatment, gave these points the name *root treatment supplementary points*. (See the section on kinds of acupuncture points and their functions in Chapter 1, page 10.)

However, it is not always the case that just because there is Liver deficiency the Liver transport point (BL-18) will be deficient. Whether to use tonification or dispersion is determined by palpation, where the basic rule is to tonify deficient points and disperse excessive points.

9.2.5 Potency of the Root and Local Treatments

When you begin to treat patients you should realize that root treatment and local treatment are but two sides of the same coin and that they blend together. In the midst of a clinical session when you are treating a patient it is pointless to be thinking that such-and-such is root treatment or such-and-such is local.

Furthermore, some people think that the root treatment is performed to bring the pulse into order, and that the local treatment is performed to alleviate the symptoms. However, the pulse can be brought into order and the symptoms alleviated just with local treatment. Conversely, the symptoms can be relieved with just the root treatment, in addition to naturally adjusting the pulse.

Speaking from the experience of the authors, the effect of the treatment will last longer if the root treatment and local treatment are combined, rather than just doing one or the other. Naturally, if the effect of the treatment lasts longer, healing will take place sooner.

The point selection principles for the root treatment explained above take Chapter 69 of the *Nan Jing* as their basis. There are, however, other selection methods mentioned in the *Nan Jing* as well as other ideas about point selection. This section summarizes these methods.

These point selection methods do not all rely simply upon the application of the five phases theory. The points selected by these methods are based upon their qualities and associated pathologies, as derived from the visceral manifestations.

9.3.1   Point Selection Method from *Nan Jing* Chapter 69

① **For deficiency, tonify the mother; for excess, disperse the child.**

This concept was explained above. According to this method: for Liver deficiency, tonify the Kidney channel; for Spleen deficiency, tonify the Pericardium channel; for Lung deficiency, tonify the Spleen channel; and for Kidney deficiency, tonify the Lung channel. Moreover, as there are points within each meridian that have the five phase characteristics, the generating cycle relationship concept should also be applied to the selection of individual points.

For dispersing excess, use the child. Thus, in the case of Liver excess, disperse the Heart channel; for Heart excess, disperse the Spleen channel; for Spleen excess, disperse the Lung channel; for Lung excess, disperse the Kidney channel; and for Kidney excess, disperse the Liver channel. This principle extends to the selection of individual five phase points within each meridian as well. However, dispersion is not necessary for all patterns of imbalance, as there will not always be an excess meridian. Moreover, it is common to select only one point for dispersion—the one thought to be the most effective. That point is usually the child point within the meridian that is excess.

② **First tonify deficiency, then disperse excess.**

Because all illnesses start from a deficiency of essential ki, as a general rule tonification of deficiency should be performed first, and then dispersal of excess if needed.

> The sixty-ninth difficult issue: The text[s] say, "For deficiency, tonify. For excess, disperse. For neither deficiency nor excess, use the [diseased] channel." What does this mean?

It means: for deficiency, tonify that [channel's] mother. For excess, disperse that [channel's] child. One must first tonify, and thereafter disperse. "For neither deficiency nor excess, use the [diseased] channel" means an illness has occurred within a regular channel by itself, and not as a result of being struck by pathogenic influences from other [channels]; hence this [diseased channel] should be used [for treatment.] That is why the [texts] say, "use the [diseased] channel". (*Nan Jing*, Chapter 69)

③ **When there is neither deficiency nor excess, treat the diseased meridian.**

Because there is no such thing as an illness that has neither deficiency nor excess, the meaning of this phrase is that if only a single meridian is diseased, the illness is not a result of the influence of deficiency or excess in any other organs or meridians. This concept is associated with the five pathogenic influences, which will be discussed later. Nevertheless, the symptom pattern is divided into either deficiency or excess, and tonification or dispersion must be given accordingly. In this case however, the channel of the mother phase is not used, rather the same phase point as the diseased meridian within that same meridian is used as the treatment point. So, for example, if the Liver channel is the diseased channel, then the wood point within the Liver channel should be used as the treatment point.

Table 9–1 below gives the appropriate points based on the selection methods just described. The following points are given as explication of this table.

- The dispersion points for the yang channels are included since the yang channel that is paired with a yin channel often becomes excess when that yin channel is deficient. Since we are following the principle that for excess the child should be dispersed, the selected points are those that correspond to the child phase of the excess channel within that same channel.

- When there is a yin channel deficiency it is possible for the yin channels that are in a controlling cycle relationship with that channel to become excess. Therefore, the table also includes the appropriate dispersion points for that excess, which again are the points corresponding to the child phase of the excess channel within the same excess channel.

- However, these points should not always be used. In considering pathology, one realizes that dispersion should naturally not be used on the Kidney channel or on the Heart channel. Because illness starts from a deficiency of yin, extreme care must be taken if a yin channel is to be dispersed.

- In the experience of the authors, the yin channels that are used for dispersion are the Liver channel and the Lung channel. In the clinic the cleft points (*geki ketsu* 郄穴) are commonly used for dispersion.

Table 9–1: Tonification and Dispersion Points of the Yin and Yang Channels							
	Yin Channel Tonification Points		**Yang Channel Dispersion Points**		**Yin Channel Dispersion Points**		**Yang Channel Tonification Points**	
Liver Deficiency Pattern	Liver Channel	LR-1 LR-8	Gallbladder Channel	GB-38	Spleen Channel	SP-5	Stomach Channel	ST-36 ST-45
	Kidney Channel	KI-1 KI-10	Bladder Channel	BL-65	Lung Channel	LU-5	Large Intestine Channel	LI-11 LI-1
Spleen Deficiency Pattern	Spleen Channel	SP-3 SP-2	Stomach Channel	ST-45	Kidney Channel	KI-1	Bladder Channel	BL-66 BL-65
	Pericardium Channel	PC-7 PC-8	Triple Warmer Channel	TW-10	Liver Channel	LR-2	Gallbladder Channel	GB-43 GB-41
			Small Intestine Channel	SI-8				
Lung Deficiency Pattern	Lung Channel	LU-8 LU-9	Large Intestine Channel	LI-2	Liver Channel	LR-2	Gallbladder Channel	GB-41 GB-38
	Spleen Channel	SP-5 SP-3	Stomach Channel	ST-45	Pericardium Channel	PC-7	Small Intestine Channel	SI-3 SI-5
							Triple Warmer Channel	TW-3 TW-6
Kidney Deficiency Pattern	Kidney Channel	KI-10 KI-7	Bladder Channel	BL-65	Pericardium Channel	PC-7	Small Intestine Channel	SI-5 SI-8
	Lung Channel	LU-5 LU-8	Large Intestine Channel	LI-2	Spleen Channel	SP-5	Triple Warmer Channel	TW-6 TW-10
							Stomach Channel	ST-41 ST-36

- As stated above, when there is a yin channel deficiency it is possible for the yin channels that are in a controlling cycle relationship with that channel to become excess. In theory the yang channels that are paired with those excess yin channels should be deficient. Therefore, the table includes the appropriate yang channel tonification points. These yang channel tonification points are used to control the yin excess, and they should be tried before the yin channel dispersion points because dispersing the yin channels can be risky. Heat can appear in the yang channels when yin becomes excess due to heat. At that time it is possible to disperse the yang channels.

- When tonifying the yang channels usually the earth points (*do ketsu* 土穴), source points (*gen ketsu* 原穴), and network points (*raku ketsu* 絡穴) are used.

- There is never a time when all the points in Table 9–1, including the yin channel tonification points, should be used. For instance, in the case of a Liver deficiency pattern, there is no need to use any more points if after tonifying KI-10 on the left side both the yin and yang pulses are brought into order. On the other hand, if tonifying KI-10 and LR-8 on both the left and right sides has brought the yin channel pulse into order, but does not adjust the yang channel pulse, or an excess Lung is not becoming calm, then at that time you should use dispersion.

9.3.2 Point Selection Method from *Nan Jing* Chapter 75

Normally the *Nan Jing* Chapter 69 point selection method is adequate, but in the case of what is called a yin excess pattern, the point selection method from Chapter 75 of the *Nan Jing* is beneficial.

This yin excess refers to Liver excess, as was previously mentioned. Yin excess is the manifestation of a condition of blood or heat stagnation and repletion. This type of excess can be verified by pathology, pulse diagnosis, or abdominal diagnosis. It does not mean that a particular pulse is simply strong.

This point selection method can be simply understood as a controlling cycle method, but the accurate interpretation is that excess arises first, and in order to control it one must treat the child channel of the deficient channel.

Thus, tonifying the Kidney channel and dispersing the Heart channel controls Liver excess. In other words, tonifying the Kidney, which is the child of the deficient Lung channel, and susequently tonifying the Lung channel can be used to subdue Liver excess. As you can see, this method is different from the tonification method described in Chapter 69 of the *Nan Jing*.

However, in regards to dispersion, the method is the same as that in Chapter 69 of the *Nan Jing*. In other words, disperse the point that corresponds to the child phase of the excess channel. So, for Liver excess, disperse the fire point (i.e., child of wood) within the Liver channel.

Lung deficiency Liver excess is treated as deficient Lung and Kidney, and excess Liver and Heart. Use tonification at LU-5 and KI-7, and dispersion at LR-2 and PC-8.

> The seventy-fifth difficult issue: The text[s] say, "If the eastern direction is excess and the western direction is deficient, disperse the southern direction and tonify the northern direction." What does this mean? It means: metal, wood, water, fire, and earth should pacify each other. The eastern direction is [associated with] wood. The western direction is [associated with] metal.
>
> If wood tends be excess, metal should pacify it.
>
> If fire tends to be excess, water should pacify it.
>
> If earth tends to be excess, wood should pacify it.
>
> If metal tends to be excess, fire should pacify it.
>
> If water tends to be excess, earth should pacify it.
>
> The eastern direction is [associated with] Liver; therefore one knows [that if the eastern direction/wood is excess] the Liver is excess. The western direction is [associated with] the Lung; therefore one knows [that if the western direction/metal is deficient] the Lung is deficient. [In this case] disperse the fire of the southern direction and tonify the water of the northern direction. The southern direction is [associated with] fire, and fire is the child of wood. The northern direction is [associated with] water, and water is the mother of wood. Water defeats fire. A child can cause excess in its mother. A mother can cause deficiency in her child. Therefore, [one] disperses the fire and tonifies the water [in order to have] metal pacify the wood. The text[s] say: If one cannot cure deficiency [by the regular method, then one] should consider if there are any other [methods]. That is [what is] meant here. (*Nan Jing*, Chapter 75)

9.3.3 Point Selection Method from *Nan Jing* Chapter 68

This method utilizes the qualities of the well points, spring points, stream points, river points, and uniting points for treating certain patterns of imbalance. The qualities of these points were already given in Section 1 of Chapter 3 (see p. 52), but they will be touched upon again here.

① **Well-wood-point(s)** *Sei-moku-ketsu* 井木穴

The well-wood points have the functional property of gathering since they are abundant in Liver ki. Therefore, these points are suitable to use as tonification points for gathering heat when there is a Liver deficiency heat pattern. In that sense it does not contradict the Chapter 69 point selection method for when there is Liver deficiency.

Furthermore, these points should definitely be used when the patient has swelling and tenderness in the subcostal region that is due to a Liver deficiency heat pattern. However, in the case of swelling and tenderness in the subcostal region that is due to Liver excess heat, LR-1 should be used as a dispersion point.

② **Spring-fire-point(s)** *Ei-ka-ketsu* 滎火穴

Because the spring-fire points have an abundance of Heart ki, they hold the functional property of stimulating yin ki and the functional property of firming. These points are good to use as tonification points when there is great heat. From the perspective of symptom pattern as well, these points control body fever (i.e., fever other than that caused by ki stagnation).

While PC-8 tends to accumulate heat, and should be used as a dispersion point when there is body fever, the other fire points should be used as tonification points to reduce heat.

③ **Stream-earth-point(s)** *Yu-do-ketsu* 俞土穴

The stream-earth points have the qualities of the Spleen and Stomach and are the source points for the yin channels. In the *Ling Shu* it says to use the source points when there is a zang organ disease. Moreover, tonifying these points improves the functioning of the Spleen and Stomach, and thereby increases the ki, blood, and fluids within the corresponding zang organ of the earth point that is tonified. Therefore, these points are good to use for any of the cold patterns, at which time both yin and yang are deficient.

Furthermore, since any pattern of imbalance, fatigue, and arthralgia (joint pain) is associated with the Spleen and Stomach, the earth points are good to use in those situations. Again, in the case of a Spleen deficiency pattern this does not contradict the point selection method from Chapter 69 of the *Nan Jing*.

④ **River-metal-point(s)** *Kei-kin-ketsu* 経金穴

The river-metal points have the functional property of releasing since they have an abundance of Lung ki. Therefore, they are good to use as tonification points when there is a stagnation of ki, or when there is an aversion to cold, fever, coughing, or asthma due to deterioration in the circulation of Lung ki. Again, there is no contradiction here to Chapter 69 of the *Nan Jing* for a case of Lung deficiency.

⑤ **Uniting-water-point(s)** *Gō-sui-ketsu* 合水穴

The uniting water points have the firming ki of the Kidney. They can subdue counter-flowing ki (hot flushes) and are good to use when there diarrhea without abdominal pain.

The uniting water points are used when there is a condition of over-relaxation or slackness due to deficient-type heat because they have the functional property of firming. In that sense this does not contradict Chapter 69 of the *Nan Jing* in using KI-10 when there is Liver deficiency.

> The sixty-eighth difficult issue: Each of the five zang organs and six fu organs has a well, spring, stream, river, and uniting [point]. What [can one] control [through] each [point]?
>
> The text[s] say, "The places where [ki] emerges are the well [points]. The places where [ki] flows are the spring [points]. The places where [ki] pours down are the stream [points]. The places where [ki] proceeds are the river [points]. The places where [ki] enters [deeper into the body] are the uniting [points].
>
> [One can] control fullness [i.e., swelling and tenderness] below the heart [through the] well [points].
>
> [One can] control body fever [through the] spring [points].
>
> [One can] control heaviness in the body and joint pain [through the] stream [points].
>
> [One can] control panting and coughing as well as chills and fever [through the] river [points].

[One can] control counterflowing ki and diarrhea [through the] uniting [points].

These are the illnesses [that can be] controlled [through] the well, spring, stream, river, and uniting [points] of the five zang and six fu organs." (*Nan Jing*, Chapter 68)

9.3.4 Five Pathogenic Influences Point Selection

This method is adapted from the Chapter 49 of the *Nan Jing* which is concerned with etiology. Some etiological factors have a tendency to affect certain organs or meridians. Other etiological factors affect all the five zang organs, producing in each a certain pathology and symptom pattern. Therefore, etiology can be thought of as the same as pathology, and can then be used in point selection.

The relationship between etiology and the five zang organs is summarized in Table 9–2 and is explicated as follows.

- Anger injures the Liver. Melancholy and worry injures the Heart. Abnormal diet and fatigue injures the Spleen. Chilling the body and imbibing cold drinks injure the Lung. Dampness ki and overindulgence in sex injure the Kidney. In such conditions where specific etiological factors influence certain zang organs, the resultant disease is known as a self-channel disease. It was to such conditions that Chapter 69 of the *Nan Jing* referred when it advised, "If there is neither deficiency nor excess treat the diseased meridian."

- There are five other etiological factors that are said to each affect all of the zang organs. For instance, wind tends to enter the Liver and cause specific symptom patterns and a specific pulse pattern. But, it can affect the other zang organs and mainly appears as a change in color. These kinds of factors are arranged in the Table 9–2 below.

- The appropriate points are listed in the table below and the phase points are listed in Table 2–3 (page 30), both of which can be used to select the correct points for this method. We will give a few examples here as an illustration.

- If Liver deficiency arises due to dampness, then you should use the water point in the Liver channel (LR-8) since dampness is the pathogenic influence associated with the Kidney.

		Liver	Heart	Spleen	Lung	Kidney
Table 9–2 Etiological Factors Affecting the Zang Organs						
Wind stroke (wood)	Color	Blue	Red	Yellow	White	Black
Swelling and tenderness in the subcostal area	Point	LR-1	PC-9	SP-1	LU-11	KI-1
Wiry pulse						
Summerheat damage (fire)	Odor	Rancid	Burnt	Fragrant	Fleshy	Rotten
Body fever	Point	LR-2	PC-8	SP-2	LU-10	KI-2
Floating and large pulse						
Abnormal diet and fatigue (earth)	Flavor	Sour	Bitter	Sweet	Spicy	Salty
Heaviness in the body; preference for lying down; lassitude in the limbs	Point	LR-3	PC-7	SP-3	LU-9	KI-3
Moderate pulse						
Cold damage (metal)	Voice	Demanding/ ordering	Delirious speech/ lying	Singing	Wailing/ weeping	Moaning/ groaning
Alternating chills and fever	Point	LR-4	PC-5	SP-5	LU-8	KI-7
Choppy pulse						
Dampness stroke (water)	Fluid	Tears	Sweat	Drool	Snivel	Saliva
Lower abdominal pain	Point	LR-8	PC-3	SP-9	LU-5	KI-10
Sinking and soggy pulse						

- If Liver deficiency arises due to cold damage, you should tonify LR-4. If it arises due to abnormal diet or fatigue, you should tonify LR-3. If it arises due to summerheat damage, you should tonify LR-2. If it arises due to wind stroke, you should tonify LR-1.

- In order to use this method it is necessary to use pulse qualities and other clues to determine which pathogenic influence caused the condition to develop. However, the pathogenic influence does not always have to cause deficiency. The Liver, for instance, easily becomes excess due to certain etiological factors. Moreover, the pulse often becomes excessive when the Heart contains extra heat. However, the Kidney has the characteristic of always showing deficiency no matter which pathogenic influence it is attacked by. Thus, in order to correctly use this method, you must think about these possibilities in terms of the six pulse positions, as illustrated in the following example.

- If deficient-type heat is generated in a Liver deficiency heat pattern, that heat can influence other organs or meridians. The Lung pulse, for instance, could become strong if the heat goes to the Lung. In such a case, since the Lung pulse is strong while the Liver is deficient, LR-4 is used, as the Liver deficiency is understood to arise from the pathogenic influence associated with the Lung. In other words, if there is an excess channel, tonify the point that belongs to the same phase as the excess channel within the deficient channel of the main pattern of imbalance. So for example in the case of Kidney deficiency Heart excess, tonify the fire point within the Kidney channel.

9.3.5 Tonification and Dispersion Points for Each Pattern of Imbalance

The preceding subsections explain principles and usages for a number of different point selection methods. In the following section, the tonification and dispersion points for each pattern of imbalance are presented. The discussion takes into consideration each of the above methods as well as point selections made by senior teachers. However, this section simply presents a standardized selection of points, and not all these points will be necessary to use during any one particular treatment, and of course there will be some differences in point selection for each patient. You need not adhere exactly to this outline in selecting points for clinical use.

The first example of a Liver deficiency heat pattern includes a simple explanation of the reasoning behind the point selection, but such explanations are left out of the other patterns.

① **Liver Deficiency Heat Pattern**

Root Treatment Points	Tonify KI-10 and LR-8.
Auxiliary Points for Specific Conditions	If the pulse is floating due to hyperactivity of deficient-type heat, tonify LR-1 and KI-1 with the purpose of stimulating the functional property of gathering. If the Heart has taken on heat, tonify KI-2 (fire point) in order to quell the heat. Otherwise disperse the Gallbladder channel using GB-38. If the pulse has a hasty quality, tonify KI-7 in order to reduce the heat in the Heart by assisting the circulation of ki. If there is abundant heat in the Gallbladder, disperse GB-38 (fire point), or the cleft points GB-36 and TW-7. If there is abundant heat in the Bladder, disperse BL-65 (wood point) or BL-63 (cleft point). For a case with signs of a condition such as cystitis, tonify LR-5. LR-5 has been traditionally used specifically for such conditions. If the Lung is excess due to taking on heat, tonify LR-4 based on the five pathogenic influences theory. Otherwise tonify LI-11 in order to subdue the excess in the Lung channel. LU-10 could also be tonified. LU-10 is the fire point within the Lung channel; tonifying it quells Lung heat. If the Lung excess cannot be brought under control by these measures, disperse the water point (LU-5) or the cleft point (LU-6). If the Spleen and Stomach have taken on heat, tonify SP-1 according to the five pathogenic influences theory. Otherwise disperse ST-36 or ST-45 in order to reduce heat in the Stomach channel.
Root Treatment Supplementary Points	LR-14, GB-24, CV-12, ST-25, CV-5, BL-17, BL-18, BL-19, BL-23.

② **Liver Deficiency Cold Pattern**

Root Treatment Points	Tonify KI-3 and LR-3.
Auxiliary Points for Specific Conditions	To tonify both yin and yang, use KI-4 and LR-5. If the Heart pulse is stronger than the other pulse positions, tonify GB-41. Tonify GB-40, TW-6, and TW-4 since there is Gallbladder channel deficiency. If there is Bladder channel deficiency, tonify BL-64, BL-59, and BL-58. If there is a Lung symptom pattern or a rapid pulse, tonify LR-4 and KI-7, reasoning that this condition developed from pathogenic cold. If there is a deficiency of the yang ki of the Stomach, tonify ST-42. If the Spleen pulse is choppy, tonify SP-1
Root Treatment Supplementary Points	CV-4, CV-5, LR-13, CV-12, GB-25, BL-18, BL-21, BL-22, BL-23.

③ **Spleen Deficiency Yang Brightness Channel Excess Heat Pattern**

Root Treatment Points	Tonify PC-8 and SP-2.
Auxiliary Points for Specific Conditions	If there is heat in the Small Intestine channel, disperse SI-7 or SI-6. If heat is in the process of developing in the Bladder channel, disperse BL-40. If heat is in the process of developing in the Lung, tonify LU-10 or disperse LU-6. If the Stomach channel is excess, disperse ST-45, ST-44, and ST-34.
Root Treatment Supplementary Points	CV-12, ST-25, BL-14, BL-20, BL-21, BL-27, BL-25.

④ Spleen Deficiency Heat Pattern

Root Treatment Points	For a Stomach excess heat pattern, tonify PC-8 and SP-2. For a Stomach deficiency heat pattern, tonify PC-7 and SP-3.
Auxiliary Points for Specific Conditions	If there is Small Intestine heat, disperse SI-3. If there is heat in the Liver or Gallbladder, disperse GB-38, GB-36, TW-5, TW-3, and LR-2. If there is heat in the Kidney and Bladder, tonify SP-9 and disperse BL-40, BL-64, and BL-63. If there is heat in the Lung, tonify LU-10 or disperse either LU-6 or LU-5. If there is excess-type heat in the Stomach, disperse ST-36, ST-37, ST-39, and BL-40. If the Lung pulse is excess, tonify PC-5, SP-5, and LU-10 or disperse LU-5 and LU-6.
Root Treatment Supplementary Points	LU-1, CV-12, ST-25, CV-4, BL-14, BL-17, BL-20, BL-21, BL-25.

⑤ Spleen Deficiency Cold Pattern

Root Treatment Points	Tonify PC-7 and SP-3.
Auxiliary Points for Specific Conditions	Tonify *luò* (network) points PC-6 and SP-4. If there is a Small Intestine symptom pattern, tonify SI-4. If there is a Lung symptom pattern, tonify SP-5. Tonify ST-42, ST-36, SI-4, and SI-5 since there is cold in the Stomach. If there is heat only in the Stomach channel, disperse ST-44. If cold has spread to the Gallbladder channel, tonify GB-40. If the yang ki of the life gate is deficient, tonify TW-4 and KI-3.
Root Treatment Supplementary Points	CV-17, CV-14, CV-12, LR-13, CV-4, BL-14, BL-20, BL-21, BL-22.

⑥ Spleen Deficiency Liver Excess Pattern

Root Treatment Points	Tonify PC-7, PC-8, SP-2, and SP-3.
Auxiliary Points for Specific Conditions	For a Liver excess heat pattern, disperse GB-38, GB-36, TW-5, TW-3, and LR-2. For a Liver excess blood stasis pattern, disperse LR-8, SP-10, and SP-6. If the etiological factor is abnormal eating, disperse LR-3. If it is pathogenic cold, disperse LR-4. If heat has spread to the Kidney and Bladder, disperse BL-40. If heat has spread to the Lung, use PC-5 and SP-5 as basic root treatment tonification points in place of the ones listed above in the root treatment points section. If there is Stomach excess, disperse ST-36, ST-37, or ST-39.
Root Treatment Supplementary Points	LR-14, GB-24, CV-12, ST-25, BL-14, BL-17, BL-18, BL-19, BL-20, BL-21, BL-22.

⑦ Lung Deficiency Heat Pattern

Root Treatment Points	Tonify SP-5 and LU-8.
Auxiliary Points for Specific Conditions	If there is Small Intestine channel heat, disperse SI-1 and SI-6. If there is Bladder channel heat, disperse BL-66 and BL-63. If there is Large Intestine channel heat, disperse LI-2 and LI-7. If there is Stomach channel heat, disperse ST-44 and ST-45.
Root Treatment Supplementary Points	CV-12, LU-1, BL-13, BL-20.

⑧ Lung Deficiency Cold Pattern

Root Treatment Points	Tonify LU-9 and SP-3.
Auxiliary Points for Specific Conditions	Tonify *luò* (network) points LU-7 and SP-4. If the Small Intestine channel has deficient-type cold, tonify SI-4. If the Bladder channel has deficient-type cold, tonify BL-64, BL-58, and BL-59. Tonify LI-11 since the Large Intestine channel has deficient-type cold. Tonify ST-42 since the Stomach channel has deficient-type cold. Tonify TW-4 since there is a deficiency of Triple Warmer source ki. If there is deficient-type cold of the lesser yin channel, tonify HT-7.
Root Treatment Supplementary Points	CV-12, LU-1, CV-4, BL-13, BL-14, BL-15, BL-22.

⑨ Lung Deficiency Liver Excess Pattern

Root Treatment Points	Tonify LU-5 and KI-7. Disperse LR-2.
Auxiliary Points for Specific Conditions	If the Heart pulse is excessive, tonify KI-2 and disperse either PC-4 or PC-8. Disperse LR-8, SP-10, and SP-6 since the Liver excess is due to blood stasis. If there is an abundance of deficient-type heat, tonfiy KI-10. LU-5 *must* be tonified if there is a profusion of water ki. For Spleen and Stomach heat use a moxa-on-the-handle needle at SP-8 and disperse ST-36. If the etiological factor is pathogenic cold, disperse LR-4. If the etiological factor is abnormal eating, disperse LR-3.
Root Treatment Supplementary Points	CV-17, CV-12, ST-25, LR-14, GB-24, CV-5, BL-13, BL-18, BL-19, BL-23, BL-26, BL-25.

⑩ Kidney Deficiency Heat Pattern

Root Treatment Points	Tonify LU-5 and KI-7.
Auxiliary Points for Specific Conditions	If there is a lot of deficient-type heat, tonify KI-1 and KI-10. If the Heart pulse is excessive, tonify KI-2 or disperse PC-4. If there is Bladder channel excess, disperse BL-65 and BL-63. If there is Large Intestine channel excess, disperse LI-2 and LI-4. If the Lung pulse is excessive, disperse LU-5 and LU-6 after tonifying KI-7, LI-11. (Note: in this case do not tonify LU-5 as given in the root treatment points section above). If the Spleen and Stomach pulses are excessive, disperse SP-8 and ST-36.
Root Treatment Supplementary Points	CV-3, CV-4, ST-25, CV-12, CV-17, CV-14, BL-13, BL-23, BL-26, BL-28, BL-25.

⑪ Kidney Deficiency Cold Pattern

Root Treatment Points	Tonify LU-9, LU-8, LU-7, KI-3, and KI-4.
Auxiliary Points for Specific Conditions	Tonify SI-4 and SI-8 since there is a tendency for deficient-type cold to appear in the Small Intestine channel. Tonify BL-64, BL-58, and BL-59 since there is deficiency in the Bladder channel. Tonify TW-4 since there is a deficiency of Triple Warmer source ki. If the etiological factor is pathogenic cold, tonify KI-7. Tonify KI-3 and ST-42 since there is a tendency for the pattern of imbalance to develop into a Spleen deficiency cold pattern.
Root Treatment Supplementary Points	CV-4, CV-5, CV-12, GB-25, LR-13, BL-13, BL-23, BL-22, BL-28, BL-20, BL-21.

Because local treatment is performed on meridians in the localized area of affliction according to deficiency or excess and heat or cold in those areas, it does not follow the same principles of point selection as the root treatment. However, that does not mean that one haphazardly selects points. The criteria for local treatment point selection are presented below.

① One should consider the meridians that flow through the area of the chief complaint to determine which need to be treated. For instance, in a case of fifty-year-old's shoulder, the meridians that flow through the shoulder joint should be examined to see which one indicates a disease pattern. Or, if the patient complains of stomachache, then one should examine the Conception Vessel and upper Stomach channel as well as the back transport points.

② The pulse diagnosis results are thought of in regards to the chief complaint. So, again in the case of a patient with fifty-year-old's shoulder who has Liver deficiency and a strong Lung pulse, sections of the Lung channel and Large Intestine channel that flow through the shoulder are considered as possible treatment areas.

③ Also consider the front alarm points and back transport points (transport points) associated with the pattern of imbalance as other possible treatment areas. As was mentioned earlier, the front alarm points and back transport points are used as root treatment supplementary points. The ones that are commonly used were given along with the root treatment points in the previous section. As one can see, they were present in each case, as they inevitably show signs in reaction to all disorders. The specific method for their selection as treatment points will be given later, but for now notice that it is not a matter, for example, of tonifying BL-18 (the Liver transport point) simply because there is Liver deficiency. Rather, if there were a heat pattern this point would tend to show excess, and would be dispersed. Nevertheless, the front alarm points and back transport points on the upper half of the body generally tend to show excess while those on the lower half of the body generally tend to show deficiency. Acupuncture points on the lower abdomen will show excess if there is blood stasis, but the alarm points on the Conception Vessel commonly show deficiency, even under such a condition.

④ When treating meridians that are associated with the chief complaint, if you have had sufficient clinical experience it is possible to treat the condition with distant points. For example, there are times when LI-6 is used to treat a toothache. However, such cases are almost always handled at the same time as the root treatment, since treatment is given based on consideration of the pathology.

⑤ The local area can also be treated without relation to the pattern of imbalance, such as in treating a sprained ankle.

Once you have figured out the meridian(s) to be treated based on the above principles, the next step is to actually select and locate the appropriate points. The standard procedure is to palpate the specific meridian and the surrounding area, searching for any pain on pressure, resistance, indurations, depressions, protuberances, moisture, dryness, coldness, or heat. Then, classify these as deficiency or excess and give tonification or dispersion accordingly.

9.4.1 Pain on Pressure

Pressing on certain meridians or acupuncture points may especially elicit pain or tenderness. This pain on pressure can be brought on by lightly pinching the skin over the meridian or by pressing with the thumb or index finger. Start by pressing with all the fingers and palm together and then switch to the thumb or finger to ascertain the precise location of the pain on pressure, trying as much as possible to narrow in on an exact point. Pain on pressure can appear on either yin channels or yang channels.

Pain on pressure that appears on yin channels is almost always related to the pattern of imbalance, and pain on pressure that appears on the yin channels along the extremities often corresponds to points selected for the root treatment.

Pain on pressure that appears on yang channels is associated with the local treatment area, and any specific acupuncture points that show pain on pressure are included in the local treatment. If pressing on the point that manifests pain on pressure feels good to the patient, that is an indication of deficient-type pain, and if discomfort is greater when pressure is applied on the point that has pain on pressure, that is an indication of excess-type pain. Points that show deficient-type pain should be tonified and those that show excess-type pain should be dispersed.

With a headache, for example, excess-type pain is indicated if simply touching the hair causes an increase in pain, while deficient-type pain would be indicated if pressing on the area of the head that hurts were to feel good.

Any points with pain on pressure that center on the alarm points or back transport points are included in the local treatment. Naturally, these are also categorized as either deficient-type pain or excess-type pain and given tonification or dispersion accordingly.

As a basic rule, areas with pain on pressure are treated with extremely shallow insertion of retained needles, but in certain conditions can be treated with direct moxibustion or intradermal needles.

9.4.2 Resistance

Resistance is a phenomenon seen more over an area rather than at a specific point. The resistance of the muscle can be felt over an area up to the size of a handprint and is often felt in the abdomen. Most of the areas on the abdomen that show resistance are what is known as accumulations, or *shaku* (積) in Japanese.

Resistance in the right subcostal area corresponds to the Lung *shaku* and indicates either a Lung deficiency Liver excess pattern or a Spleen deficiency Liver excess pattern. Resistance in the left subcostal area corresponds to the Liver *shaku* and indicates a Liver deficiency heat pattern. Cone moxibustion or moxa-on-the-handle needles are good to use for these conditions. Retention of extremely shallow needles can also be used.

These *shaku* normally show only resistance and not pain on pressure. Since without pain on pressure it can be difficult to limit and determine the treatment area, treatment should be given at points within the center of the area of resistance or at the area that shows the strongest resistance. In the subcostal area, for example, LR-14 or ST-19 would be taken as treatment points.

Resistance in the lower abdomen is related to blood stasis. Pressing on these areas invariably reveals pain on pressure. Any pain on pressure should be classified as either deficiency or excess and treated accordingly.

These areas of resistance are useful references for helping to determine the pattern of imbalance, but they can also be used as local treatment areas in connection with the pattern of imbalance. Moreover, even if blood stasis in the lower abdomen does not seem to be related to the pattern of imbalance, it can still be used as a local treatment area if it is associated with a chief complaint of tending to get cold easily.

9.4.3 Indurations

Indurations are smaller than areas of resistance, and can range from being as hard as a rock to being soft like a clump of fat. Moreover, the size can vary from the size of a grain of rice to the size of an egg yolk.

Indurations are frequently accompanied by pain on pressure. Since most cases of indurations can be thought of as excess, they are commonly treated with dispersion. Of course, indurations can be thought of as acupuncture points.

Extremely shallow retention needles can be used for indurations. Direct moxibustion can also be applied until it feels hot.

9.4.4 Depressions and Protuberances

Depressions can be used as treatment areas. There are two different kinds to note.

Rather than an actual depression, one kind feels more like there is no strength at the superficial level of the skin, and is an area of ki and blood deficiency. Such areas naturally appear on the back, but can also appear at root treatment points such as PC-7, LU-9, KI-3, and KI-7. These points are tonified when used either as root treatment points or local treatment points since they almost never are accompanied by pain on pressure. Contact needling is appropriate.

The other kind is raised but then caves in when pressed to reveal a point about the size of a guide tube or the tip of one's finger. The point is raised and blocked off due to an abundance of deficient-type heat. The point can be treated after pressing reveals it.

These kinds of points can appear on the extremities at root treatment points such as KI-10 or LR-8, but they are most common at local treatment points on the back. These points have a deficiency of nutritive blood and therefore are frequently accompanied by pain on pressure. But, they should be tonified whether they are root treatment or local treatment points.

9.4.5 Dampness and Dryness

When palpating the skin pay attention to any damp or dry areas as this information is used to help determine the pattern of imbalance. Such areas can also be used for local treatment.

Generally, damp skin is due to an abundance of deficient-type heat. If the dampness is apparent only in certain areas, press the acupuncture points in those areas to check for pain on pressure, indurations, or depressions and designate appropriate local treatment points. Note that it is also possible for the dampness to be caused by sweat leaking from pores that are not closed properly due to a deficiency of yang ki.

Dry skin is almost always caused by blood stasis, in which case there will be resistance due to blood stasis deep in the abdomen and pain on pressure. An example of this would be pain on pressure found along the upper edge of the groin and near the pubic bone. If this condition is related to the pattern of imbalance, this area can be used as a local treatment area. As might be expected, extremely shallow retained needles are appropriate, and moxa-on-the-handle needles are good for blood stasis beside or below the navel. The prognosis is not good if the patient is thin and weak and has dry skin.

9.4.6 Cold and Heat

During palpation, check also for cold and heat, and use their detection as a reference to help determine the pattern of imbalance. If there is a connection with the pattern of imbalance, then acupuncture points in these areas can be used as local treatment points.

The lower abdomen, especially around CV-4, CV-5, and CV-6, is commonly cold. At such a time *o-kyū* moxibustion should be used at these points. There will usually be little pain on pressure or resistance. The points will be mostly depressed. Of course this is a condition of ki and blood deficiency.

A feeling of heat is common at CV-17 and along the governing vessel and the paravertebral points. All of these points can be used as treatment points. They will usually reveal pain on pressure.

9.4.7 Concluding Remarks

This section has presented the standard methods of point selection for the local treatment. There is no other way to learn it than by practicing to make the palm and fingers sensitive. In order to do that it is best to calm the mind and just feel what there is to feel.

As was previously mentioned, when one is able to perform a good examination and determine the pattern of imbalance, the selection of the root treatment points as well as the local treatment points naturally follows through. Moreover, relying on the name of an illness or the chief complaint and then looking only for pain on pressure cannot be called Meridian Therapy.

Since treating pain on pressure markedly raises the effectiveness of the treatment, it is easy to be enticed by the lure of pain on pressure points even though one says they are practicing Meridian Therapy. Great care must be taken about this matter. As many senior teachers have said, healing is slow when treatment is given without performing the root treatment.

9.5   Types of Treatment   治療法の種類

After determining the pattern of imbalance and selecting the points to be treated one is still faced with the problem of what kind of treatment to give. Acupuncture necessarily involves tonification and dispersion for the treatment of deficiency and excess, and therefore any treatment method will fall within the bounds of tonification or dispersion. Yet there are many variations, from the type of needle to the insertion method, and from the kind of moxibustion to the method of using it.

9.5.1 Tonification and Dispersion Techniques

In this section are tables of the tonification and dispersion techniques presented by Inoue Keiri in *Oriental Medical Journal* (*Tōhō Igakushi*), along with some further explanation.

Table 9–3: Yin/Yang Tonification and Dispersion Techniques			
Type	**Tonification**	**Dispersion**	**Comments**
Yin & Yang	Used mainly for yin diseases, deficiency patterns, and on the yin channels.	Used mainly for yang diseases, excess patterns, and on the yang channels.	Yin diseases are often seen in deficiency patterns, and are treated on the yin channels. Yang diseases are often seen in excess patterns, and are treated on the yang channels. Because yin excess and yang deficiency are not normal illnesses, they need a different treatment approach.

The term "yin diseases" refers to cold patterns. The root treatment for cold patterns consists only of tonification, and the local treatment is mainly tonification. The term "deficiency diseases" has two meanings: yin channel deficiency and deficiency in the overall pathological condition. Tonification of the yin channels is used as the root treatment for such conditions. Local treatment also focuses on tonification (using shallow insertion) at various places around the body. Tonification is the primary treatment method for the yin channels; they are only rarely dispersed.

The term "yang diseases" refers to a heat pattern or a yang excess pattern. For either pattern, tonification of the yin channels is performed first, followed by dispersion. It is also common to use dispersion for the local treatment. The term "excess patterns" refers to yang excess or yin excess, as well as to overall excess. Dispersion can be added to the root treatment for such conditions, but dispersion (using slightly deep insertion) is the primary treatment method for the local treatment. Dispersion is often used on the yang channels since they tend to accumulate stagnated heat.

Table 9–4: Insertion Methods for Tonification and Dispersion			
Type	**Tonification**	**Dispersion**	**Comments**
Deep and shallow insertion for male and female	Use deep insertion after strongly pressing the point for females, as they are yin and their ki is internal. Use shallow insertion after lightly pressing the point for males, as their ki is superficial.	Use shallow insertion on both men and women for yang excess and deep insertion on both men and women for yin excess.	The rule is to start treatment on the left for men and on the right for women.

Females tend to have a lot of blood stasis, thus they also tend to require deep needling. Males who are white-collar workers tend to have ki that is sensitive to needle stimulation and manual laborers tend to have good circulation of ki. Therefore shallow insertion is used for men. This is the rough guideline for local treatment.

A long tonification time with shallow needling is the primary treatment method for elderly patients. A short tonification time with shallow needling is good for children, but sometimes they also require dispersion.

Shallow, gentle needling is appropriate for patients with weak, pale skin. Deep needling is appropriate for patients with dark, thick skin. Gentle tonification is the primary treatment method for patients with flaccid flesh, while deep needling or dispersion is more common for patients with stocky flesh. This is also a rough standard for local treatment.

Although Inoue says to start treatment on the left for males and on the right for females, it is not our experience that it is critical to do so.

Table 9–5: Inhalation and Exhalation for Tonification and Dispersion			
Type	Tonification	Dispersion	Comments
Inhalation & Exhalation	Insert needles during exhalations and remove needles during inhalations.	Insert needles during inhalations and remove needles during exhalations.	The body becomes deficient during exhalations and excess during inhalations due to the incomings and outgoings of ki with the breath.

Some practitioners insert needles while having the patient exhale and remove needles while having the patient inhale. This method is fine for the root treatment but is inconvenient for the local treatment. If the patient's breathing is calm (you may have them rest a little and then perform a *sanshin* technique on the abdomen before starting the main treatment), you can adjust your needling to the rhythm of the patient's inhalations and exhalations of ki, and can then naturally tonify with the patient's exhalations and disperse with their inhalations without being overly conscious of their breath.

Additionally, there is a theory that says tonification is done by inserting and removing the needles during exhalation, and dispersion is done by inserting and removing the needles during inhalation.

Table 9–6: Size and Temperature of Needles for Tonification and Dispersion			
Type	Tonification	Dispersion	Comments
Size and Temperature of Needles	Use thin needles. Warm the tips of the needles.	Slightly thick needles can be used. Bloodletting needles can be used. Insert the needles without warming the tips.	Tonification is used to prevent decreases in ki. Dispersion is used to let out pathogenic ki. Warming needles prevent decreases in ki.

These days, the most commonly used needle is the *gōshin* needle (毫鍼 filiform needle). This needle comes in a few varieties, such as gold, silver, stainless steel, and iron, and also in various gauges. Of course, gold is the softest, followed by silver, then stainless steel, and then iron. The softer needles are more suitable for tonification. But if the practitioner taps it strongly, a soft needle will bend the instant it breaks the skin, so the softer needle must be tapped very slowly and gently many times in order to make it penetrate the skin. The same is true when inserting a needle without an insertion tube; the needle will bend unless inserted very slowly. The initial contact between the needle and the skin must also be very gentle.

The #00 gauge *gōshin* needle is the thinnest. Presently, many Meridian Therapy practitioners commonly use gauges #0 to #3 depending on the situation, although they sometimes use thicker (larger gauge) needles. They also use moxa-on-the-handle needles (灸頭鍼 *kyūtōshin*) and intradermal needles (皮内鍼 *hinaishin*) when appropriate.

In the classics, the use of warmed needles is called tonification (supplementation) and the use of needles without warming them is called dispersion. In the olden days people used to warm the needles in their mouth. As this is an unhygienic practice in modern times, there are no practitioners who do this nowadays.

Since a professional practitioner's hands are filled with ki when held in the *oshide* (押し手 supporting hand) and *sashide* (刺し手 inserting hand) positions, they should be warm. Simply handling the needles with such warm hands should naturally make them warm.

Table 9–7: Stroking and Closing Techniques for Tonification and Dispersion			
Type	**Tonification**	**Dispersion**	**Comments**
Stroking and closing the point	Insert the needle after gathering ki to the area by stroking with the fingers over the acupoint (in the direction of the flow of the meridian). After removing the needle, quickly press the needle hole to close it.	Insert the needle after sinking channel ki by stroking with the fingers over the acupoint (in the opposite direction of the flow of the meridian). After removing the needle, do not press the needle-hole to close it.	This is done to tonify and augment ki (channel ki) and avert its leakage, and to expel pathogenic ki and prevent its reentry.

These are the most commonly employed techniques for tonification and dispersion. They are associated with the angle of insertion and flicking, which are also techniques for tonification and dispersion. These will be covered later. Be sure you understand that although both these tonification and dispersion techniques use stroking, the tonification technique is done so as to gather ki and the dispersion technique is done so as to sink (i.e., calm) ki. The principle is that tonification is achieved by stroking in the direction of the flow of the meridians and dispersion is achieved by stroking against the flow. But, the manner (or intention) behind the use of the hands is different for each of each of these.

In order to gather as much ki as possible for tonification, the hands must be used very gently. In other words, the hands must not chase ki away. Therefore, rather than saying "press" the hands onto the skin, as is done in Japanese, it is probably more correct to just say "touch" the acupuncture point with the palm, thumb, and index finger. The reason for this is because this is a tonification technique for defensive ki.

Inoue used the verb *shizumeru* (沈める), which means "to sink," to describe the dispersion of channel ki. However, this is probably a mixup with the verb *shizumeru* (鎮める), meaning "to calm." For dispersion you should rub or massage the area in order to disperse even a little excess heat-ki (i.e., defensive ki), which will make it easier to disperse with the needle.

Table 9–8: Angle of Needle for Tonification and Dispersion			
Type	**Tonification**	**Dispersion**	**Comments**
Angle	Insert the needle in the direction of the flow of the meridian.	Insert the needle in the direction opposite to the flow of the meridian.	This is done to make channel ki flow and to block the movement of pathogenic ki.

The reason for inserting the needle in the direction of the flow of the meridian is to further improve the flow of the meridian. Conversely, the reason for inserting the needle in the direction opposite to the flow of the meridian is to plug up and stop the flow of channel ki in that meridian.

However, this technique is difficult to perform with an insertion tube, because it is always necessary to tilt the insertion tube while inserting the needle so that the needle goes with or against the flow of the meridian. The tilting makes it difficult to get the end of the tube flush with the skin. If the tube is not flush with the skin, inserting the needle can be painful, and ki can easily leak out. To prevent this you should take care in preparing the point for insertion by gently massaging it.

Table 9–9: Timing of Needle Removal for Tonification and Dispersion			
Type	**Tonification**	**Dispersion**	**Comments**
Removal Timing	Make the channel ki circulate. When it becomes full and is flowing well, that is the signal to remove the needle.	Remove pathogenic ki. Calm naturally excessive ki. Clear blood stagnation. Make channel ki flow. The disappearance of pathogenic ki is the sign to remove the needle.	[Recognizing the] movement of ki requires the most practice.

Common sense tells us that the indication of the effectiveness of treatment is a noticeable change in the symptoms. But, not all illnesses show such improvement immediately after treatment. Therefore, in some cases the practitioner must determine the effectiveness of the treatment and the prognosis by checking the pulse and abdomen as well as other observable signs. Before that, however, a primary concern is to know how deep to insert the needles and when to remove them and finish the treatment. This is impossible without being able to sense the movement of ki.

Table 9–10: Speed of Insertion and Removal of Needle for Tonification and Dispersion			
Type	**Tonification**	**Dispersion**	**Comments**
Insertion and Removal Speed	Slowly insert the needle so that it does not hurt, and slowly remove the needle.	Quickly insert the needle and quickly remove it.	Hasty insertion injures the blood, and rapid removal injures ki. "Quickly" is a little different from hasty and rapid.

There are various theories about the speed of insertion and removal. The technique for tonification is to slowly insert the needle and slowly remove the needle while maintaining a well-formed supporting hand (*oshide*). Chapter 1 of the *Ling Shu* describes this idea of tonification speed as being similar to the parting of lovers when they do not want the other person to leave. Hurried technique is the worst technique to have. There is a theory that says the needle should be removed very quickly in order to prevent leakage of ki from an open supporting hand. But if one has a well-formed supporting hand it is good to slowly remove the needle. Hurried removal on the other hand can cause the problem of ki leakage and inflict pain, which does not produce good results.

Concerning quick insertion and removal for dispersion, Chapter 1 of the *Ling Shu* described the movement as being similar to the reaction of reaching for something in hot water.

Table 9–11: Pressing and Flicking Techniques for Tonification and Dispersion			
Type	**Tonification**	**Dispersion**	**Comments**
Flicking & Fingernail Pressing	In order to gather ki to the point to be needled, press it, or flick it with a fingernail, or press a fingernail into it. After inserting the needle, flick the handle in order to gather ki [to the area].	Use the same techniques as for tonification in order to separate healthy ki from pathogenic ki, to sink (calm) healthy ki, and to stop the flow of pathogenic ki. After inserting the needle, relax the supporting hand, flick the needle, and sway the supporting hand.	Flicking can be done after stroking. Flicking the needle after insertion increases the effectiveness of the tonification or dispersion technique.

This technique is very similar to stroking. But, stroking is a technique used for defensive ki whereas flicking is a technique used for nutritive ki (blood). Both are considered examples of preparing the point for insertion.

The purpose of the flicking and fingernail pressing tonification technique is to expose acupuncture points that are hidden due the flesh being puffed up—that is, areas that are deficient in nutritive ki (blood). Thus the fingernails are sometimes pressed into the skin, but for the most part pressing with the pad of the index finger or thumb is used to find the point. It is good to sway the fingers while they are firmly in contact with the skin. The swaying motion should not just be back and forth movement of the fingers, but should follow the flow of the meridian.

In the case of dispersion, Inoue said to separate healthy ki and pathogenic ki. This refers to locating indurations. Indurations are created by the stagnation of nutritive ki (blood). First, locate any indurations by gently stroking the surface of the skin, but take care not to cause a loss of defensive ki. Next, feel the induration to determine the acupuncture point by pressing the finger deeper into the skin. This should be done with the intention of grasping the pathogenic ki.

Inoue also wrote that one should vibrate the needle after insertion so as to gather ki to the area. This is generally a widely used technique. However, it is not a matter of only vibrating the needle. This technique must be performed while constantly feeling the ki with the supporting hand. For tonification, use graceful, slow vibrations. Of course, the supporting hand must be maintained in a well-formed position. For dispersion, the supporting hand is relaxed so as to let ki leak out from the needled point.

Table 9–12: Needle Twisting Techniques for Tonification and Dispersion			
Type	**Tonification**	**Dispersion**	**Comments**
Twisting the needle clockwise or counter clockwise	With the patient in the prostrate position twist the needle clockwise when needling the left side of the body and counterclockwise when needling the right side of the body.	Do the opposite of tonification: twist the needle clockwise when needling the right side of the body and counterclockwise when needling the left side of the body.	Since the direction of twisting depends on the left or right side of the body, when needling the abdomen the direction will be opposite that when needling the back.

Taking the midsagital plane of the patient as the dividing line, for needling on the back, tonification is accomplished by twisting the needle counterclockwise when needling on the right side of the body (the side with the patient's right hand) and clockwise when needling on the left side of the body (the side with the patient's left hand). Dispersion is accomplished by twisting the needle clockwise when needling on the right side of the body and counterclockwise when needling on the left side of the body. For needling on the abdomen, tonification is accomplished by twisting the needling counterclockwise when needling on the left side of the body (the side with the patient's left hand) and clockwise when needling on the right side of the body (the side with the patient's right hand). Dispersion is accomplished by twisting the needle clockwise when needling on the left side of the body and counterclockwise when needling on the right side of the body.

Twisting the needle does *not* imply a full rotation, but could mean a half turn or even one third of a turn. Quick and short twisting is used more for tonification, while large and slow twisting should be used for dispersion.

Another theory proposes that twisting the needle counterclockwise when using the right hand and clockwise when using the left hand results in tonification; and that twisting the needle clockwise when using the right hand and counterclockwise when using the left hand results in dispersion.

Table 9–13: Needle Vibrating Techniques for Tonification and Dispersion			
Type	**Tonification**	**Dispersion**	**Comments**
Vibrating	After inserting the needle, gently vibrate the needle with the inserting hand in order to gather ki to the area.	After inserting the needle, quiver the needle with the supporting hand in such a way as to cause the leakage of ki.	For tonification, perform the technique while needling, and make sure to preserve ki at the moment of needle removal. For dispersion, vibration is used to cause leakage of pathogenic ki while removing the needle, but is sometimes also used during needling.

Vibrating and flicking are commonly used needle techniques. They help ki to gather to the area and also make it easy to cause leakage of ki. Be careful to avoid accidentally turning an intended tonification technique into one that disperses.

Table 9–14: Use of Cold and Heat for Tonification and Dispersion			
Type	**Tonification**	**Dispersion**	**Comments**
Cold and Heat	Tonification is used against cold with the purpose of warming the insides. Sometimes the needles are retained.	Insert the needle many times in order to reduce the heat. Use the *sanshin* technique.	For a cold condition, the technique is like not wanting someone to leave. For a heat condition, the technique is like reaching for something in hot water.

Cold patterns occur when there is deficiency of yang or of both yin and yang. It goes without saying that tonification will be used in such situations, but there is a slight difference in the techniques depending on whether the cold pattern is acute or chronic.

For an acute cold pattern, focus on using touch needling or shallowly inserted needles in order to tonify the defensive ki, while taking care to preserve ki. Sugiyama Waichi said that one should needle "with the mind set on tonification."

In a chronic cold pattern, both ki and blood are deficient. For that reason it is often necessary to retain needles for a long time.

In a heat pattern there could be deficient-type heat or excess-type heat. In either case the heat must be reduced. Whether there is an acute or chronic case, this is done by shallowly inserting the needle many times using a quick insertion/quick removal technique. However, for chronic heat patterns or for patients who constitutionally tend to have a heat pattern, there are times when deeply inserted needles are retained for a long time.

Table 9–15: Shallow and Deep Insertion for Tonification and Dispersion			
Type	**Tonification**	**Dispersion**	**Comments**
Shallow and Deep Insertion	First insert the needle shallowly and then later insert it deeper. For yin deficiency, insert the needle shallowly and send yang ki to the yin level.	First insert the needle deeply and then later make it shallow. For yang excess, disperse pathogenic ki after tonifying the yin deficiency. Therefore, two methods are performed on one point.	Yang ki is present in many cases of yin deficiency. Yang excess is caused by yin deficiency. However, there are different ways to treat this condition.

According to Chapter 70 of the *Nan Jing*, since autumn and winter are cold the practitioner must transmit "one yang."[11] Considering this, the yin deficiency mentioned under tonification should correspond to a cold pattern. Since both yin and yang must be tonified in a cold pattern, one must tonify the yin channels, picking points along them that

---

[11] Translator's note: This is based on the yin and yang theory of the *I Ching*, or *Book of Changes*, in which trigrams and hexagrams represent the different changes or phases through which yin and yang pass. The symbol 陷 corresponds to yin and the symbol 陙 corresponds to yang. In this case the text is referring to the one yang at the top of the trigram 陬.

will increase the blood and the source ki of the Triple Warmer. However, the implication is that one should first shallowly insert the needle to gather yang ki, and then send that ki to the yin level. This will improve the production and circulation of ki and blood and thus tonify both yin and yang.

Concerning dispersion the *Nan Jing* says that since the spring and summer are warm the practitioner must transmit "one yin." [12] Therefore, this dispersion technique is one that is used when there is an abundance of heat, such as in a deficient-type heat pattern or an excess-type heat pattern. Illness starts from deficiency in the yin channels whether it results in deficient-type heat or excess-type heat, and it is common practice to first tonify the yin channels and then disperse the heat. The technique explained here is one in which both of these are performed together at the same point. First, insert the needle deeply to invigorate the yin ki, and then pull the yin ki up to the yang level, thereby causing dispersion. This technique, known as transport dispersion (輸瀉 *yusha*), is used instead of the regular dispersion technique.

Table 9–16: Treatment Order for Deficiency and Excess			
Type	**Tonification**	**Dispersion**	**Comment**
Treatment order for deficiency and excess of yin and yang	For yin exuberance, if there is yang deficiency, first tonify the yang and then disperse the yin to harmonize yin and yang. For yin deficiency, if there is yang abundance, first tonify the yin and then disperse pathogenic ki from the yang to harmonize yin and yang. When giving treatment, first pay attention to the channel ki and then remove the pathogenic ki.		These rules should be followed for all tonification and dispersion techniques.

---

[12] Translator's note: Again, this is based on the yin and yang theory of the *I Ching*, or *Book of Changes*, in which trigrams and hexagrams represent the different changes or phases through which yin and yang pass. The trigram in question here is 陦.

The phrase "yin exuberance" in the text corresponds to yin excess. However, because yin exuberance is accompanied by an abundance of cold, dispersion should not be used.

The rule here is first to tonify deficiency then disperse excess.

Table 9–17: Degree of Needling Stimulation for Tonification and Dispersion			
Type	**Tonification**	**Dispersion**	**Comments**
Degree of Stimulation	There is no need to question [i.e., limit] the dosage if ki has not reached [i.e., has not been effective or is not detected by the practitioner] the intended purpose when needling. Do not needle again once ki has reached the intended purpose after needling.		Techniques should be used in accord with deficiency or excess and in each case attention must be given to the degree of needling stimulation.

As was previously mentioned, a major concern in acupuncture is determining the depth of needle insertion and how long to needle. This is difficult to determine without being able to sense the arrival of ki. Yet, this skill is one of the most important mysteries that lie at the heart of the art, and as such is a topic that acupuncture practitioners must spend a lifetime studying.

Table 9–18: Tonification and Dispersion with Moxibustion		
Type	**Tonification**	**Dispersion**
Tonification and Dispersion with Moxibustion	The fire of moxa can strengthen original yang [channel ki]. Using moxibustion on areas that are cold can warm and tonify channel ki. Softly twist the moxa. Gently apply it to the skin. Burn the moxa on top of the ash of the previous cone. Allow the moxa to burn by itself without blowing on it. Use soft, slow-burning moxa. Use tiny cones.	If there is pathogenic cold, use the fire of moxa to release it. If there is heat on the surface of the body, use moxa to expel it. Tightly twist the moxa. Firmly press it onto the skin. Burn [the moxa] after removing the ash [of the previous cone]. Blow on the lit moxa to make it burn faster. Use moxa that burns intensely. Use medium to large size cones.

9.5.2 Needling Techniques

This section presents modern-day needling techniques and the methods for using them for tonification and dispersion.

① Scattering Needle *Sanshin* 散鍼

Needles	*Gōshin* #0 to #3.
Purpose	The *sanshin* technique is used for tonification or dispersion of defensive ki during the local treatment. It can be used for tonification of deficient defensive ki in a cold pattern, or for dispersion of excess defensive ki in a heat pattern.
Tonification	The *sanshin* tonification technique is used to treat cold in the external areas of the body without being particular about specific acupuncture points. There are two methods to choose from when using an insertion tube: manipulation of the needle while it is still in the insertion tube, or quick single-handed reinsertion of the needle into the tube while performing the *sanshin* technique. If performing *sanshin* without an insertion tube, do it slowly, making sure to always employ the technique with a well-formed supporting hand. In all cases, the tip of the needle should barely touch the skin without causing the slightest pain. The area on which the *sanshin* technique is performed should turn red, or it should become moist and feel warm to the patient. Gently stroke the area before and after performing *sanshin*.
Dispersion	The technique is basically the same as for tonification except that for dispersion you perform it as if lightly bouncing the supporting hand or gently pinching. In other words, use the stroking dispersion technique. For dispersion it is fine if the patient feels a little pain. The heat-ki should disappear after doing this technique.

② Single Needle Technique *Tanshi* 単刺

Needles	40 mm *gōshin*. Decide the gauge based on the deficiency or excess of the area to be needled as well as on the overall deficiency and excess
Purpose	The *tanshi* technique is used during the root treatment for tonification or dispersion of defensive ki or nutritive ki.
Tonification for Defensive Ki	Areas that are deficient in defensive ki lack strength and are depressed and cold. Or, they could be very soft and lack strength when pressed. Locate the point within this area and then perform the stroking technique in order to gather ki to this spot. At this time care must be taken not to press more than necessary on this area since doing so can cause a loss of yang ki. It is best to just lightly touch the supporting hand to the area with the acupuncture point. Next, touch the tip of the needle to the skin, pointing in the direction of the flow of the meridian. Hold that position for a few breaths until the meridians and acupuncture point become warm and stronger. You must not try too hard to insert the needle. It should feel more like the needle just naturally slips in. Of course you must not cause any pain.
Tonification for Nutrititve Ki	Areas that are deficient in nutritive ki (blood) usually show a protuberance. Use the flicking and fingernail pressing techniques to reveal (open) the acupuncture point at this spot. Place the insertion tube (or needle tip if not using an insertion tube) against the skin and insert the needle. Only insert the needle to the depth to which it gently penetrates, and then wait for the count of a few breaths while the needled area becomes filled with ki. However, if there is no feeling of ki filling the area, try twisting the needle in the direction for tonification as explained in Table 9–12 (page 319) or try vibrating it. Remove the needle when it feels heavy, as this is an indication of the arrival of ki.
Dispersion for Defensive Ki	The technique for the dispersion of defensive ki is basically the same as the *sanshin* technique that is used for the dispersion of defensive ki except that specific acupuncture points are used for the single needle technique, as well as slight insertion of about 1mm. This technique is used on the yang channels. The patient should feel a prick as if bitten by a mosquito.

Dispsersion for Nutritive Ki	The technique used for the dispersion of nutritive ki (blood) is used on indurations. First thoroughly palpate the selected area to determine the location of indurations and then insert a needle into the center of each induration. But, do not skewer them. When indurations are needled the needle should start to feel heavy. Hold this position for a few breaths. However, if it seems to be taking a long time to make the indurations disappear, try using a pecking technique: a light and quick thrusting motion like that of a sparrow. If that does not work, try the pecking technique with a thicker needle.

③ Retained Needle *Chishin* 置鍼

Needles	*Gōshin* #0 to #3 needles are typically used when needle retention is called for, but slightly thicker needles can be used if the condition warrants it.
Purpose	Retained needles are used for tonification and dispersion of nutritive ki (blood) during the local treatment. Recently there are many people who retain the needles during the root treatment, but in such cases the practitioner needs to always pay close attention to the movements of the patient's ki. For those who cannot feel ki, they should determine any adjustments to the retention time by observing the pulse. If needles are retained for too long, ki will be lost rather than gathered. Because this can happen particularly when treating the hands or feet, it is not advisable to retain needles there.
Tonification	For tonification, #0 to #2 *gōshin* needles are retained on the abdomen or back. The points to focus on are those that are opened or revealed by pressing, or in other words, those points that are deficient in nutritive ki (blood). Consider using gold or silver needles for elderly patients who have weak bodies. The insertion depth should be about 1mm so that the needle falls over to the side. The number of needles should be adjusted according to the pathological condition. But, for the abdomen use at least four needles and

	not more than eight, and for the back use at least two and not more than 20. The needles should be retained for 10 to 30 minutes. Generally, gentle tonification is used when there are acute symptoms and more needles and longer retention time is used for chronic problems.
Dispersion	If the patient is constitutionally a yang-type person or constitutionally tends to have blood stasis, needles are retained at indurations both on the abdomen and back. Vary the depths from 2mm to more than 1cm. Thin *gōshin* needles are usually used, but thicker needles can also be used if needed. The number of needles and the duration of retention are the same as for tonification, but should of course be adjusted according to the hardness and number of the indurations.

④ Moxa-on-the-Handle Needle *Kyūtōshin* 灸頭鍼

Needles	*Gōshin* #3 or larger gauge needles specially made for *kyūtōshin* are used. Use 40mm to 60mm needles, depending on the need. Because poor-quality moxa may fall off the needle when burning, a semi-pure quality moxa should be used.
Purpose	*Kyūtōshin* is used to relieve pain due to longstanding coldness.
Technique	Because *kyūtōshin* has a fundamentally warming effect it is most often used for tonification. But it is also effective when used for indurations, and thus over time has come to be used for both tonification and dispersion. *Kyūtōshin* is used at areas of deficient nutritive ki (blood), at areas of chronic pain such as on the lower back, buttocks, thighs, and around the shoulder joints, and at areas in the abdomen that show resistance or pain on pressure due to blood stasis. *Kyūtōshin* is surprisingly suitable for use on many patients. However, this is not the same as saying that the illnesses of all such patients will be cured. Because *kyūtōshin* feels good to the patent, there is a risk that practitioners will get into the habit of giving *kyūtōshin* just for the comfort of the patient. However, it should be used with a clear purpose in mind based on a sound determination of the pattern of imbalance.

⑤ **Intradermal Needle** *Hinaishin* 皮内鍼

Needles	There are many types of intradermal needles.
Purpose	Intradermal needles are used to treat defensive ki in a similar manner to the *sanshin* technique, and are effective for giving a light dispersion.
Technique	Intradermal needles are generally used when there is pain in the muscles or at areas where there is severe soreness when palpating on the trunk (e.g., the back transport points).

⑥ **Long Needle and Big Needle** *Chōshin tō Taishin* 長鍼と大鍼

Needles	These needles are longer than 20cm. The thickness of the handle is about that of a match and the thickness of the needle is about that of the lead of a mechanical pencil. These needles are hard to get unless you have them specially made. Long Chinese needles can be used as a substitute.
Purpose	These needles are used for deep pain due to long-term coldness of the body. They are typically used between the lower back and buttocks.
Technique	Naturally, these needles are used for dispersion. In order to insert a big needle, first find the location of the acupuncture point and then press the thumbnail into it. Then bring the needle up against the nail and let it touch the skin. Next, take note of the timing of the patient's breath, and then insert the needle while relaxing the tension in your fingers. In most cases the needle is inserted horizontally to the body. This technique was the forte of Yanagiya Sorei.

9.5.3 Moxibustion Techniques

Moxibustion treatment includes direct application; *chinetsukyū* (cone moxibustion, in which the moxa is removed when it begins to feel warm); and *kakubutsukyū* (indirect moxibustion, in which a sliver of ginger or garlic is placed between the skin and the moxa).

① Direct Moxibustion (also known as Scarring Moxibustion) *Tōnetsukyū* 透熱灸

Moxa	Use good quality, very dry bleached moxa. Standard cones are half-rice-grain size.
Purpose	Direct moxibustion is used during the local treatment to treat nutritive ki (blood) deficiency.
Technique	When there is a deficiency of nutritive ki (blood), some acupuncture points will develop depressions or indurations. Acute disorders that are accompanied by heat and that suppurate are also caused by nutritive ki (blood) deficiency. Moxibustion is appropriate in any of these cases. The effectiveness of direct moxibustion is most dramatically seen when employed on indurations. The first three cones should feel hot, and afterwards the feeling of heat from the moxa will be lost. The moxa treatment should end when the moxa feels hot again. At this time the symptoms of the illness should have diminished. Press the patient's skin to locate depressions that should be used as treatment points. When burning moxa on these points the patient should feel a comfortable heat soaking into them. If the moxa is not exactly on the acupuncture point then it will just feel hot. For suppurations, apply thread moxa. One or two pieces should be burned at a number of spots around the suppuration. Because this should be performed as a dispersion technique the moxa should be tightly twisted.

② Cone moxibustion *Chinetsukyū* 知熱灸

Moxa	Use slightly coarse moxa. High quality moxa will burn too quickly, leaving the goal unattained.
Purpose	Cone moxibustion is used to induce the release of yang ki and fluids from areas that are excess.
Technique	Cone moxibustion is a dispersion technique. In addition to other signs, the effect of cone moxibustion can be judged from the fact that it causes sweating and reduces heat. Based on such results, cone moxibustion is appropriate for use on areas that feel warm, have indurations, are tense, or have edema.

③ Indirect Moxibustion *Kakubutsukyū* 隔物灸

Moxa	Use coarse moxa. Burn a suitably sized cone on top of salt or ginger or garlic that is placed on the treatment point.
Purpose	Indirect moxibustion is used to treat coldness or pain.
Technique	Indirect moxibustion is used to tonify yang ki through the addition of heat. However, it must not be allowed to get so warm that it causes sweating, as this will result in the undesired effect of further coldness.

9.5.4 Fundamentals and the Judgment of Results of Treatment

This subsection touches on the topics of treatment fundamentals and the issue of "ki," which we have put off until now.

① Attitude During Treatment

In his book *Meridian Therapy and the Mystery of Acupuncture*, Okada Meiyu described the state of mind one should have during needling.

> Chapter 9 of the *Ling Shu* says, "When needling, one should not look, not listen, not speak, and not move, but should rather focus the intention, direct the mind to the needle tip, and wait for the coming and going of ki," warns that while needling in the clinic one must be in a state of oneness of mind, as the art of acupuncture, based on maintaining extreme attention, requires an almost meditative concentration [i.e., a state of oneness of mind and body reached by entering into a perfect state of stillness], putting strength into the *tanden* (丹田), and emptying the self, all without disrupting the spirit.

> This involves always maintaining the humble attitude of being given the honor of adjusting the patient's ki through acupuncture, perceiving the essence of acupuncture, properly and moreover affectionately being present in the moment with a pure heart, and evoking in the patient the longed-for feeling of relief. The practitioner must be deeply conscious of these facts and must master the innermost secrets of the true way of acupuncture.

In essence, his point is that good treatment cannot be given if the practitioner has such impure thoughts as speculating about acquiring more patients and earning more money if they boast about themselves and achieve renown for giving quick cures.

② Ki and Judging the Results of Treatment

Feeling the coming and going of ki allows the practitioner to ascertain when the treatment should be finished and is also related to judging the results of treatment.

In his book *Japanese Classical Acupuncture: Introduction to Meridian Therapy*, Shudō Denmei listed the following indications to use for judging the results of treatment.

A. Has the pulse strength at different positions become more balanced?

B. Has the pulse quality (of the basic pulses) changed?

C. Have cold hands and feet warmed up?

D. Was the arrival of ki clearly felt during needling?

E. Were there changes in the abdominal signs?

F. Has pain on pressure along the meridians been reduced?

G. Were there improvements in the subjective symptoms of the patient?

H. Was there an increase in skin luster?

I. Were there abdominal sounds during needling?

These indications are all useful for judging the results of treatment. But, as was previously mentioned, the most difficult thing is deciding just when enough tonification has been given. Consequently, beginners should start by tonifying until they think they have given enough and then check the pulse for confirmation. However, the most preferable method is of course to be able to perform the treatment while feeling the movements of ki.

When ki arrives during needling, in the case of tonification, there is a feeling of warmth in the meridian and acupuncture point and the point becomes full. In the case of dispersion, the feeling of warmth decreases and indurations disappear. These sensations can be felt with either the supporting hand or the insertion hand. The patient may indicate that his or her hands or feet warmed up or that they feel good. Shudō Denmei also put it as getting a feeling that the treatment "worked." This is hard to understand without experiencing it firsthand, but in short, a feeling of "now," or "it's better," or "this is enough" will just come to you. This feeling will come without a clear reason when you earnestly perform treatment with an empty or clear mind.

Afterword

Until now English translations of traditional Japanese medicine (TJM) books have been limited to Fukushima Kodo's *Meridian Therapy* and Shudo Denmei's *Japanese Classical Acupuncture: Introduction to Meridian Therapy*, both of which are books written from the perspective of a single author. However, this publication is not the work of a single author. It is the product of discussions among leading Japanese clinicians who were brought together by the Society of Traditional Japanese Medicine, which serves as the backbone of traditional medicine in Japan and is noteworthy for making clear the fundamentals (standards) of traditional Japanese acupuncture. It should be understood as a summarization of the traditional acupuncture treatment that is practiced in Japan.

On a global scale, traditional Japanese medicine is less well known than traditional Chinese medicine (TCM). The reason for this, I believe, is not due to an inferiority of TJM in comparison to TCM, but is rather a historical problem. Traditional Chinese medicine was born as a national project with Mao Zedong's directive to form collaboration between Chinese and Western medicines. It then quickly spread throughout the world in conjunction with the export to Western countries of instructors, textbooks, and equipment as single packages after President Nixon's visit to China. In comparison, because TJM had a history of antagonism with the Japanese government's modernization and democratization policies, there was no possibility of establishing a national project around TJM. Thus, there was no choice but to popularize it around the world through individual and private sector group efforts.

It may be a touch long, but I would here like to mention the history of TJM.

East Asian medicine was introduced to Japan from China in 562B.C.E. In 701 a medical administration system and an educational system for doctors who would practice East Asian medicine were established. Thereafter, East Asian medicine was at the center of the medical establishment in Japan until the end of the Meiji period (1867) and developed in tune with the Japanese climate and lifestyle. However, in 1874, after entering the Meiji period, the government placed an outright ban on East Asian medicine, thinking that it was a holdover from the previous feudal period, and instituted a policy of a common medical system based on modern Western medicine in order to help achieve its goals of modernizing Japan and increasing its wealth and military power. The people then repeatedly held restoration movements for East Asian medicine, but the government only recognized *anma* massage, acupuncture, and moxibustion therapy as professions for the blind, and even then, the textbooks made for use in schools for the blind were based on modern medicine. Thus, acupuncture was recognized in a form that did not conflict with modern medicine. Traditional East Asian medicine, which had continued in an unbroken line up through the Edo period, was completely denied by the government. In the early part of the Showa period (1933), when the light of traditional acupuncture therapy was on the verge of being extinguished, Yanagiya Sorei, Okabe Sodō, and Inoue Keiri became the pivotal leaders of a movement to follow the traditional East Asian medical theories and use the traditional techniques that had accumulated during and prior to the Edo period. Thus the resurgence movement to traditional acupuncture that was later to be called Meridian Therapy was developed, and its long-awaited therapeutic method quickly spread throughout the acupuncture world.

However, in 1947, as part of its reforms of the medical system, General Headquarters, which was governing the defeated Japan after World War II, required the Japanese Ministry of Health and Welfare to issue an order banning acupuncture. The reasons given by the Department of Public Health and Welfare, which was headed by C.F. Sams, were that acupuncture was a holdover from militaristic Japan, was barbaric and unsanitary, and was incompatible with Western medicine. Once again the government tried to prohibit traditional East Asian medicine as a feudal era relic. Naturally, movements for the survival of acupuncture and moxibustion arose. General Headquarters and the Ministry of Health and Welfare came to understand that acupuncture and moxibustion were widely instilled throughout the Japanese populace and were supported by the people as a form of general medicine and that they had no relation to militaristic Japan. Thus, on December 10, 1947, a law of status was established for acupuncture and moxibustion, giving it the first official recognition as a medical treatment since 1868, which brings us up to the present.

As is clear from this historical review, modern Western medicine is still central to the Japanese medical system, and East Asian medicine is not given an active role as a form of medical treatment. Thus, from the beginning there was no room for the government to plan a project for introducing and popularizing TJM around the globe. Regardless of this, the fact that TJM enjoys widespread support among the people can be attributed not only to its long record of achieving clinical results in treating illnesses and maintaining health and to its traditional status, but as well as to recent movements that view traditional medicine as a modality that can successfully overcome the risks and limitations of modern Western medicine.

In studying this book you have taken a first step toward learning TJM. Since in all probability many readers have already learned TCM, I hope you will keep the differences between TJM and TCM in mind as you read (or reread) this book. After you understand the theoretical framework of TJM, the next step is to learn the clinical form. I imagine that many people will be surprised at the numerous differences between TJM and TCM when they first observe the clinical practice of TJM. I believe that TJM offers much that you can absorb, and that this will broaden your possibilities for helping patients with individually tailored treatments.

East Asian medicine is a *clinical* medicine. I believe that careers as superb clinicians are awaiting many people of the English-speaking world who go on to master the theories presented in this book and learn clinical practice under the direction of a good TJM instructor.

Finally, I would like to express my great appreciation to Kuwahara Koei's group and all the people in America who were involved in preparing this English translation.

Aizawa Ryō
Board Member
Society of Traditional Japanese Medicine

Selected East Asian Medical Terminology
東 洋 医 学 用 語 の 選 択

The "Other Common English" column is meant to offer English translations that either are or might be in use by other translators, thereby giving the readers a reference tool for different works with different terminology.

漢字	English Translation	Japanese	Chinese	Other Common English Translations
経穴	acupuncture point	keiketsu	jīng xué	point; acupoint; channel point; meridian point
甘味	sweetness	kanmi/amami	gān wèi	sweetness
望証	observational signs	bōshō	wàng zhèng	inspection
病因	etiology	byōin	bìng yīn	cause of disease
病証	symptom pattern	byōshō	bìng zhèng	disease pattern
中風	wind stroke	chūfū	zhòng fēng	wind stroke
中湿	dampness stroke	chūshitsu	zhòng shī	
怒	anger	do	nù	anger
風	wind	fū	fēng	wind
外因	exogenous factors	gai'in	wài yīn	external cause
内因	endogenous factors	nai'in	nèi yīn	internal cause
不内外因	non-endogenous/ non-exogenous factors	funaigai'in	bù nèi wài yīn	neutral cause [of disease]; miscellaneous factors
弦脉	wiry pulse (quality)	gen myaku	xián mài	stringlike pulse
煩熱	heat vexation	hannetsu	fán rè	heat vexation
悲	sorrow	hi	bēi	sadness; grief
飲食	food	inshoku	yǐn shí	food and drink
邪気	pathogenic ki	jaki	xié qì	evil ki/qi
火	fire	ka	huǒ	fire
寒	cold	kan	hán	cold
鹹味	saltiness	kanmi/ shiokarami	xián wèi	saltiness
辛味	spiciness	shinmi/karami	xīn wèi	pungency; acridity
経脈	channel(s)	keimyaku	jīng mài	channel
経絡	meridian(s)	keiraku	jīng luò	channels and network vessels; meridian and collateral
経絡治療	Meridian Therapy	keiraku chiryō	jīng luò zhì liaó	
経隧	conduit	keisui	jīng suì	channel passages
喜	joy	ki	xǐ	joy
恐	fear	kyō	kǒng	fear

漢字	English Translation	Japanese	Chinese	Other Common English Translations
驚	fright	kyō	jīng	fright
苦味	bitterness	kumi/nigami	kǔ wèi	bitterness
絡脈	network vessel(s)	rakumyaku	luò mài	network vessel; collateral
労倦	fatigue	rōken	laó juàn	taxation fatigue; overexertion
酸味	sourness	sanmi	suān wèi	sourness
思	pensiveness	shi	sī	thought; worry
四診	four examinations	shishin	sì zhěn	four examinations
湿	dampness	shitsu	shī	dampness
暑	summerheat	sho	shǔ	summerheat
証	pattern (of imbalance)	shō	zhèng	sign; disease pattern; symptom complex
傷寒	cold damage	shōkan	shāng hán	cold damage
傷暑	summerheat damage	shōsho	shāng shǔ	summerheat damage
燥	dryness	sō	zào	dryness
素因	predisposing factors	soin	sù yīn	predisposition; constitutional factors
孫脈	grandchild vessel	sonmyaku	sūn mài	grandchild vessel
孫絡	grandchild network vessel	sonraku	sūn luò	grandchild network vessel; grandchild collateral
憂	grief	yū	yōu	anxiety; melancholy
蔵象	visceral manifestation	zōshō	zàng xiàng	Physiology; image of the organs
浮脉	floating pulse (quality)	fu myaku	fú mài	floating pulse
芤脉	hollow pulse (quality)	kō myaku	kōu mài	scallion-stalk pulse
洪脉	flooding pulse (quality)	kō myaku	hóng mài	surging pulse
滑脉	slippery pulse (quality)	katsu myaku	huá mài	slippery pulse
数脉	rapid pulse (quality)	saku myaku	shòu mài	rapid pulse
促脉	hasty pulse (quality)	soku myaku	cù mài	skipping pulse
緊脉	tight pulse (quality)	kin myaku	jǐn mài	tight pulse
沈脉	sinking pulse (quality)	chin myaku	chén mài	submerged pulse; sunken pulse
伏脉	hidden pulse (quality)	fuku myaku	fú mài	hidden pulse
革脉	leathery pulse (quality)	kaku myaku	gé mài	drumskin pulse
実脉	excess pulse (quality)	jitsu myaku	shí mài	replete pulse
実	excess/excessive	jitsu	shí	repletion
微脉	minute pulse (quality)	bi myaku	wēi mài	faint pulse
濇脉	choppy pulse (quality)	shoku myaku	sè mài	rough pulse; hesitant pulse
細脉	thin pulse (quality)	sai myaku	xì mài	fine pulse
軟脉	soft pulse (quality)	nan myaku	ruǎn mài	soft pulse

漢字	English Translation	Japanese	Chinese	Other Common English Translations
弱脉	weak pulse (quality)	jaku myaku	ruò mài	weak pulse
虚脉	deficient pulse (quality)	kyo myaku	xū mài	vacuous pulse
虚	deficiency/deficient	kyo	xū	vacuity/vacuous
散脉	scattered pulse (quality)	san myaku	sàn mài	dissipated pulse; scattered pulse
緩脉	moderate pulse (quality)	kan myaku	huǎn mài	moderate pulse
遅脉	slow pulse (quality)	chi myaku	chí mài	slow pulse
結脉	knotted pulse (quality)	ketsu myaku	jié mài	bound pulse; slow regularly interupted pulse
代脉	intermittent pulse (quality)	tai myaku	dài mài	intermittent pulse; regularly interrupted pulse
動脉	moving pulse (quality)	dō myaku	dòng mài	stirred pulse
硬結	induration(s)	kōketsu	yìng jié	induration(s)
挾脊穴	paraverterbal (points)	kyōsekiketsu	jiā jí xué	paraverterbal points (i.e., Hua Tuo's paravertebral points)
殿圧	gluteal tender point	den'atsu	diàn yà	
水滞	water stagnation	suitai	shuǐ zhì	water stagnation
圧痛	pressure pain	attsū	yà tòng	tender point(s); sore points
按圧する	(apply) pressure	anatsu (suru)		
単刺	single needle technique	tanshi	dān cì	lightly needle
刺絡	bloodletting	shiraku	cì luò	prick the network vessel; pricking
子午	midday-midnight (treatment)	shigo	zǐ wǔ	midday-midnight (point selection); stem and branch (point selection)
（治療）過剰	over stimulation [of/during] (treatment)	(chiryō) kajō		
運動鍼	motor-response needling	undōshin	yùn dòng zhēn	
皮膚鍼	touch needle	hifushin	pí fū zhēn	cutaneous needle
接触鍼	touch needle	sesshokushin	jiē chù zhēn	contact needle
胸脇苦満	tightness and pain in the thoracic rib cage area	kyōkyō kuman	xiōng xié kǔ mǎn	chest and rib-side fullness
痰飲	phlegm retention	tan'in	tán yǐn	phlegm-rheum
透熱灸	direct moxibustion	tōnetsukyū	tòu rè jiǔ	
灸頭鍼	moxa-on-the-handle needle	kyūtōshin	jiǔ tóu zhēn	
知熱灸	cone moxibustion	chinetsukyū	zhī rè zhēn	
雀啄	pecking technique	jakutaku	què zhuō	pecking sparrow [moxibustion]
脇下満痛	light swelling and pain in the subcostal area	kyōka mantsū	xié xià mǎn tòng	pain and fullness in the rib-side
身熱	body fever	shinnetsū	shēn rè	generalized heat [effusion]
口苦	bitter taste in the mouth	kōku	kǒu kǔ	bitter taste in the mouth
腹満	abdominal distention	fukuman	fù mǎn	abdominal fullness

漢字	English Translation	Japanese	Chinese	Other Common English Translations
身重	heaviness in the body	shinjū	shēn zhòng	generalized heaviness; heavy body
悪風	aversion to wind	ofū	wù fēng	aversion to wind
喘	pant (and puff), gasp	zen	chuǎn	panting
小便不利	urinary difficulty	shōben furi	xiǎo biàn bù	inhibited urination
小便自利	copious urination	shōben jiri	xiǎo biàn zì lì	uninhibited urination
口渇	dry mouth	kōkatsu	kǒu kě	thirst; hydrodipsia
喘咳	wheezing and coughing	zengai	chuǎn ké	panting and cough
弾石脉	striking pulse (quality)	dankoku myaku	tán shí mài	stone flicking pulse
湿病	dampness disease	shitsubyō	shī bìng	dampness disease
痰飲病	phlegm retention disease	tan'inbyō	tán yǐn bìng	phlegm-rheum disease
水気病	water-ki disease	suikibyō	shuǐ qì bìng	water qi disease
そわそわ	restless, fidgety, nervous	sowasowa		
煩躁	irritable restlessness	hansō	fán zào	vexation and agitation
濡脉	soggy pulse (quality)	nan myaku	rú mài	soggy pulse
大腹	upper abdomen	taifuku	dà fù	greater abdomen
少腹	lower abdomen	shōfuku	shào fù	lesser abdomen
脱汗	leaky sweating	dakkan	tuō hàn	desertion sweating
正邪	primary pathogenic influence	seija	zhèng xié	regular evil
虚邪	deficient-type pathogenic influence	kyoja	xū xié	vacuity evil
賊邪	bandit pathogenic influence	zokuja	zéi xié	bandit evil
微邪	weak-pathogenic influence	bija	wēi xié	mild evil
実邪	excess-type pathogenic influence	jitsuja	shí xié	repletion evil
逆上せる	have hot flushes	noboseru		
冷えのぼせ	chills in the lower limbs and hot flushes in the upper body	hienobose		
四肢収まらず	lassitude in the limbs	shishi osamarazu		
悪寒	aversion to cold	okan	wù hán	aversion to cold
哭	wail (as in mourning)	koku	kū	wailing
呻	to groan; to moan	shin	shēn	groaning
無汗	absence of sweating	mukan	wú hàn	absence of sweating
譫言	delirious utterances	uwagoto	zhān yán	delirious speech
頭項強痛	stiffness and pain in the nape of the neck	zukō kyōtsū	tóu xiàng qiáng tòng	headache and painful stiff nape

漢字	English Translation	Japanese	Chinese	Other Common English Translations
陰盛内寒	yin exuberance internal cold	insei naikan	yīn shèng nèi hán	exuberant internal yin cold
陰盛	yin exuberance	insei	yīn shèng	exuberant yin
発散	release or diffusion	hassan	fā sàn	effuse and dissipate
収斂	gather(ing)	shūren	shōu liǎn	astringe; promote contraction
亡血	blood collapse	bōketsuō	wáng xuè	blood collapse
盗汗	night sweats	tōkan	dào hàn	night sweating
遺溺	enuresis	ijō	yí niào	enuresis
耳聾	deafness	jirō	ěr lóng	deafness
自汗	unnaturally profuse sweating	jikan	zì hàn	spontaneous sweating
湯液治療	herbal treatment	tōeki chiryō	tāng yè zhì liaó	
痞（え）	obstruction	tsuka(e); hi	pǐ	glomus
不消化下痢	lientery	fushōka geri	bù xiaō huà xià lì	diarrhea containing incompletely digested material
喘逆	dry heaving	zengyaku	chuǎn nì	panting counterflow
裏急後重	diarrhea that afterwards leaves a dull ache in the lower abdomen and rectum	rikyūkōjū	lǐ jí hòu zhòng	abdominal urgency and heaviness in the rectum; tenesmus
脇下	subcostal area	kyōka	xié xià	below the rib-side
脇	anterior inferior aspect of the rib cage	waki/kyō	xié	rib-side
貴豚気病	running piglet	hontonkibyō	bēn tún qì bìng	running piglet
督脈	governing vessel	tokumyaku	dū māi	governing vessel
任脈	conception vessel	ninmyaku	rèn mài	controlling vessel
衝脈	penetrating vessel	shōmyaku	chōng mài	thoroughfare vessel
帯脈	girdling vessel	taimyaku	dài mài	girdling vessel
陽蹻脈	yang heel vessel	yōkyōmyaku	yáng qiaō mài	yang springing vessel
陰蹻脈	yin heel vessel	inkyōmyaku	yīn qiaō mài	yin springing vessel
陽維脈	yang linking vessel	yōimyaku	yáng wéi mài	yang linking vessel
陰維脈	yin linking vessel	in'imyaku	yīn wéi mài	yin linking vessel
瘧病	malarial disease	gyaku byō	nüè bìng	malaria
人中	philtrum	jinchū	rén zhōng	philtrum
疾脈	racing pulse (quality)	shitsu myaku	jí mài	racing pulse
牢脈	firm pulse (quality)	rō myaku	laó mài	confined pulse; prison pulse
心下満	swelling and tenderness in the hypochondriac region	shinkaman	xīn xià mǎn	fullness below the heart
鍼灸	acupuncture	shinkyū	zhēn jǐu	acumoxatherapy; acupuncture and moxibustion

漢字	English Translation	Japanese	Chinese	Other Common English Translations
漢方	kampo	kanpō	hàn fāng	Japanese herbal medicine
古典治療	classical therapy	koten chiryō	gǔ diǎn zhì liaó	
経穴（的）治療	acupoint therapy	keiketsu (teki) chiryō	jīng xué (de) zhì liaó	
補瀉	tonification and dispersion	hosha	bǔ xiè	supplementation and drainage
脉位脉状診	pulse position/pulse quality diagnosis	myakui myakujō shin	mài wèi mài zhuàng zhěn	
軽按	superficial level [for pulse diagnosis]	kcian	qīng àn	
重按	deep level [for pulse diagnosis]	jūan	zhòng àn	
脉状診	pulse quality diagnosis	myakujōshin	mài zhuàng zhěn	
脉差診	pulse strength comparison diagnosis	myakusashin	mài chā zhěn	
六部定位脉診	six-position pulse diagnosis	rokubu teii myakushin	liù bù dìng wèi mài zhěn	
改正孔穴	revised acupuncture points	kaisei kōketsu	gǎi zhèng kǒng xué	
新人弥生会	Yayoi Freshman Group	shinjin yayoi kai	xīn rén mí shēng huì	
経絡治療学会	Society of Traditional Japanese Medicine	Keiraku Chiryō Gakkai	jīng luò zhì liaó xué huì	
東邦医学誌	Oriental Medical Journal	tōhō igakushi	dōng bāng yī xué zhì	
毫鍼	filiform needle	gōshin	haó zhēn	fine needle; filiform needle
大鍼	big needle	taishin	dà zhēn	large needle
長鍼	long needle	chōshin	cháng zhēn	long needle
鍉鍼	blunt needle	teishin	bǎi zhēn	spoon needle
員利鍼	round-sharp needle	enrishin	yuán lì zhēn	rounded sharp needle; sharp round needle
三稜鍼	three-edged needle	sanryōshin	sān léng zhēn	three-edged needle
長柄鍼	long-handled needle	chōheishin	cháng bǐng zhēn	long-handled needle
鑱鍼	chisel needle	zanshin	qiàn zhēn	arrow-headed needle; shear needle
員鍼	round needle	enshin	yuán zhēn	round-headed needle
鋒鍼	lance needle	hōshin	fēng zhēn	sharp-edged needle
鈹鍼	sword needle	hishin	pī zhēn	sword-shaped needle
温灸	warming moxibustion	onkyū	wēn jǐu	warming moxibustion
隔物灸	indirect moxibustion	kakubutsukyū	gé wù jǐu	indirect moxibustion
鍼管	insertion tube	shinkan	zhēn guǎn	guide tube
刺鍼（法）	needling (method)	shishin(hō)	cì zhēn (fǎ)	needle insertion; pricking

漢字	English Translation	Japanese	Chinese	Other Common English Translations
管鍼法	needling with an insertion tube	kanshinhō	guǎn zhēn fǎ	tube insertion
燃鍼法	needling without an insertion tube	nenshinhō	rán zhēn fǎ	
腹診	abdominal diagnosis	fukushin	fù zhěn	abdominal examination
脉診	pulse diagnosis	myakushin	mài zhěn	pulse examination
積	accumulation	shaku	jī	accumulation
取穴	point location	shuketsu	qǔ xué	point location
選穴	point selection	senketsu	xuǎn xué	point selection
五行	five phases	gogyō	wǔ xíng	five phases
臓	zang organ	zō	zàng	viscera; viscus
腑	fu organ	fu	fǔ	bowel(s)
臓腑	organs	zōfu	zàng fǔ	bowels and viscera
寸	distal position [in pulse diagnosis]	sun	cùn	inch; first position
関	middle position [in pulse diagnosis]	kan	guān	bar; second position
尺	proximal position [in pulse diagnosis]	shaku	chǐ	cubit; third position
肝虚熱証	Liver deficiency heat pattern	kan-kyo nesshō	gān xū rè zhèng	liver-vacuity heat pattern
肝虚寒証	Liver deficiency cold pattern	kan-kyo kanshō	gān xū hán zhèng	liver-vacuity cold pattern
脾虚熱証	Spleen deficiency heat pattern	hi-kyo nesshō	pí xū rè zhèng	spleen-vacuity heat pattern
脾虚寒証	Spleen deficiency cold pattern	hi-kyo kanshō	pí xū hán zhèng	spleen-vacuity cold pattern
脾虚陽明経実熱証	Spleen deficiency yang brightness channel excess heat pattern	hi-kyo yōmeikei-jitsu nesshō	pí xū yáng míng jīng shí rè zhèng	spleen-vacuity yang ming channel repletion heat pattern
脾虚胃実熱証	Spleen deficiency Stomach excess heat pattern	hi-kyo i-jitsu nesshō	pí xū wèi shí rè zhèng	spleen-vacuity stomach-repletion heat pattern
脾虚胃虚熱証	Spleen deficiency Stomach deficiency heat pattern	hi-kyo i-kyo nesshō	pí xū wèi xū rè zhèng	spleen-vacuity stomach-vacuity heat pattern
脾虚肝実熱証	Spleen deficiency Liver excess heat pattern	hi kyo kan-jitsu nesshō	pí xū gān shí rè zhèng	spleen-vacuity liver-repletion heat pattern
脾虚肝実証	Spleen deficiency Liver excess pattern	hi-kyo kan-jitsu shō	pí xū gān shí zhèng	spleen-vacuity liver-repletion pattern
肺虚陽経実熱証	Lung deficiency yang channel excess heat pattern	hai-kyo yōkei-jitsu nesshō	fèi xū yáng jīng shí rè zhèng	lung-vacuity yang channel repletion heat pattern
肺虚寒証	Lung deficiency cold pattern	hai-kyo kanshō	fèi xū hán zhèng	lung-vacuity cold pattern
肺虚肝実	Lung deficiency Liver	hai-kyo	fèi xū gān shí	lung-vacuity liver-repletion pattern

漢字	English Translation	Japanese	Chinese	Other Common English Translations
証	excess pattern	kan-jitsu shō	zhèng	
腎虚熱証	Kidney deficiency heat pattern	jin-kyo nesshō	shèn xū rè zhèng	kidney-vacuity heat pattern
腎虚寒証	Kidney deficiency cold pattern	jin-kyo kanshō	shèn xū hán zhèng	kidney-vacuity cold pattern
気血津液	ki, blood, and fluids	ki ketsu shin'eki	qì xuè jīn yè	qi, blood, (body) fluids
木	Wood	moku	mù	wood
土	Earth	do	tǔ	earth
金	Metal	kin/kon	jīn	metal
水	Water	sui	shuǐ	water
相生	generative cycle	sōsei	xiāng shēng	engendering cycle; creative cycle
相剋	controlling cycle	sōkoku	xiāng kè	restraining cycle; checking cycle
衛気	defensive ki	eki	wèi qì	defense qi; protective qi
栄気	nutritive ki	eiki	róng qì	another term for constructive ki
精	essence	sei	jīng	essence; (also) semen
神	spirit	shin/kami	shén	spirit
皮毛	skin (and hair)	himō	pí maó	skin and [body] hair
肌肉	flesh	kiniku	jī ròu	flesh
虚熱	deficient-type heat	kyonetsu	xū rè	vacuity heat
壮火	vigorous fire	sōka	zhuàng huǒ	vigorous fire
外邪	external pathogen(s)	gaija	wài xié	external evil
腠理	pore(s)	sōri	còu lǐ	interstice
臊	rancid [odor]	sō/aburakusai	saō	animal [odor]
焦	burnt [odor]	shū/kogekusai	jiaō	burnt [odor]
香	fragrant [odor]	kō/kaorikusai	xiāng	fragrant [odor]
腥	fleshy [odor]	sei/namagusai	xīng	fishy [odor]
腐	rotten [odor]	fu/kusarekusai	fǔ	putrid [odor]
魂	ethereal soul	kon/tamashii	hún	ethereal soul
意智	intention and wisdom	ichi	yì zhì	reflection and wisdom
魄	corporeal soul	haku	pò	corporeal soul; animal soul
精志	will	seishi	jīng zhì	
血脈	blood vessel(s)	ketsumyaku	xuè mài	blood vessel(s)
筋膜	sinews and fascia	kinmaku	jīn mó	sinew membrane
宗気	ancestral ki	sōki	zōng qì	ancestral qi
心	Heart	shin	xīn	heart
肝	Liver	kan	gān	liver

漢字	English Translation	Japanese	Chinese	Other Common English Translations
脾	Spleen	hi	pí	spleen
腎	Kidney	jin	shèn	kidney
胆	Gallbladder	tan	dǎn	gallbladder
胃	Stomach	i	wèi	stomach
大腸	Large Intestine	daichō	dà cháng	large intestine
小腸	Small Intestine	shōchō	xiǎo cháng	small intestine
肺	Lung	hai	fèi	lung
心包	Pericardium	shinpō	xīn bāo	pericardium
三焦	Triple Warmer	sanshō	sān jiāo	triple burner
原気	source ki	genki	yuán qì	source ki
神気	spirit ki	shinki	shén qì	spirit qi
精気	essential ki	seiki	jīng qì	essential qi
先天	prenatal	senten	xiān tiān	earlier heaven; congenital constitution
後天	postnatal	kōten	hòu tiān	later heaven; acquired constitution
命門	life gate	meimon	mìng mén	life gate
陽気	yang ki	yōki	yáng qì	yang qi
陰気	yin ki	inki	yīn qì	yin qi
五穀	five grains	gokoku	wǔ gǔ	five grains
糟粕	dregs [i.e. a chyme-like substance]	sōhaku	zāo pò	waste
三隧	three paths	sansui	sān suì	
膀胱	Bladder	bōkō	páng guāng	urinary bladder
君火	sovereign fire	kunka	jūn huǒ	sovereign fire
相火	ministerial fire	sōka	xiàng huǒ	ministerial fire
熱性	heat-type	nessei	rè xìng	hot-natured
寒性	cold-type	kansei	hán xìng	cold-natured
五臓六腑	five zang organs and six fu organs	gozōroppu	wǔ zàng liù fǔ	five viscera and six bowels
水穀	food and drink	suikoku	shuǐ gǔ	food; grain and water
肝血	Liver blood	kanketsu	gān xuè	liver blood
気虚	ki deficiency	kikyo	qì xū	qi vacuity
肺気	Lung ki	haiki	fèi qì	lung qi
表裏(関係)	paired (relationship)	hyōri(kankei)	biào lì (guān xì)	exterior-interior (relationship)
内攻	strike inward	naikō	nèi gōng	
本治法	root treatment	honchihō	běn zhì fǎ	

漢字	English Translation	Japanese	Chinese	Other Common English Translations
本治法補助穴	root treatment supplementary points	honchihō hojoketsu	běn zhì fǎ bǔ zhù xué	
標治法	local treatment	hyōchihō	biaō zhì fǎ	
募穴	alarm point(s)	boketsu	mù xué	alarm point(s)
背部兪穴	back transport point(s)	haibu yuketsu	bèi bù shū xué	back transport point(s)
五行穴	five phase points	gogyōketsu	wǔ xíng xué	five phase points
井穴	well point	sei-ketsu	jǐng xué	well point
榮穴	spring point	ei-ketsu	yíng xué	brook point
兪穴	stream point	yu-ketsu	shū xué	stream point
経穴	river point	kei-ketsu	jīng xué	river point; channel point
合穴	uniting point	gō-ketsu	hé xué	uniting point
井木穴	well-wood-point	sei'moku'ketsu	jǐng mù xué	
榮火穴	spring-fire-point	ei'ka'ketsu	yíng huǒ xué	
兪土穴	stream-earth-point	yu'do'ketsu	shū tǔ xué	
経金穴	river-metal-point	kei'kin'ketsu	jīng jīn xué	
合水穴	uniting-water-point	gō'sui'ketsu	hé shuǐ xué	
手（の）太陰肺経	hand greater yin Lung channel	te (no) taiin haikei	shǒu tài yīn fèi jīng	hand tai yin lung channel
手（の）少陰心経	hand lesser yin Heart channel	te (no) shōin shinkei	shǒu shào yīn xīn jīng	hand shao yin heart channel
手（の）厥陰心包経	hand reverting yin Pericardium channel	te (no) ketsuin shinpōkei	shǒu jué yīn xīn baō jīng	hand jue yin pericardium channel
手（の）陽明大腸経	hand yang brightness Large Intestine channel	te (no) yōmei daichōkei	shǒu yáng míng dà cháng jīng	hand yang ming large intestine channel
手（の）太陽小腸経	hand greater yang Small Intestine channel	te (no) taiyō shōchōkei	shǒu tài yáng xiāo cháng jīng	hand tai yang small intestine channel
手（の）少陽三焦経	hand lesser yang Triple Warmer channel	te (no) shōyō sanshōkei	shǒu shào yáng sān jiaō jīng	hand shao yang triple burner channel
足（の）太陰脾経	foot greater yin Spleen channel	te (no) taiin hikei	zú tài yīn pí jīng	foot tai yin spleen channel
足（の）少陰腎経	foot lesser yin Kidney channel	ashi (no) shōin jinkei	zú shào yīn shèn jīng	foot shao yin kidney channel
足（の）厥陰肝経	foot reverting yin Liver channel	ashi (no) ketsuin kankei	zú jué yīn gān jīng	foot jue yin liver channel
足（の）少陽胆経	foot lesser yang Gallbladder channel	ashi (no) shōyō tankei	zú shào yáng dǎn jīng	foot shao yang gallbladder channel
足（の）少陽胆経	foot lesser yang Gallbladder channel	ashi (no) shōyō tankei	zú shào yáng dǎn jīng	foot shao yang gallbladder channel
足（の）少陽胆経	foot lesser yang Gallbladder channel	ashi (no) shōyō tankei	zú shào yáng dǎn jīng	foot shao yang gallbladder channel

漢字	English Translation	Japanese	Chinese	Other Common English Translations
奇経	extraordinary vessel(s)	kikei	qí jīng	extraordinary vessel(s)
脾の大絡	great network vessel of the Spleen	hi no tairaku	pí zhī dà luò	great network vessel of the spleen
経別	divergent channel(s)	keibetsu	jīng bié	channel divergence
経筋	channel sinews	keikin	jīng jīn	channel sinew
経水	water channel(s)	keisui	jīng shuǐ	channel water; also menstruation
気門	ki gate	kimon	qì mén	qi gate
気穴	ki point	kikctsu	qì xué	qi point
五兪穴	five transport points	goyuketsu	wǔ shū xué	five transport points
原穴	source point	genketsu	yuán xué	source point
郄穴	cleft point	gekiketsu	xì xué	accumulation point
絡穴	network point	rakuketsu	luò xué	network point
八会穴	eight meeting points	hassōketsu	bā huì xué	eight meeting points
四総穴	four command points	shisōketsu	sì zǒng xué	four command points
上焦	upper warmer	jōshō	shàng jiāo	upper burner
中焦	middle warmer	chūshō	zhōng jiāo	center burner; middle burner
下焦	lower warmer	geshō	xià jiāo	lower burner
五精	five essences	gosei	wǔ jīng	
五主	five principle parts	goshu	wǔ zhǔ	five governings
五官	five orifices	gokan	wǔ guān	five offices
五志	five minds	goshi	wǔ zhì	five minds
五華	five accessory parts	goka	wǔ huá	five blooms
五味	five flavors	gomi	wǔ wèi	five flavors
五臭	five odors	goshū	wǔ xiù	five odors
五声	five voices	gosei	wǔ shēng	five voices
胃口	cardia (噴門 funmon) or pylorus (幽門 yūmon)	ikō	wèi kǒu	
膈	diaphragm	kaku	gé	diaphragm
魚	thenar eminence of the palm	gyo	yú	
心主	heart governing (Pericardium channel)	shinshu	xīn zhǔ	that which the heart governs…
寸口	radial pulse	sunkō	cùn kǒu	wrist pulse; inch opening
季脇	free ribs	kiroku	jì xié	free rib (region)
外踝	lateral malleolus	gaika	wài huái	lateral malleolus
内踝	medial malleolus	naika	nèi huái	mcdial mallcolus
瘀血	blood stasis	oketsu	yū xuè	static blood
宗筋	ancestral sinews/sexual	sōkin	zōng jīn	ancestral sinew

漢字	English Translation	Japanese	Chinese	Other Common English Translations
	organs			
目の内眥	inner canthus [of the eye]	me no naishi	mù nèi zì	
鋭眥	outer canthus [of the eye]	eishi	ruì zì	outer canthus [of the eye]
顔面のシミ	discolored patch on the face	ganmen no shimi		
頬が腫れる	swollen cheeks	hoho ga hareru		
顎が腫れる	swollen jaw	ago ga hareru		
虚満	deficient-type distention	kyoman	xū mǎn	vacuity distention
陰茎硬直症	priapism	inkei kōchokushō	yīn jīng yìng zhí zhèng	persistent erection
心痛	heart pain	shintsū	xīn tòng	heart pain
胸痛	chest pain	kyōtsū	xiōng tòng	chest pain
熱性病	febrile disease	nesseibyō	rè xìng bìng	hot-natured disease
置鍼	retained needle	chishin	zhì zhēn	
表	exterior/yang-type	hyō	biào	exterior
裏	interior/yin-type	ri	lì	interior
望診	looking	bōshin	wàng zhěn	inspection; looking examination; visual examination
聞診	listening (and smelling)	bunshin	wén zhěn	listening and smelling; audio-olfactory examination
問診	questioning	monshin	wèn zhěn	inquiry
尺膚	cubit skin	shakufu	chǐ fū	cubit skin
腰眼穴	yao yan point	yōganketsu	yāo yǎn xué	lumbar eye point
人迎気口診	carotid pulse diagnosis	jinkei kikō shin	rén yíng qì kǒu zhěn	pulse [taking at] man's prognosis
祖脉診	six-basic-pulses diagnosis	somyakushin	zǔ mài zhěn	
平脉	normal pulse	heimyaku	píng mài	normal pulse
水毒	water toxin	suidoku	shuǐ dú	water toxin
温鍼	warming needle	onshin	wēn zhēn	warm needle
導引	massage	dōin	dāo yǐn	
栄血	nutritive blood	eiketsu	róng xuè	
押し手	supporting hand	oshide	yā shǒu	
刺し手	inserting hand	sashide	cì shǒu	
提按	stroking	teian	tí àn	lifting and pressing
迎随	angle [of needling]	geizui	yíng suí	directional [needling method]
弾爪	flicking and fingernail pressing	dansō	tán zhāo	needle flicking and nail-press [needling method]

漢字	English Translation	Japanese	Chinese	Other Common English Translations
搓転	twisting [the needle]	saten	cuō zhuǎn	[needle] twisting
揺動	vibrating [the needle]	yōdō	yáo dòng	[needle] waggling
輸瀉	transport dispersion	yusha	shū xiè	
暴気	fulminant ki	bōki	bào qì	
心下痞	feeling of fullness and oppression below the heart	shinkahi	xīn xià pǐ	glomus below the heart
脉象	pulse picture	myakushō	mài xiàng	pulse manifestation
足裏の煩熱	heat vexation in the soles of the feet	sokuri no hannetsu	zú lǐ fán rè	
足腰が冷える	cold feet and lower back	ashi-koshi ga hieru		
胃気の脉	Stomach ki pulse	iki no myaku	wèi qì mài	
陰中の陰	yin within yin	inchū no in	yīn zhōng zhī yīn	yin within yin
陰中の至陰	most extreme yin within yin	inchū no shi'in	yīn zhōng zhì zhì yīn	
陰中の陽	yang within yin	inchū no yō	yīn zhōng zhī yáng	yang within yin
陽中の陰	yin within yang	yōchū no in	yáng zhōng zhī yīn	yin within yang
陽中の陽	yang within yang	yōchū no yō	yáng zhog1 zhī yáng	yang within yang
陰陽とも虚	deficiency of both yin and yang	inyō tomo kyo	yīn yáng liǎng xū	dual vacuity of yin and yang
鬱状態	state of emotional depression	utsu jōtai	yù zhuàng tài	
鬱病	(emotional) depression	utsubyō	yu bing	
逆気	counter-flowing ki	gyakki	nì qì	counterflow qi
悪心	nausea	oshin	ě xīn	nausea
形と色	physique and color	katachi to iro	xíng hé sè	physical body and complexion
下腹部瘀血	blood stasis in the lower abdomen	kafukubu oketsu	xià fù bù yū xuè	blood stasis in the lower abdomen
髪	hair [on the head]	kami	fà	hair
気の医学	ki medicine	ki no igaku	qì de yī xué	
脚弱	weak legs	kyakujaku	jiāo ruò	weak legs
中寒	cold stroke	chūkan	zhòng hán	cold stroke
痺	numbness (bi syndrome)	hi	bì	impediment
営気	constructive ki	eiki	yíng qì	construction qi; another term for nutritive ki
正気	correct ki	seiki	zhèng qì	right qi
死脉	death pulse (quality)	shi myaku	sǐ mài	
長脉	long pulse (quality)	chō myaku	cháng mài	long pulse

漢字	English Translation	Japanese	Chinese	Other Common English Translations
短脉	short pulse (quality)	tan myaku	duǎn mài	short pulse
大脉	large pulse (quality)	dai myaku	dà mài	large pulse
小脉	small pulse (quality)	shō myaku	xiāo mài	small pulse
正経自病	self-channel disease	seikei jibyō	zhèng jīng zì bìng	
熱気	heat-ki	nekki	rè qì	hot qi
実熱	excess-type heat	jitsu netsu	shí rè	repletion heat
元陽	original yang	gen'yō	yuán yáng	original yang
経気	channel ki	keiki	jīng qì	channel qi
雀啄法	pecking technique	jakutakuhō	què zhuō fǎ	pecking sparrow moxibustion
糸状灸	thread moxa	shijōkyū	sī zhuàng jiǔ	
七情	seven affects	shichijō	qī qíng	seven affects
真寒仮熱	true cold false heat	shinkan kanetsu	zhēn hán jiǎ rè	true cold and false heat
変動穴	traveling point	hendōketsu	biàn dòng xué	
脇下硬	subcostal tension	kyōkakō	xié xià yìng	hardness below the rib-side

Selected Japanese Modern Medical Terminology

現代医学用語の選択

日本語	English	Japanese
打撲	bruise, contusion	daboku
体質	(physical) constitution	taishitsu
膠原病	a collagen disease	kōgenbyō
円形脱毛症	alopecia areata	enkei datsumōshō
動脈瘤	aneurysm	dōmyakuryū
口角炎	angular cheilitis	kōkakuen
尿閉	anuria	nyōhei
虫垂炎	appendicitis	chūsuien
不整脈	arrhythmia	fuseimyaku
関節痛	arthralgia	kansetsutsū
関節炎	arthritis	kansetsuen
喘息	asthma	zensoku
（目が）充血	bloodshot eyes	(me ga) jūketsu
体臭	body odor	taishū
逆子	breech birth	sakago
気管支	bronchial tubes	kikanshi
カリエス	caries	kariesu
白内障	cataract	hakunaishō
細胞病理学	cellular pathology	saibō byōrigaku
胆嚢炎	cholecystitis	tannōen
胆石症	cholelithiasis [gallstones]	tansekishō
愁訴	complaint	shūso
結膜炎	conjunctivitis	ketsumakuen
クローン病	Crohn's disease	kurōn byō
膀胱炎	cystitis	bōkōen
痴呆	dementia	chihō
陥下	depression(s)	kange
錯乱	derangement	sakuran
皮膚病	dermatosis	hifubyō
適応症	diseases for which a medicine is efficacious	tekōshō
立ちくらみ	dizziness/faintness on standing up	tachikurami

鈍痛	dull pain	dontsū
十二指腸潰瘍	duodenal ulcer	jūnishichō kaiyō
湿疹	eczema	shisshin
浮腫	edema	fushu
蓄膿症	empyema	chiku'nōshō
癲癇	epilepsy	tenkan
眼底出血	eyegrounds hemorrhage	gantei shukketsu
熱感	feverish	netsukan
五十肩	fifty-year-old's shoulder [i.e. stiff and painful shoulders due to age]	gojūkata
歯齦炎	gingivitis	shigin'en
緑内障	glaucoma	ryokunaishō
舌炎	glossitis	zetsuen
臀部痛	gluteal pain	denbutsū
婦人科疾患	gynecological problems	fujinka shikkan
難聴	hardness of hearing	nanchō
痔疾	hemorrhoids	jishitsu
肝硬変	hepatic cirrhosis	kankōhen
肝炎	hepatitis	kan'en
蕁麻疹	hives, nettle rash	jinmashin
麦粒腫	hordeolum	bakuryūshu
腸骨稜	iliac crest	chōkotsuryō
疳（の）虫	irascibility bug	kan no mushi
黄疸	jaundice	ōdan
角膜炎	keratitis	kakumakuen
硬結	induration(s)	kōketsu
帯下	leukorrhea	koshike
舌乳頭	lingual papilla	zetsunyūtō
局所	local [symptomatic/painful] area	kyokusho
食欲不振	loss of appetite	shokuyoku fushin
梨状筋部	lower buttocks	rijōkinbu
光沢	luster	kōtaku
リンパ節炎	lymphadenitis	rinpasen'en
躁病	mania	sōbyō
気鬱	melancholy, depression	kiutsu
更年期障害	menopausal syndrome	kōnenki shōgai
経絡治療	Meridian Therapy	keiraku chiryō
偏頭痛	migraine headache	henzutsū

現代医学	modern medicine, contemporary medicine	gendai igaku
腎炎	nephritis	jin'en
骨粗鬆症	osteoporosis	kotsusoshōshō
触診	palpation	shokushin
動悸	palpitations	dōki
膵炎	pancreatitis	suien
不随	paralysis	fuzui
既往症	past (previous) illness(es)	kiōshō
病理	pathology	byōri
会陰部	perineum	einbu
吹き出物	pimples or small boils	fukidemono
胸膜炎	pleurisy	kyōmakuen
肺炎	pneumonia	haien
多発性関節リウマチ	polyarticluar rheumatism	tahatsusei kansetsu riumachi
前立腺炎	prostatitis	zenritsusen'en
前立腺肥大	prostatomegaly	zenritsusenhidai
隆起	protuberance	ryūki
膨隆	protuberance(s)	bōryū
肺気腫	pulmonary emphysema	haikishu
下剤	purgative	gezai
腎盂炎	pyelitis	jin'uen
呼吸器疾患	respiratory disease	kokyūki shikkan
鼻炎	rhinitis	bien
蛔虫	roundworm	kaichū
唾液	saliva	daeki
坐骨神経痛	sciatica	zakotsu shinkeitsū
側彎症	scoliosis	sokuwanshō
疼痛	sharp, stabbing pain	tōtsū
息切れ	shortness of breath	ikigire
副作用	side effects	fukusayō
痙攣	spasm, cramp	keiren
拘攣	spasm, twitch	kōren
自発痛	spontaneous pain	jihatsutsū
胸鎖乳突筋	sternocleidomastoid muscle	kyōsanyū tokkin
口内炎	stomatitis	kōnaien
頸部リンパ腺腫	swollen cervical lymph glands	keibu rinpasenshu

甲状腺	thyroid gland	kōjōsen
甲状腺炎	thyroiditis	kōjōsen'en
扁桃炎	tonsillitis	hentōen
逆まつげ	trichiasis	sakamatsuge
三叉神経痛	trigeminal neuralgia	sansashinkeitsū
結核	tuberculosis	kekkaku
中耳炎	tympanitis	chūjien
潰瘍性大腸炎	ulcerative colitis	kaiyōsei daichōen
意識不明	unconsciousness	ishikifumei
尿道炎	urethritis	nyōdoen
静脈瘤	varicose veins	jōmyakuryū
蜘蛛状血管腫	vascular spiders	kumojō kekkanshu
疣	wart(s)	ibo
アトピー性の皮膚炎	atopic dermatitis	atopiisei no hifuen
口唇ヘルペス	herpes labialis	kōshin herupesu
ベーチェット病	Behcet's Syndrome	beechetto byō
結節性紅班	erythema nodosum	kessetsusei kōhan
経産婦	mulitparous woman	keisanpu
神経症	neurosis	shinkeishō
胆嚢疾患	cholecystopathy	tannō shikkan
寒冷	frigidity	kanrei
腸閉塞	intestinal obstruction, ileus	chōheisoku
アキレス腱痛	pain in the calcaneal tendon	akiresukentsū
咽喉痛	sore throat	inkōtsū
胃痛	stomachache	itsū
嘔吐	vomiting	ōto
外傷	trauma	gaishō
下肢の浮腫	edema of the lower limbs	kashi no fushu
過食	overeating	kashoku
下腹部痛	lower abdominal pain	kafukubutsū
廻盲部痛	pain in the ileocecum	kaimōbutsū
飢餓	starvation	kiga
ネフローゼ	nephrosis	nefurōze

Point Names

経 穴

English Alpha-Numeric	Japanese Romaji	経穴	Chinese PinYin	English Name
BL-1	seimei	睛明	jīng míng	Bright Eyes
BL-2	sanchiku	攢竹	zǎn zhú	Bamboo Gathering
BL-3	bishō	眉衝	meí chōng	Eyebrow Ascension
BL-4	kyokusa	曲差	qū chā	Deviating Turn
BL-5	gosho	五処	wǔ chù	Fifth Place
BL-6	shōkō	承光	chéng guāng	Light Guard
BL-7	tsūten	通天	tōng tiān	Celestial Connection
BL-8	rakkyaku	絡却	luò què	Declining Connection
BL-9	gyokuchin	玉枕	yù zhěn	Jade Pillow
BL-10	tenchū	天柱	tiān zhù	Celestial Pillar)
BL-11	daijo	大杼	dà zhù	Great Shuttle
BL-12	fūmon	風門	fēng mén	Wind Gate
BL-13	haiyu	肺兪	fèi shū	Lung Transport
BL-14	ketsuin'yu	厥陰兪	jué yīn shū	Reverting Yīn Transport
BL-15	shin'yu	心兪	xīn shū	Heart Transport
BL-16	tokuyu	督兪	dū shū	Governing Transport
BL-17	kakuyu	膈兪	gé shū	Diaphragm Transport
BL-18	kan'yu	肝兪	gān shū	Liver Transport
BL-19	tan'yu	胆兪	dǎn shū	Gallbladder Transport
BL-20	hiyu	脾兪	pí shū	Spleen Transport
BL-21	iyu	胃兪	wèi shū	Stomach Transport
BL-22	sanshōyu	三焦兪	sān jiāo shū	Triple Burner Transport
BL-23	jin'yu	腎兪	shèn shū	Kidney Transport
BL-24	kikaiyu	気海兪	qì hǎi shū	Sea-of-Qì Transport
BL-25	daichōyu	大腸兪	dà cháng shū	Large Intestine Transport

BL-26	kangen'yu	関元俞	guān yuán shū	Pass Head Transport
BL-27	shōchōyu	小腸俞	xiǎo cháng shū	Small Intestine Transport
BL-28	bōkōyu	膀胱俞	páng guāng shū	Bladder Transport
BL-29	chūryoyu	中膂俞	zhōng lǚ shū	Central Backbone Transport
BL-30	hakkan'yu	白環俞	bái huán shū	White Ring Transport
BL-31	jōryō	上髎	shàng liáo	Upper Bone-Hole)
BL-32	jiryō	次髎	cì liáo	Second Bone-Hole
BL-33	chūryō	中髎	zhōng liáo	Central Bone-Hole
BL-34	geryō	下髎	xià liáo	Lower Bone-Hole
BL-35	eyō	会陽	huì yáng	Meeting of Yáng
BL-36	shōfu	承扶	chéng fú	Support
BL-37	inmon	殷門	yīn mén	Gate of Abundance)
BL-38	fugeki	浮郄	fú xī	Superficial Cleft
BL-39	iyō	委陽	wěi yáng	Bend Yáng
BL-40	ichū	委中	wěi zhōng	Bend Center
BL-41	fubun	附分	fù fēn	Attached Branch
BL-42	hakko	魄戸	pò hù	Pò Door
BL-43	kōkō	膏肓	gāo huāng shū	Gāo Huāng Transport
BL-44	shindō	神堂	shén táng	Spirit Hall
BL-45	iki	譩譆	yī xǐ	Yi Xi
BL-46	kakukan	膈関	gé guān	Diaphragm
BL-47	konmon	魂門	hún mén	Hún Gate
BL-48	yōkō	陽綱	yáng gāng	Yáng Headrope
BL-49	isha	意舎	yì shè	Reflection Abode
BL-50	isō	胃倉	wèi cāng	wèi cāng
BL-51	kōmon	肓門	huāng mén	Huāng Gate
BL-52	shishitsu	志室	zhì shì	Will Chamber
BL-53	hōkō	胞肓	bāo huāng	Bladder Huang
BL-54	chippen	秩辺	zhì biān	Sequential Limit
BL-55	gōyō	合陽	hé yáng	Yáng Union
BL-56	shōkin	承筋	chéng jīn	Sinew Support
BL-57	shōzan	承山	chéng shān	Mountain Support

BL-58	hiyō	飛揚	fēi yáng	Taking Flight
BL-59	fuyō	跗陽	fū yáng	Instep Yáng
BL-60	konron	昆侖	kūn lún	Kūnlún Mountains
BL-61	bokushin	僕参	pú cān	Subservient Visitor
BL-62	shinmyaku	申脈	shēn mài	Extending Vessel
BL-63	kinmon	金門	jīn mén	Metal Gate
BL-64	keikotsu	京骨	jīng gǔ	Capital Bone
BL-65	sokkotsu	束骨	shù gǔ	Bundle Bone
BL-66	(ashi no) tsūkoku	(足)通谷	(zú) tōng gǔ	(Foot) Valley Passage
BL-67	shi'in	至陰	zhì yīn	Reaching Yīn
CV-1	ein	会陰	huì yīn	Meeting of Yīn
CV-2	kyokkotsu	曲骨	qū gǔ	Curved Bone
CV-3	chūkyoku	中極	zhōng jí	Central Pole
CV-4	kangen	関元	guān yuán	Pass Head
CV-5	sekimon	石門	shí mén	Stone Gate
CV-6	kikai	気海	qì hǎi	Sea of Qì
CV-7	inkō	陰交	yīn jiāo	Yīn Intersection
CV-8	shinketsu	神闕	shén què	Spirit Gate Tower
CV-9	suibun	水分	shuǐ fēn	Water Divide
CV-10	gekan	下脘	xià wǎn	Lower Stomach Duct
CV-11	kenri	建里	jiàn lǐ	Interior Strengthening
CV-12	chūkan	中脘	zhōng wǎn	Central Stomach Duct
CV-13	jōkan	上脘	shàng wǎn	Upper Stomach Duct
CV-14	koketsu	巨闕	jù què	Great Tower Gate
CV-15	kyūbi	鳩尾	jīu wěi	Turtledove Tail
CV-16	chūtei	中庭	zhōng ting	Center Palace
CV-17	danchū	膻中	dàn zhōng	Chest Center
CV-18	gyokudō	玉堂	yù táng	Jade Hall
CV-19	shikyū	紫宮	zǐ gōng	Purple Palace
CV-20	kagai	華蓋	huá gài	Florid Canopy
CV-21	senki	璇璣	xuán jī	Jade Swivel
CV-22	tentotsu	天突	tiān tú	Celestial Chimney

CV-23	rensen	廉泉	lián quán	Ridge Spring
CV-24	shōshō	承漿	chéng jiāng	Sauce Receptacle
GB-1	dōshiryō	瞳子髎	tóng zǐ liáo	Pupil Bone-Hole
GB-2	chōe	聴会	tīng huì	Auditory Convergence
GB-3	jōkan	上関	shàng guān	Upper Gate
GB-4	gan'en	頷厭	hàn yàn	Forehead Fullness
GB-5	kenro	懸顱	xuán lú	Suspended Skull
GB-6	kenri	懸釐	xuán lí	Suspended Tuft
GB-7	kyokubin	曲鬢	qū bìn	Temporal Hairline Curve
GB-8	sokkoku	率骨	shuài gǔ	Valley Lead
GB-9	tenshō	天衝	tiān chòng	Celestial Hub
GB-10	fuhaku	浮白	fú bái	Floating White
GB-11	atama no kyōin	頭竅陰	tóu qiào yīn	Head Orifice Yīn
GB-12	kankotsu	完骨	wán gǔ	Completion Bone
GB-13	honshin	本神	běn shén	Root Spirit
GB-14	yōhaku	陽白	yáng bái	Yáng White
GB-15	atama no rinkyū	頭臨泣	tóu lín qì	Head Overlooking Tears
GB-16	mokusō	目窓	mù chuāng	Eye Window
GB-17	shōei	正営	zhèng yíng	Upright Construction
GB-18	shōrei	承霊	chéng líng	Spirit Support
GB-19	nōkū	脳空	nǎo kōng	Brain Hollow
GB-20	fūchi	風池	fēng chí	Wind Pool
GB-21	kensei	肩井	jiān jǐng	Shoulder Well
GB-22	en'eki	淵腋	yuān yè	Armpit Abyss
GB-23	chōkin	輒筋	zhé jīn	Sinew Seat
GB-24	jitsugetsu	日月	rì yuè	Sun and Moon
GB-25	keimon	京門	jīng mén	Capital Gate
GB-26	taimyaku	帯脈	dài mài	Girdling Vessel
GB-27	gosū	五枢	wǔ shū	Fifth Pivot
GB-28	idō	維道	weí dào	Linking Path
GB-29	kyoryō	居髎	jū liáo	Squatting Bone-Hole
GB-30	kanchō	環跳	huán tiào	Jumping Round

GB-31	fūshi	風市	fēng shì	Wind Market
GB-32	chūtoku	中瀆	zhōng dú	Central River
GB-33	hiza no yōkan	膝陽関	xī yáng guān	Knee Yáng Joint
GB-34	yōryōsen	陽陵泉	yáng líng quán	Yáng Mound Spring
GB-35	yōkō	陽交	yáng jiāo	Yáng Intersection
GB-36	gaikyū	外丘	wài qiū	Outer Hill
GB-37	kōmei	光明	guāng míng	Bright Light
GB-38	yōho	陽輔	yáng fǔ	Yáng Assistance
GB-39	kenshō	懸鍾	xuán zhōng	Suspended Bell
GB-40	kyūkyo	丘墟	qiū xū	Hill Ruins
GB-41	ashi no rinkyū	足臨泣	zú lín qì	Foot Overlooking Tears
GB-42	chigoe	地五会	dì wǔ huì	Earth Fivefold Convergence
GB-43	kyōkei	侠谿	xiá xī	Pinched Ravine
GB-44	ashi no kyōin	足竅陰	zú qiào yīn	Foot Orifice Yīn
GV-1	chōkyō	長強	cháng qiáng	Long Strong
GV-2	yōyu	腰俞	yāo shū	Lumbar Transport
GV-3	koshi no yōkan	腰陽関	yāo yáng guān	Lumbar Yáng Pass
GV-4	meimon	命門	mìng mén	Life Gate
GV-5	kensū	懸枢	xuán shū	Suspended Pivot
GV-6	sekichū	脊中	jǐ zhōng	Spinal Center
GV-7	chūsū	中枢	zhōng shū	Central Pivot
GV-8	kinshuku	筋縮	jīn suō	Sinew Contraction
GV-9	shiyō	至陽	zhì yáng	Extremity of Yáng
GV-10	reidai	霊台	líng tá	Spirit Tower
GV-11	shindō	神道	shén dào	Spirit Path
GV-12	shinchū	身柱	shēn zhù	Body Pillar
GV-13	tōdō	陶道	táo dào	Kiln Path
GV-14	daitsui	大椎	dà zhuī	Great Hammer
GV-15	amon	瘂門	yǎ mén	Mute's Gate
GV-16	fūfu	風府	fēng fǔ	Wind Mansion
GV-17	nōko	脳戸	nǎo hù	Brain's Door
GV-18	kyōkan	強間	qiáng jiān	Unyielding Space

GV-19	gochō	後頂	hòu dǐng	Behind the Vertex
GV-20	hyakue	百会	bǎi huì	Hundred Convergences
GV-21	zenchō	前頂	qián dǐng	Before the Vertex
GV-22	shin'e	囟会	xìn huì	Fontanel Meeting
GV-23	jōsei	上星	shàng xīng	Upper Star
GV-24	shintei	神庭	shén tíng	Spirit Court
GV-25	soryō	素髎	sù liáo	White Bone-Hole
GV-26	suikō	水溝	shuǐ gōu	Water Trough
GV-27	datan	兌端	duì duān	Extremity of the Mouth
GV-28	ginkō	齦交	yín jiāo	Gum Intersection
HT-1	kyokusen	極泉	jí quán	Highest Spring
HT-2	seirei	青霊	qīng líng	Green-Blue Spirit
HT-3	shōkai	少海	shào hǎi	Lesser Sea
HT-4	reidō	霊道	líng dào	Spirit Pathway
HT-5	tsūri	通里	tōng lǐ	Connecting Li
HT-6	ingeki	陰郄	yīn xī	Yīn Cleft
HT-7	shinmon	神門	shén mén	Spirit Gate
HT-8	shōfu	少府	shào fǔ	Lesser Mansion
HT-9	shōshō	少衝	shào chōng	Lesser Surge
KI-1	yūsen	湧泉	yǒng quán	Gushing Spring
KI-2	nenkoku	然谷	rán gǔ	Blazing Valley
KI-3	taikei	太谿	tài xī	Great Ravine
KI-4	daishō	大鍾	dà zhōng	Large Goblet
KI-5	suisen	水泉	shuǐ quán	Water Spring
KI-6	shōkai	照海	zhào hǎi	Shining Sea
KI-7	fukuryū	復溜	fù līu	Recover Flow
KI-8	kōshin	交信	jiāo xìn	Intersection Reach
KI-9	chikuhin	築賓	zhú bīn	Guest House
KI-10	inkoku	陰谷	yīn gǔ	Yīn Valley
KI-11	ōkotsu	横骨	héng gǔ	Pubic Bone
KI-12	daikaku	大赫	dà hè	Great Manifestation
KI-13	kiketsu	気穴	qì xué	Qì Point

KI-14	shiman	四満	sì mǎn	Fourfold Fullness
KI-15	chūchū	中注	zhōng zhù	Central Flow
KI-16	kōyu	肓兪	huāng shū	Huāng Transport
KI-17	shōkyoku	商曲	shāng qū	Shāng Bend
KI-18	sekikan	石関	shí guān	Stone Pass
KI-19	into	陰都	yīn dū	Yīn Metropolis
KI-20	(hara no) tsūkoku	(腹)通谷	(fù) tōng gǔ	(Abdominal) Open Valley
KI-21	yūmon	幽門	yōu mén	Dark Gate
KI-22	horō	歩廊	bù láng	Corridor Walk
KI-23	shinpō	神封	shén fēng	Spirit Seal
KI-24	reikyo	霊墟	líng xū	Spirit Ruins
KI-25	shinzō	神蔵	shén cáng	Spirit Storehouse
KI-26	ikuchū	彧中	yù zhōng	Lively Center
KI-27	yufu	兪府	shū fǔ	Transport Mansion
LI-1	shōyō	商陽	shāng yáng	Shāng Yáng
LI-2	jikan	二間	èr jiān	Second Space
LI-3	sankan	三間	sān jiān	Third Space
LI-4	gōkoku	合谷	hé gǔ	Union Valley
LI-5	yōkei	陽谿	yáng xī,	Yáng Ravine
LI-6	henreki	偏歴	piān lì	Veering Passageway
LI-7	onryū	温溜	wēn līu	Warm Dwelling
LI-8	geren	下廉	xià lián	Lower Ridge
LI-9	jōren	上廉	shàng lián	Upper Ridge
LI-10	te no sanri	手三里	shǒu sān lǐ	Arm Three Lǐ
LI-11	kyokuchi	曲池	qū chí	Pool at the Bend
LI-12	chūryō	肘髎	zhǒu liáo	Elbow Bone-
LI-13	te no gori	手五里	shǒu wǔ lǐ	Arm Five Lǐ
LI-14	hiju	臂臑	bì nào	Upper Arm
LI-15	kengū	肩髃	jiān yú	Shoulder Bone
LI-16	kokotsu	巨骨	jù gǔ	Great Bone
LI-17	tentei	天鼎	tiān dǐng	Celestial Tripod
LI-18	futotsu	扶突	fú tú	Protuberance Assistant

LI-19	karyō	禾髎	hé liáo	Grain Bone-Hole
LI-20	geikō	迎香	yíng xiāng	Welcome Fragrance
LR-1	daiton	大敦	dà dūn	Large Pile
LR-2	kōkan	行間	xíng jiān	Moving Between
LR-3	taishō	太衝	tài chōng	Supreme Surge
LR-4	chūhō	中封	zhōng fēng	Mound Center
LR-5	reikō	蠡溝	lǐ gōu	Woodworm Canal
LR-6	chūto	中都	zhōng dū	Central Metropolis
LR-7	shitsukan	膝関	xī guān	Knee Joint
LR-8	kyokusen	曲泉	qū quán	Spring at the Bend
LR-9	inpō	陰包	yīn bāo	Yīn Bladder
LR-10	ashi no gori	足五里	zú wǔ lǐ	Foot Five Lǐ
LR-11	inren	陰廉	yīn lián	Yīn Corner
LR-12	kyūmyaku	急脈	jí mài	Urgent Pulse
LR-13	shōmon	章門	zhāng mén	Camphorwood Gate
LR-14	kimon	期門	qī mén	Cycle Gate
LU-1	chūfu	中府	zhōng fǔ	Central Treasury
LU-2	unmon	雲門	yún mén	Cloud Gate
LU-3	tenpu	天府	tiān fǔ	Celestial Storehouse
LU-4	kyōhaku	侠白	xiá bái	Guarding White
LU-5	shakutaku	尺沢	chǐ zé	Cubit Marsh
LU-6	kōsai	孔最	kǒng zuì	Collection Hole
LU-7	rekketsu	列缺	liè quē	Broken Sequence
LU-8	keikyo	経渠	jīng qú	Channel Ditch
LU-9	taien	太淵	tài yuān	Great Ab
LU-10	gyosai	魚際	yú jì	Fish Border
LU-11	shōshō	少商	shào shāng	Lesser Shang
PC-1	tenchi	天池	tiān chí	Celestial Pool
PC-2	tensen	天泉	tiān quán	Celestial Spring
PC-3	kyokutaku	曲沢	qū zé	Marsh at the Bend
PC-4	gekimon	郄門	xī mén	Cleft Gate
PC-5	kanshi	間使	jiān shǐ	Intermediary Courier

PC-6	naikan	内関	nèi guān	Inner Pass
PC-7	dairyō	大陵	dà líng	Great Mound
PC-8	rōkyū	労宮	láo gōng	Palace of Toil
PC-9	chūshō	中衝	zhōng chōng	Central Hub
SI-1	shōtaku	少沢	shào zé	Lesser Marsh
SI-2	zenkoku	前谷	qián gǔ	Front Valley
SI-3	gokei	後谿	hòu xī	Back Ravine
SI-4	wankotsu	腕骨	wàn gǔ	Wrist Bone
SI-5	yōkoku	陽谷	yáng gǔ	Yáng Valley
SI-6	yōrō	養老	yǎng lǎo	Nursing the Aged
SI-7	shisei	支正	zhī zhèng	Branch to the Correct
SI-8	shōkai	小海	xiǎo hǎi	Small Sea
SI-9	kentei	肩貞	jiān zhēn	True Shoulder
SI-10	juyu	臑俞	nào shū	Upper Arm Transport
SI-11	tensō	天宗	tiān zōng	Celestial Gathering
SI-12	heifū	秉風	bǐng fēng	Grasping the Wind
SI-13	kyokuen	曲垣	qū yuán	Crooked Wall
SI-14	kengaiyu	肩外俞	jiān wài shū	Outer Shoulder Transport
SI-15	kenchūyu	肩中俞	jiān zhōng shū	Central Shoulder Transport
SI-16	tensō	天窓	tiān chuāng	Celestial Window
SI-17	ten'yō	天容	tiān róng	Celestial Countenance
SI-17	kanryō	顴髎	quán liáo	Cheek Bone-Hole
SI-19	chōkyū	聴宮	tīng gōng	Auditory Palace
SP-1	inpaku	隠白	yǐn bái	Hidden White
SP-2	daito	大都	dà dū	Great Metropolis
SP-3	taihaku	太白	tài bái	Supreme White
SP-4	kōson	公孫	gōng sū	Yellow Emperor
SP-5	shōkyū	商丘	shāng qīu	Shāng Hill
SP-6	san'inkō	三陰交	sān yīn jiāo	Three Yīn Intersection
SP-7	rōkoku	漏谷	lòu gǔ	Leaking Valley
SP-8	chiki	地機	dì jī	Earth's Crux
SP-9	inryōsen	陰陵泉	yīn líng quán	Yīn Mound Spring

SP-10	kekkai	血海	xuè hǎi	Sea of Blood
SP-11	kimon	箕門	jī mén	Winnower Gate
SP-12	shōmon	衝門	chōng mén	Surging Gate
SP-13	fusha	府舍	fǔ shè	Bowel Abode
SP-14	fukketsu	腹結	fù jié	Abdominal Bind
SP-15	daiō	大横	dà hèng	Great Horizontal
SP-16	fukuai	腹哀	fù āi	Abdominal Lament
SP-17	shokutoku	食竇	shí dòu	Food Hole
SP-18	tenkei	天谿	tiān xī	Celestial Ravine
SP-19	kyōkyō	胸郷	xiōng xiāng	Chest Village
SP-20	shūei	周栄	zhōu róng	All-Round Flourishing
SP-21	daihō	大包	dà bāo	Great Embracement
ST-1	shōkyū	承泣	chéng qì	Tear Container
ST-2	shihaku	四白	sì bái	Four Whites
ST-3	koryō	巨髎	jù liáo	Great Bone-Hole
ST-4	chisō	地倉	dì cāng	Earth Granary
ST-5	daigei	大迎	dà yíng	Great Reception
ST-6	kyōsha	頬車	jiá chē	Cheek Carriage
ST-7	gekan	下関	xià guān	Below the Joint
ST-8	zui	頭維	tóu weí	Head Corner
ST-9	jingei	人迎	rén yíng	Man's Prognosis
ST-10	suitotsu	水突	shuǐ tú	Water Prominence
ST-11	kisha	気舎	qì shè	Qì Abode
ST-12	ketsubon	缺盆	quē pén	Empty Basin
ST-13	kiko	気戸	qì hù	Qì Door
ST-14	kobō	庫房	kù fáng	Storeroom
ST-15	okuei	屋翳	wū yì	Roof
ST-16	yōsō	膺窓	yīng chuāng	Breast Window
ST-17	nyūchū	乳中	rǔ zhōng	Breast Center
ST-18	nyūkon	乳根	rǔ gēn	Breast Root
ST-19	fuyō	不容	bù róng	Not Contained
ST-20	shōman	承満	chéng mǎn	Assuming Fullness

ST-21	ryōmon	梁門	liáng mén	Beam Gate
ST-22	kanmon	関門	guān mén	Pass Gate
ST-23	tai'itsu	太乙	tài yǐ	Supreme Unity
ST-24	katsunikumon	滑肉門	huá ròu mén	Slippery Flesh Gate
ST-25	tensū	天枢	tiān shū	Celestial Pivot
ST-26	gairyō	外陵	wài líng	Outer Mound
ST-27	daiko	大巨	dà jù	Great Gigantic
ST-28	suidō	水道	shuǐ dào	Waterway
ST-29	kirai	帰来	guī lái	Return
ST-30	kishō	気衝	qì chōng	Qì Thoroughfare
ST-31	hikan	髀関	bì guān	Thigh Joint
ST-32	fukuto	伏兔	fú tù	Crouching Rabbit
ST-33	inshi	陰市	yīn shì	Yīn Market
ST-34	ryōkyū	梁丘	liáng qiū	Beam Hill
ST-35	tokubi	犢鼻	dú bí	Calf's Nose
ST-36	ashi no sanri	足三里	zú sān lǐ	Leg Three Lǐ
ST-37	jōkokyo	上巨虚	shàng jù xū	Upper Great Hollow
ST-38	jōkō	条口	tiáo kǒu	Ribbon Opening
ST-39	gekokyo	下巨虚	xià jù xū	Lower Great Hollow
ST-40	hōryū	豊隆	fēng lóng	Bountiful Bulge
ST-41	kaikei	解谿	jiě xī	Ravine Divide
ST-42	shōyō	衝陽	chōng yáng	Surging Yáng
ST-43	kankoku	陷谷	xiàn gǔ	Sunken Valley
ST-44	naitei	内庭	nèi tíng	Inner Court
ST-45	reida	厲兌	lì duì	Severe Mouth
TW-1	kanshō	関衝	guān chōng	Passage Hub
TW-2	ekimon	液門	yè mén	Humor Gate
TW-3	chūsho	中渚	zhōng zhǔ	Central Islet
TW-4	yōchi	陽池	yáng chí	Yáng Pool
TW-5	gaikan	外関	wài guān	Outer Pass
TW-6	shikō	支溝	zhī gōu	Branch Ditch
TW-7	esō	会宗	huì zōng	Convergence and Gathering

TW-8	san'yōraku	三陽絡	sān yáng luò	Three Yáng Connection
TW-9	shitoku	四瀆	sì dú	Four Rivers
TW-10	tensei	天井	tiān jǐng	Celestial Well
TW-11	seireien	清冷淵	qīng lěng yuān	Clear Cold Abyss
TW-12	shōreki	消濼	xiāo luò	Dispersing Riverbed
TW-13	jue	臑会	nào huì	Upper Arm Convergence
TW-14	kenryō	肩髎	jiān liáo	Shoulder Bone-Hole
TW-15	tenryō	天髎	tiān liáo	Celestial Bone-Hole
TW-16	ten'yū	天牖	tiān yǒu	Celestial Window
TW-17	eifū	翳風	yì fēng	Wind Screen
TW-18	keimyaku	瘈脈	qì mài	Tugging Vessel
TW-19	rosoku	顱息	lú xī	Skull Rest
TW-20	kakuson	角孫	jiǎo sūn	Angle Vertex
TW-21	jimon	耳門	ěr mén	Ear Gate
TW-22	waryō	和髎	hé liáo	Harmony Bone-Hole
TW-23	shichikukū	糸竹空	sī zhú kōng	Silk Bamboo Hole

About the Authors

(in alphabetical order after Okabe Somei)

Okabe Somei, M.D.　　　　　　　　岡部素明

Born in Tokyo, 1936, the eldest son of Okabe Sodō. Passed away March 25, 2000.

Graduate, Radiology Department, Showa University Graduate School of Medicine

Clinical Experience: 29 years

After engaging in research and clinical practice using radiation therapy for the treatment of cancer at the Showa University Hospital, Dr. Okabe took up a post at Kitazato University as Head of the Acupuncture and Moxibustion Department of the Research Center for East Asian Medicine, which he helped establish.

In 1984, following the death of his father, Okabe Sodō (then President of the Society of Traditional Japanese Medicine), Okabe Somei assumed the office of President of the Society, and at the same time founded the Okabe Clinic and Institute of Traditional Japanese Medicine. He was active in organizing the Society of Traditional Japanese Medicine and in the popularization and development of Meridian Therapy.

Positions Held at Time of Death:

President, Society of Traditional Japanese Medicine
Director, Seiwadō Okabe Clinic
Director, Institute of Traditional Japanese Medicine

Aizawa Ryō

相澤良

Born in Tokyo, 1949

Graduate, Faculty of Law, Chūō University

Graduate, Japan School of Acupuncture, Moxibustion and Physiotherapy

Clinical Experience: 24 years

Present Positions:

>Board Member, Society of Traditional Japanese Medicine
>
>Instructor, Department of Teacher Training, Tokyo Therapeutic Institute
>
>Assistant Director, Institute of Traditional Japanese Medicine

Higuchi Hideyoshi

樋口秀吉

Born in Miyagi Prefecture, 1953

Graduate, Tōhoku Gakuin University

Graduate, Akamon Acupuncture Moxibustion and Japanese Bone Setting School

Clinical Experience: 24 years

Present Positions:

>Instructor, Meridian Therapy Summer College
>
>Vice President, Society of Traditional Japanese Medicine
>
>Instructor, Akamon Acupuncture Moxibustion and Japanese Bone Setting School
>
>Instructor, Sendai Nursing and Midwifery School of the Sendai National Hospital
>
>Standing Director and International Affairs Department Chief, Japan Acupuncture and Moxibustion Association
>
>President, Miyagi Acupuncture and Moxibustion Association
>
>Councilor, Japan Traditional Acupuncture & Moxibustion Society
>
>Clinic Director, Higuchi Acupuncture & Moxibustion
>
>Clinic Director, Acupuncture & Moxibustion Higuchi Shiseido

Ikeda Masakazu

池田政一

Born in Ehime Prefecture, 1945

Graduate, Acupuncture and Moxibustion Department of Meiji East Asian Medical Academy

Clinical Experience: 35 years

Present Positions:

> Director of Education and International Affairs, Society of Traditional Japanese Medicine
> President, Kampo In Yō Society
> Adviser, Kampo Hari Society
> Director, Traditional Medicine Training Center

Publications:

> *Handbook Series for the Classics*. Ido no Nippon
> *The Traditional Acupuncture Approach to Therapy*. Ido no Nippon
> *Pulse Classic*. Taniguchi Shoten
> And many more.

Kuwahara, T. Koei

桑原浩榮

Born in Kagoshima Prefecture, 1956

Graduate, Tokyo Therapeutic Institute

Clinical Experience: 24 years

Present Positions:

> Assistant Professor, New England School of Acupuncture
> President, Hari Society
> Director, Ki Science Institute
> Director, Culia Ki Clinic
> Instructor, Boston Shiatsu School
> Special Lecturer, Meridian Therapy Summer College

Okada Akizō 岡田明三

Born in Tokyo, 1948

Graduate, Faculty of Letters, Kokugakuin University

Graduate, ToyoShinkyu College of Oriental Medicine

Clinical Experience: 32 years

Present Positions:

President, Society of Traditional Japanese Acupuncture

Senior Counselor, Japan Traditional Acupuncture & Moxibustion Society

Instructor, Department of Teacher Training, Tokyo Therapeutic Institute

Instructor, ToyoShinkyu College of Oriental Medicine

Instructor, Tokyo Eisei Academy

Assistant Director, Jingumae Acupuncture Center

Shudō Denmei 首藤傳明

Born in Oita Prefecture, 1932

Passed the high school equivalency examination, and received acupuncture license under the old licensure system.

Clinical Experience: 43 years

Present Positions:

Instructor, Meridian Therapy Summer College

President, Japan Traditional Acupuncture & Moxibustion Society

Director, Gensai Jyuku

Advisor, Acupuncturist Society of Oita Prefecture (NPO)

Books:

Recommendation of Meridian Therapy. Ido no Nippon (English version translated by Stephen Brown. *Japanese Classical Acupuncture: Introduction to Meridian Therapy*. Eastland Press)

INDEX

ST-38, 63, 365
ST-39, 63, 66, 303-304, 365
ST-4, 60, 62, 98, 364
ST-40, 56, 63-64, 365
ST-41, 30, 63, 293, 365
ST-42, 30, 63, 267-268, 302-303, 305-306, 365
ST-43, 30, 63, 365
ST-44, 30, 63, 66, 142, 302-304, 365
ST-45, 30, 63, 293, 301-302, 304, 365
ST-5, 62-63, 89, 364
ST-6, 62, 89, 364
ST-7, 62, 364
ST-8, 62, 74, 364
ST-9, 63, 98, 364
Stagnation, 34, 41, 78, 91, 99, 131, 134, 147, 156, 158, 160, 166, 169-170, 172, 176, 181, 185-186, 188, 192-193, 230, 233, 241-242, 244-245, 250, 254-256, 258, 262, 265, 274, 294, 296-297, 317-318, 339
Stagnation of blood, 41, 78, 131, 147, 156, 158, 170, 176, 193, 241, 262
Stagnation of heat, 42, 151, 169, 242, 254, 256, 262, 265
Stagnation of ki, 134, 255, 258, 297
Stagnation of lung ki, 134
Stagnation of nutritive ki, 318
Stagnation of water, 181-182, 185
Stagnation of yang ki, 78, 99, 166, 186, 188
Stasis pattern, 177, 304
Sticky sputum, 217
Stiff lumps, 58, 257
Stiffness, 78, 86, 91, 121, 131, 167, 169, 172, 177, 180, 187-188, 195, 216, 218, 231, 286, 340
Stiff shoulders, 62, 74, 78, 87, 91, 125, 127, 165, 187, 200, 210-211, 216
Stomach cancer, 140
Stomach deficiency, 15, 53, 126, 170, 182-183, 202, 220, 228, 268-269, 303, 343
Stomach deficiency heat, 15, 126, 170, 182-183, 202, 220, 228, 268-269, 303, 343
Stomach excess, 15, 126, 167, 182-183, 192, 202, 205, 208, 219-220, 222, 227, 262, 267-268, 303-304, 343
Stomach excess heat, 15, 126, 167, 182-183, 192, 202, 205, 208, 219-220, 222, 227, 262, 267-268, 303, 343
Stomach heat, 140, 183, 202-203, 215, 305
Stomach ki, 35, 54, 115, 247-250, 256, 258, 260-261, 264, 287, 349
Stomach ki pulse, 247-248, 349
Stomach problems, 193
Stomach pulse, 247, 264, 270, 275, 306
Stomach yang ki, 32

Stool leakage, 189
Stream-earth-point, 296, 346
Striking pulse, 154, 269, 340
Stroking dispersion technique, 324-325
Strong appetites, 126
Strong pulse, 253
Stuffy nose, 118, 188, 192, 215
Subarachnoid hemorrhage, 214
Subjective feeling of alternating chills, 173
Subjective feeling of fever, 160, 215, 219
Sudden deafness, 214
Sudden loss of yang ki, 161
Sudden noises, 186
Sudden onset, 54, 202, 217
Sugiyama Waichi, 321
Summer doyo, 19
Summerheat, 123, 148-149, 152-154, 254, 299-300, 338
Summerheat damage, 149, 299-300, 338
Summerheat fire, 148-149, 152
Summer kidney deficiency, 212
Summer pulse, 248
Summer yang ki, 248
Su Wen, 1, 9, 16-17, 21-22, 25, 36, 40, 45, 50-51, 95-96, 99-101, 105-111, 114-119, 121, 124, 131-135, 137-139, 143, 150, 168-171, 193, 201, 206, 235, 246
Sweat leaking, 311
Sweaty hands, 186
Sweet foods, 138, 141
Sweet grains, 140
Sweet herbs, 114
Sweet medicine, 114
Swollen cervical lymph glands, 4, 353
Swollen jaw, 180, 348
Swollen neck, 189
Swollen tonsils, 128

T

Takeyama Shin'ichiro, 1, 5, 8, 105
Teeth sound, 207
Temperature of needles, 314
Thin pulse, 243, 258, 338
Thread moxa, 329, 350
Tight pulse, 242, 256, 338
Trigeminal neuralgia, 94, 177, 216, 354
Triple warmer pulse, 264
Triple warmer source ki, 53, 122, 305-306
True cold false heat, 168, 188, 200, 350
True ki, 21, 32-33, 133
TW-1, 30, 84, 365
TW-10, 30, 84, 87, 293, 366
TW-11, 84, 366
TW-12, 84, 366
TW-13, 61, 84, 87, 366
TW-14, 84, 366

TW-15, 85, 88, 103, 366
TW-16, 85-86, 366
TW-17, 85, 87, 89, 214, 287, 366
TW-18, 85, 366
TW-19, 85, 366
TW-2, 30, 84, 365
TW-20, 85, 88, 366
TW-21, 85, 366
TW-22, 85, 366
TW-23, 366
TW-3, 30, 84, 293, 303-304, 365
TW-4, 30, 84, 240, 302-303, 305-306, 365
TW-5, 56, 84-85, 87, 303-304, 365
TW-6, 30, 84, 293, 302, 365
TW-7, 56, 84, 301, 365
TW-8, 84, 365
TW-9, 84, 366
Twelve divergent channels, 47

U

Ulceration of the genitals, 215
Ulceration of the mouth, 215
Ulcerative colitis, 174, 354
Unbalanced diet, 136, 176
Unbalanced fluid signs, 42
Uniting-water-point, 297, 346
Unstable neurosis, 177
Unstable psyche, 35
Uranaitei, 142
Urethritis, 173, 177, 202, 220, 230, 354
Urinary abnormalities, 32, 121, 184
Urinary difficulty, 74, 78, 152, 168, 175, 191, 194, 220, 266, 340

V

Vascular spiders, 205, 354
Vexation, 150, 152-155, 163, 170-173, 190-191, 193, 337, 340, 349
Viral warts, 182

W

Wagi Tessai, 4
Warming moxibustion, 11, 342
Warming needles, 253, 314
Water accumulation, 158, 184
Water channels, 48
Water-ki disease, 156, 158-159, 190, 340
Water ki syndrome, 48
Water retention, 156, 159, 191, 205, 229
Water retention obesity, 156, 159
Water stagnation, 160, 233, 245, 250, 339
Water toxin, 250, 253, 348
Watery bowel movements, 42
Weakness of the legs, 78
Weak pulse, 14, 243, 246, 259, 339
Weak voices, 128

Traditional Japanese Acupuncture: Fundamentals of Meridian Therapy